Milestones in Drug Therapy
MDT

Atypical Antipsychotics

Edited by B.A. Ellenbroek, A.R. Cools

Birkhäuser Verlag
Basel · Boston · Berlin

Editor

Dr. Bart A. Ellenbroek
Dr. Alexander R. Cools
Dept. of Psychoneuropharmacology
University of Nijmegen
P.O. Box 9101
NL-6500 Nijmegen
The Netherlands

Library of Congress Cataloging-in-Publication Data

Atypical antipsychotics / edited by B.A. Ellenbroek, A.R. Cools.
p. ; cm. – (Milestones in drug therapy)
Includes bibliographical references and index.
ISBN 376435948X (hard cover : alk. paper)
1. Antipsychotic drugs. 2. Clozapine – Therapeutic use. 3.
Schizophrenia – Chemotherapy. I. Ellenbroek, B.A. (Bart A.), 1958- II. Cools,
Alexander Rudolf, 1941- III. Series
[DNLM: 1. Antipsychotic Agents – therapeutic use. 2. Antipsychotic Agents – pharmacology.
3. Clozapine – therapeutic use. 4. Schizophrenia – drug therapy.
QV 77.9 A887 2000]
RM333.5 .A89 2000
616.89'18 – dc21

Deutsche Bibliothek – CIP Einheitsaufnahme

Atypical antipsychotics / ed. by B.A. Ellenbroek ; A.R. Cools. –
Basel ; Boston ; Berlin : Birkhäuser, 2000
(Milestones in drug therapy)
ISBN 3-7643-5948-X

ISBN 3-7643-5948-X Birkhäuser Verlag, Basel – Boston – Berlin

Printed on acid-free paper produced from chlorine-free pulp. TCF ∞
Printed in Germany
ISBN 3-7643-5948-X

9 8 7 6 5 4 3 2 1

Contents

List of Contributors

Jørn Arnt, Department of Psychopharmacology, Psychopharmacological Research, H. Lundbeck A/S, Ottiliavej 9, DK-2500 Copenhagen-Valby, Denmark; e-mail: ja@lundbeck.com

Alexander R. Cools, Department of Psychoneuropharmacology, University of Nijmegen, Geert Grooteplein N21, P.O. Box 9101, NL-6500 HB Nijmegen, The Netherlands; e-mail: A.Cools@pnf.kun.nl

Johan A. Den Boer, Department of Biological Psychiatry, University of Groningen, P.O. Box 30001, NL-9700 RB Groningen, The Netherlands

Bart A. Ellenbroek, Department of Psychoneuropharmacology, University of Nijmegen, Geert Grooteplein N21, P.O. Box 9101, NL-6500 HB Nijmegen, The Netherlands; e-mail: A.Ellenbroek@pnf.kun.nl

Christian Haasen, Universitäts-Krankenhaus Eppendorf, Klinik für Psychiatrie und Psychotherapie, Martinistrasse 52, D-20246 Hamburg, Germany

Josée E. Leysen, Department of Biochemical Pharmacology, Janssen Research Foundation, Turnhoutseweg 30, B-2340 Beerse, Belgium; e-mail: jleysen2@janbe.jnj.com

Jakob Korf, Department of Biological Psychiatry, University of Groningen, P.O. Box 30001, NL-9700 RB Groningen, The Netherlands

Peter F. Liddle, Department of Psychiatry, University of British Columbia, 2255 Wesbrook Mall, Vancouver, BC, V6T 2A1, Canada; e-mail: liddle@interchange.ubc.ca

Herbert Y. Meltzer, Department of Psychiatry, Vanderbilt University School of Medicine, Suite 306, 1601 23rd Avenue S, Nashville, TN 37215, USA; e-mail: herbert.meltzer@mcmail.vanderbilt.edu

Dieter Naber, Universitäts-Krankenhaus Eppendorf, Klinik für Psychiatrie und Psychotherapie, Martinistrasse 52, D-20246 Hamburg, Germany

Christian Perro, Universitäts-Krankenhaus Eppendorf, Klinik für Psychiatrie und Psychotherapie, Martinistrasse 52, D-20246 Hamburg, Germany

John F. Quinn, Stanley Foundation Research Unit, St. Davnet's Hospital, Monaghan, Ireland and Department of Clinical Pharmacology, Royal College of Surgeons in Ireland, St. Stephen's Green, Dublin 2, Ireland

Frank Sams-Dodd, Department of Psychopharmacology, Pharmacological Research, H. Lundbeck A/S, Ottiliavej 9, DK-2500 Copenhagen-Valby, Denmark

Darius K. Shayegan, Department of Psychiatry, University of California San Diego and Clinical Neuroscience Research Center, 8899 University Center Lane, Suite 130, San Diego, CA 92122, USA; e-mail: dshayega@ucsd.edu

Stephen M. Stahl, Department of Psychiatry, University of California San Diego and Clinical Neuroscience Research Center, 8899 University Center Lane, Suite 130, San Diego, CA 92122, USA

John L. Waddington, Department of Clinical Pharmacology, Royal College of Surgeons in Ireland, St. Stephen's Green, Dublin 2, Ireland and Stanley Foundation Research Unit, St. Davnet's Hospital, Monaghan, Ireland; e-mail: jwadding@rcsi.ie

Preface

The introduction of chlorpromazine in 1953, and haloperidol in 1958, into clinical practice dramatically altered the therapy of schizophrenic patients. Although representing by no means a cure for this severe psychiatric illness, it allowed, for the first time, to adequately control the severe hallucinations and delusional beliefs which prevent these patients from leading a more or less independent life. Indeed these antipsychotics (and the many congeners that were to follow) significantly reduced the number of chronic schizophrenic inpatients in psychiatric clinics all over the world.

However soon after their introduction it became clear that, like all other available drugs, antipsychotics were by no means miracle drugs. In fact, two major problems appeared. First, the antipsychotics had very little effect on the so-called negative or defect symptoms, like social isolation, apathy and anhedonia, and secondly virtually all antipsychotics produced a number of side-effects, of which the neurological (often called extrapyramidal) side-effects were the most troublesome. Especially the tardive dyskinesia, which occurred in about 15 to 20% of the patients after prolonged treatment, represented a major problem in the treatment of schizophrenic patients.

In the early 1960s, Arvid Carlsson and his collaborators [1] suggested that the catecholamines may play an important role in the mode of action of antipsychotic drugs. Using biochemical techniques, these authors found that drugs such as chlorpromazine and haloperidol enhanced the levels of dopamine and noradrenaline metabolites in the brains of mice. However, it was Jac van Rossum who first launched the dopamine hypothesis of schizophrenia, in his famous paper "The significance of dopamine-receptor blockade for the mechanism of action of neuroleptic drugs" [2], based predominantly on behavioural evidence. After this paper, many years passed before it became clear that, like acetylcholine and noradrenaline, dopamine also binds to more than one receptor. Based on the original work of Struyker-Boudier and collaborators in the snail *Helix aspersa*, Cools and van Rossum proposed the existence of two types of dopamine receptors termed DA_i and DA_e, through which dopamine respectively inhibited and enhanced cell firing [3]. This concept was accepted for many years, until a new subdivision (primarily based on binding studies) emerged separating dopamine receptors in D_1 and D_2. Interestingly, in the same years as the paper by Cools and van Rossum, two research groups independently found that the affinity of antipsychotics for the radioactively labelled dopamine receptors was correlated with the clinical daily dose, thus strengthening the dopamine hypothesis [4, 5].

A second major breakthrough occurred in the 1980s with the renewed interest in clozapine. This drug, introduced in the early 1960s appeared to be virtually free of extrapyramidal side-effects (therefore often referred to as an atypical antipsychotic). It was removed from the market in the 1970s after reports of increased risk of agranulocytosis. The studies in the 1980s showed that clozapine could also relieve negative symptoms and was especially effective in therapy resistance. However, the heightened risk of agranulocytosis prevented a wide scale reintroduction of this drug in clinical practice. The studies nevertheless proved that certain antipsychotics may have a substantially better effect than others and that dopamine blockade alone cannot adequately describe antipsychotic action. Although the mechanism of action of clozapine is still not completely understood, two papers published independently in 1984, showed that all antipsychotics affected the firing of the mesolimbic dopamine cells, but drugs such as haloperidol and chlorpromazine, but not clozapine, also affected the firing rate of nigrostriatal system [6, 7]. This has led to the so-called regional selectivity hypothesis of antipsychotic drugs.

The renewed interest in clozapine has set the stage for a potential third breakthrough. In the last few years a number of new potentially atypical antipsychotics have been introduced in clinical practice, and several others will be introduced within the next few years. These new drugs may have an important impact on the therapy and especially the well being of schizophrenic patients.

These data show that the advances in our understanding of the actions of antipsychotic drugs have been obtained from many sources, including behavioural, biochemical, electrophysiological and clinical studies. The present book represents an attempt to present the current status of our knowledge on all these fields of research. It is written by experts on the field of schizophrenia both from a clinical and from a preclinical point of view. Given the rapid introduction of a series of the new atypical antipsychotics, this book may be of great importance for the practising psychiatrist who want a quick update of the clinical effects of these atypical drugs. However, since the book also has a large introductory section on schizophrenia and antipsychotics, it is also of value for the medical student. Moreover, since a large section is devoted to the neurochemical, neurophysiological and behavioural aspects of antipsychotic drugs, this book may also prove to be of general value for the neuroscientist. Finally, the book includes an overview of the most recent animal models for schizophrenia, making it a valuable source of information for neuroscientists working in the pharmaceutical industry.

The book is subdivided into three sections. Section one gives a general introduction on schizophrenia (Liddle), antipsychotics (Waddington and Quinn) and animal models (Ellenbroek and Cools). Section 2 is dedicated to the preclinical effects of atypical antipsychotics. It represents chapters on the receptor profiles of antipsychotics (Leysen), on regional selectivity of antipsychotics (Ellenbroek and Cools), on screening models for atypical antipsychotic (Arnt) and on simulation models for schizophrenia

(Ellenbroek et al.). The third section is devoted to the clinical effects of atypical antipsychotic. After an introductory chapter on clozapine (Naber et al.), there are chapters on selective dopamine receptor ligands (Den Boer and Korf), and multireceptor antipsychotic drugs (Meltzer). The book finishes with a highly speculative chapter on the possible new strategies for obtaining novel antipsychotic drugs (Stahl and Shayegan).

References

1 Carlsson A, Lindqvist M (1963) Effects of chlorpromazine or haloperidol on formation of 3-methoxytyramin and normetanephrine in mouse brain. *Acta Pharmacol Toxicol* 20: 140–144
2 Van Rossum J (1966) The significance of dopamine-receptor blockade for the mechanism of action of neuroleptic drugs. *Arch Intern Pharmacodyn Ther* 160: 492–494
3 Cools A, van Rossum J (1976) Excitation-mediating and inhibition-mediating dopamine receptors: a new concept towards a better understanding of electrophysiological, biochemical, functional and clinical data. *Psychopharmacol* 45: 243–254
4 Creese I, Burt D, Snyder S (1976) Dopamine receptor binding predicts clinical and pharmacological potenties of antischizophrenic drugs. *Science*, 192: 481–483
5 Seeman P, Lee T, Choa-Wong M, Wong K (1976) Antipsychotic drug doses and neuroleptic/dopamine receptors. *Nature* 261: 717–719
6 Chiodo L, Bunney B (1983) Typical and atypical neuroleptics: Differential effects of chronic administration on the activity of A9 and A10 midbrain dopaminergic neurons, *J Neurosci* 3: 1607–1619
7 White FJ, Wang RY (1983) Differential effects of classical and atypical antipsychotic drugs on A9 and A10 dopamine neurons. *Science* 211: 1054–1056

Bart A. Ellenbroek
Alexander R. Cools
September 1999

A general introduction

Atypical Antipsychotics
ed. by B.A. Ellenbroek and A.R. Cools

Introduction to schizophrenia

Peter F. Liddle

Department of Psychiatry, University of British Columbia, 2255 Wesbrook Mall, Vancouver, BC, V6T 2A1, Canada

Introduction

Schizophrenia is a complex disorder that affects virtually all domains of mental function, including perception, thought, emotion, will, judgement and execution of voluntary motor action. Although the course of the illness varies greatly between individuals, the characteristic time-course includes episodes of florid illness superimposed upon a level of chronic disability. The degree of chronic disability ranges from a relatively mild reduction in ability to cope with stress, to severe difficulties in initiating and organising voluntary activity that render the person unable to take care of him or herself.

The essential characteristic that defines schizophrenia remains elusive. Kraepelin [1] who provided the first comprehensive description of the condition, designated it "dementia praecox" denoting onset in young adult life with subsequent deterioration of mental function. Bleuler [2] assigned the name schizophrenia to denote the fragmentation of mental activity that characterises the condition. The tendency for remorseless deterioration implied by Kraepelin's use of the term dementia has not been confirmed by subsequent long-term studies, which show that many cases exhibit at least partial recovery over a period of several decades [3]. Nonetheless, onset before middle age, deterioration of function over a sustained period, and fragmentation of mental activity remain central features of the concept of schizophrenia.

The operational criteria for diagnosis of schizophrenia defined in the 10th edition of the *International Classification of Diseases* (ICD-10) [4], demand that symptoms from a specified set of characteristic symptoms are clearly present for most of the time for at least 1 month. The criteria defined in the 4th edition of the *Diagnostic and Statistical Manual of the American Psychiatric Association* (DSM-IV) [5] specify that symptoms from a similar set must be present for a significant proportion of the time throughout a period of 1 month, and in addition require that there is marked impairment of social or occupational functioning, and continuous signs of disturbed mental function for at least 6 months. According to both the ICD-10 and DSM-IV, a diagnosis of schizophrenia should not be made if the clinical features can be accounted for by mood disorder, overt brain disease, a general medical condition, or toxic substances.

Symptoms

The symptoms of schizophrenia embrace the full range of mental symptoms (see Table 1). They include particularly characteristic symptoms such as delusions, hallucinations, formal thought disorder, bizarre behaviour, flattening of affect and poverty of speech. These symptoms are given considerable weight in making a diagnosis, though they can occur in other psychotic illnesses. Other symptoms, such as depression, excitation and anxiety, which are more characteristic of affective or neurotic disorders, are nonetheless prevalent in schizophrenia.

In the 1980s, several studies that examined the correlations between the characteristic symptoms of schizophrenia [6–11] found that the characteristic symptoms segregated into three syndromes as shown in Table 1. The first group of symptoms, the reality distortion syndrome, comprises delusions and hallucinations, and reflects a failure of the ability to evaluate the reality of ideas and perceptions. The second group of symptoms, the disorganisation syndrome, reflects a disruption of the connections between the elements of thought, emotion and action, and is manifest as disjointed or irrelevant speech, affect and behaviour. The third group, the psychomotor poverty syndrome, reflects a diminution in the amount of thought, emotion and voluntary motor activity.

These three groups of characteristic schizophrenic symptoms constitute three distinguishable dimensions of a single illness rather than representing distinct sub-types of illness. It is common to find symptoms of more than one of the three syndromes co-existing in an individual case [7], though within an individual case the severity of the three syndromes tends to

Table 1. The symptoms of schizophrenia

Characteristic syndromes	*Affective syndromes*
Reality distortion	Depression
Delusions	Low mood
Hallucinations	Low self-esteem
Disorganization	Hopelessness
Formal thought disorder	Suicidality
Inappropriate affect	Psychomotor Excitation
Disorganized or bizarre behaviour	Irritability
Psychomotor Poverty	Pressure of speech
Flat affect	Motor agitation
Poverty of speech	*Non-specific symptoms*
Decreased voluntary motor activity	Anxiety
	Coenesthesia

vary almost independently over time [12]. There is a substantial body of evidence indicating that each of the three syndromes is associated with a specific pattern of neuropsychological impairments, and with a specific pattern of aberrant cerebral activity [13, 14].

Reality distortion

Reality distortion, which is manifest as hallucinations and/or delusions, is the hallmark of psychosis. In schizophrenia, hallucinations in any modality can occur, but auditory hallucinations are the most characteristic. The delusions that occur in schizophrenia can have almost any type of content. Persecutory delusions and delusions of reference are the most common, though these types of delusion are also common in other psychotic disorders. Bizarre or non-understandable delusions are also common, and are more specific to schizophrenia, though there is no specific type of delusion that is pathognomic of the illness.

In an attempt to identify clinical features with high specificity to schizophrenia, Schneider [15] identified a group of delusional and hallucinatory experiences that are usually known as first rank symptoms of schizophrenia. Several of these items appear to reflect a loss of the sense of ownership or control of one's own mental and physical activity. These include phenomena such as thought insertion, made actions and made affect. The first rank symptoms also include third person auditory hallucinations, and primary or autothonous delusions that arise without any understandable relationship to prior mental events. First rank symptoms occur in about 70% of schizophrenic patients and can also occur bipolar disorder. Nonetheless, there is some evidence that if the symptoms are defined very rigorously, the specificity to schizophrenia is quite high [16].

Studies using factor analysis [7] demonstrate that reality distortion actually consists of two distinguishable but nonetheless correlated groups of symptoms: disintegrative reality distortion, which includes Schneiderian first rank symptoms and other bizarre delusions; and integrative reality distortion, which comprises of paranoid features such as delusions of persecution and delusions of reference. The phenomena of integrative reality distortion are also common in other psychotic disorders, and appear to reflect a relatively understandable attempt to deal with circumstances in a way that preserves the sense of self. Disintegrative reality distortion is uncommon in any other condition. Thus, it appears that in schizophrenia, as in other psychotic illnesses, there is a defect of the cerebral mechanism for evaluating reality. However, in schizophrenia this defect tends to be more profound, causing more extraordinary ideas to be accepted as true. Furthermore, in a substantial proportion of cases of schizophrenia there is also a defect of the mechanism for identifying the source of one's own mental activity.

Reality distortion symptoms are especially prominent during florid episodes of illness, but often resolve as the acute episode resolves. However in a substantial minority of cases, they persist despite antipsychotic treatment.

Disorganisation

Disorganisation, which includes positive formal thought disorder and inappropriate affect, reflects the fragmentation of mental activity implied by the name schizophrenia. Disorganisation is associated with impairment in a diverse range of cognitive tasks, especially attentional tasks [13]. The common feature of these various cognitive tasks is the need to select between competing mental activities, and to suppress inappropriate responses. For example, many studies have reported an association between the symptoms of disorganisation and impaired performance in the Stroop task, in which the subject is required to name the ink colour when presented with a colour word printed in an incongruent colour [17–19].

Disorganisation can be a major feature of florid episodes of illness, though in many cases a more subtle form of disorganisation, characterised by vague speech, odd affect and poorly organised behaviour, persists even after the florid episode has resolved [20]. Chronic disorganisation is associated strongly with poor social and occupational performance [7].

Psychomotor poverty

Psychomotor poverty embraces the core negative symptoms of schizophrenia: blunted affect, poverty of speech, and decreased spontaneous movement. These symptoms reflect a diminution in amount of mental and motor activity. Like disorganisation, psychomotor poverty is associated with impairment of a range of cognitive tasks. In particular, it is associated with slowing of mental activity and with difficulty planning and initiating mental activity. For example, severity of psychomotor poverty is correlated with decreased rate of word production in word generation tasks [17, 21]. Chronic psychomotor poverty is associated with impaired social function, especially with lack of relationships with friends and peers [7].

Psychomotor poverty is usually persistent. Bleuler [2] noted “when the affects disappear, the illness becomes chronic”. However psychomotor poverty can also increase in severity during florid episodes of illness, and decrease as the florid episode clears [22]. At least in part, the increase in severity of psychomotor poverty symptoms that occurs during florid exacerbations of the illness might be secondary to factors such as depression, social withdrawal in response to hallucinations, or a manifestation of the akinesia that can arise from treatment with dopamine blocking antipsychotics. However, the observation that even during relatively brief treatment trials, atypical antipsychotics produce a reduction in negative symptoms that cannot be accounted for by change in other symptoms of the illness or extrapyramidal side-effects [23], suggests that at least part of the increase in psychomotor poverty occurring during florid episodes is a direct expression of the pathophysiology of the florid relapse.

Furthermore, several studies have reported that core negative symptoms change in parallel with changes in plasma levels of the dopamine metabolite, homovanillic acid, suggesting that these symptoms can be associated with dopaminergic hyperactivity [24]. If this is indeed the case, it presents an enigma. The similarity between psychomotor-poverty and neuroleptic induced akinesia strongly suggests that psychomotor-poverty is associated with dopamine hypo-activity. The issue of whether or not intrinsic psychomotor poverty is associated with dopaminergic hyper- or hypo-activity remains a significant question in considering the pharmacological treatment of the illness.

The positive-negative symptom dichotomy

Alternatively, the characteristic symptoms of schizophrenia can be classified on conceptual grounds, into positive and negative clusters. Positive symptoms are those that reflect the presence of a mental process that is not present in normal individuals. These include delusions, hallucinations, formal thought disorder, bizarre behaviour and inappropriate affect. Positive symptoms embrace the symptoms of both the reality distortion and disorganisation syndromes. Negative symptoms are symptoms that reflect a decrease or absence of mental activity that is present in normal individuals. These symptoms include poverty of speech, flat affect, and decreased amount of voluntary activity. These negative symptoms correspond to the symptoms of psychomotor poverty. The positive-negative symptom dichotomy forms the basis of Crow's [25] influential type 1/type 2 formulation of the pathophysiology of schizophrenia, which we shall consider in greater detail below.

While the evidence that reality distortion and disorganisation are associated with quite different patterns of association of neuropsychological impairment [13, 17, 19, 21] indicates that these two clusters of positive symptoms reflect different patterns of brain malfunction, nonetheless these two syndromes do appear to share some features of their pathophysiology. In particular, both positive syndromes respond relatively well to treatment with dopamine blocking medication. In contrast, negative symptoms respond less well to treatment with antipsychotics [26]. One of the major goals in the development of novel antipsychotics in the final two decades of the 20th century has been to achieve effective treatment of negative symptoms.

When interpreting studies of the treatment of negative symptoms in schizophrenia, it is important to be aware that different investigators employ differing definitions of negative symptoms. For example, the set of symptoms that Crow [25, 27] defined as negative is almost identical to the group of symptoms that comprise the psychomotor poverty syndrome as illustrated in Table 1, whereas the symptoms included by Andreasen [28] in the widely used Scale for the Assessment of Negative Symptoms embrace a much broader range of phenomena, including attentional impairment and anhedonia. The negative symptoms defined in the Positive and Negative Syndrome Scale (PANSS) [29], and also in the Brief Psychiatric Rating Scale (BPRS) [30] correspond moderately closely to the concept of negative symptoms proposed by Crow [25,27], though in both of these scales, inappropriate affect is included within the blunted affect item.

Affective symptoms

In addition to the symptoms that are characteristic of schizophrenia, other symptoms that are usually regarded as more characteristic of affective disorder, are also prevalent. Depression, manifest as lowering of mood, lowered self-esteem, pessimism. and hopelessness, can occur during any phase of the illness. It is a common prodromal feature, occurring even before the first psychotic episode. Depression often increases during florid episodes and resolves as the psychosis resolves [31]. It occurs independently of psychotic features during stable phases of illness [32]. In addition depression is a recognised feature of the post-psychotic phase. The risk of suicide is substantial, especially in the early years of the illness, even after psychotic symptoms have resolved.

The causes of depression in schizophrenia are probably multifactorial. In some instances it appears to be an understandable psychological reaction to the illness. Furthermore, dopamine blocking antipsychotic medication can produce dysphoria that resembles depression. Nonetheless it is likely that much of the depression is an intrinsic part of the pathophysiology of schizophrenia. The speculation that a multiplicity of factors contribute to depression in schizophrenia is supported by path analysis of the factors contributing to resolution of depression in treatment trials. The antidepressant affect of atypical antipsychotics can be accounted for in part by reduction in positive symptoms of schizophrenia, negative symptoms of schizophrenia and extrapyramidal side-effects, but 60% of the reduction cannot be accounted for by changes in these variables [33].

A state of psychomotor excitation resembling that occurring in mania often occurs during the florid phase of schizophrenia. This excitation is characterised by motor over-activity, agitation and irritability. In some instances, it is accompanied by hostility.

The high prevalence of affective symptoms in schizophrenia raises the issue of the relationship between schizophrenia and bipolar affective disorder. Kraepelin [1] initially separated these two disorders on the basis of the greater tendency for a sustained deterioration in schizophrenia. Typically in schizophrenia, there is some deterioration of affect. Episodes of excitation or depression are set against a background of more persistent blunted or inappropriate affect, whereas in bipolar affective disorder, a normal, lively affect is usually preserved between episodes. Nonetheless, these differences are a matter of degree, raising the possibility that schizophrenia and bipolar disorder lie at opposites end of a continuum, with schizoaffective cases, which exhibit features characteristic of both disorders, lying near the mid-point.

Cognitive deficits

The majority of schizophrenic patients exhibit overt defects in cognitive function. Virtually all aspects of cognition can be affected, though the defects in memory, executive functions, motor co-ordination and attention are the most marked. In monozygotic twins discordant for schizophrenia, the ill twin usually exhibits poorer cognitive performance than the well twin, even when both perform within the normal range [34], suggesting that in virtually all cases, there is a failure to achieve the potential that might have been expected in the absence of the illness. Furthermore, this finding indicates that non-genetic factors contribute to the cognitive deficits in schizophrenia. However, cognitive deficits are also observed in first degree relatives of patients. For example, nearly 50% of first degree relatives show evidence of impairment in spatial working memory task [35], suggesting that at least some of the cognitive impairments are a manifestation of the inherited predisposition to the illness. Cognitive deficits are detectable prior to onset of the illness [36, 37], and tend to be persistent. There is a growing body of evidence indicating that atypical antipsychotics, which block serotonin $5HT_2$ receptors in addition to blocking dopamine D_2 receptors, are effective in alleviating the cognitive deficits, especially the impairments of executive function and working memory [38].

Time course of schizophrenia

The earliest signs of schizophrenia are discernible in infancy, at least in some cases. Video recordings of children who later develop schizophrenia show noticeable motor incoordination when compared with their siblings [39]. The likelihood that a child who subsequently develops schizophrenia in adult life, will have failed to acquire speech by age two, is approximately five times greater than for their peers [36]. When tested at age 7 years and at age 11 years, these pre-schizophrenic children show impaired language and mathematical skills relative to their classmates [36, 37]. Their most significant behavioural anomalies are shyness and inconsequential behaviours [37].

When this evidence of developmental delay and cognitive impairment is added to the large body of evidence demonstrating an association between schizophrenia and birth difficulties [40], minor physical anomalies of developmental origin [41], and evidence of aberrant migration of neurons, especially in frontal and temporal lobes [42], there can be no doubt that schizophrenia is associated with abnormalities of neuro-development. Whether or not such neuro-developmental anomalies are merely a non-specific predisposing factor, or play a specific role in the pathophysiology of schizophrenia, has yet to be clearly established. The fact that the behavioural disturbances include features such as inconsequential behaviours which bear a similarity to the disorganisation syndrome, suggests that the relationship might be specific.

In adolescence it is common for social withdrawal and other evidence of negative symptoms to develop. During this prodromal phase it is quite common for episodes of depressive symptoms to occur as well. Typically, at the end of adolescence or early in adult life, the first psychotic episode occurs. There is a well established gender difference, with the peak onset being several years earlier in males than in females. It should also be noted that despite onset in young adult life being the norm, in a minority of cases the illness does not emerge until after age 35 and occasionally the onset is not until after age 50.

The course subsequent to the first episode is very variable. A minority, perhaps 10–15%, make a complete recovery [43] but in the majority, there is a period of several decades during which there are intermittent episodes of florid psychosis super-imposed upon a background of enduring disability. During the florid episodes, the most noticeable features are excitement, delusions, hallucinations and formal thought disorder. Psychomotor excitation is common, although, paradoxically, a substantial number of cases show an increase in psychomotor poverty during this phase. In the chronic phase, disorganisation is expressed as vague wandering speech, oddities of manner and disjointed volitional behaviour. Psychomotor poverty often becomes pronounced in this phase of the illness. Cognitive impairments usually persist during the chronic phase of the illness. In a significant minority of cases, delusions and hallucinations can also persist, although this is not the norm. In some patients, non-specific symptoms such as anxiety and coenesthesia (abnormal somatic perceptions) are common in this phase.

The long-term outcome of the illness is variable. About 10% of cases suffer persisting, severe disability throughout life, though the majority show improvement in middle age. Even among populations who suffer severe illness in the early phases, over 50% are functioning quite well 30 years later [3]. It is noteworthy that duration of psychosis prior to first treatment is a strong predictor of subsequent outcome, suggesting that psychosis itself damages the brain [44].

The heterogeneity of schizophrenia

The heterogeneity of symptoms and of time-course in schizophrenia have prompted many attempts to identify a satisfactory division of the illness into different sub-types.

The classical sub-types

According to the classical sub-typing, derived from clinical descriptions provided by Kraepelin [1] and Bleuler [2], there are four sub-types:

1) paranoid schizophrenia, characterised by reality distortion symptoms with relatively good preservation of personality;
2) hebephrenia, which usually presents in adolescence or early adult life and is characterised by silly behaviour, fatuous affect, formal thought disorder and fragmented delusions;
3) catatonia, which is dominated by episodic disorders of voluntary motor activity;
4) simple schizophrenia, characterised by gradual deterioration in function over a period of more than a year, without florid symptoms.

The classical subtyping has been retained in ICD-10 [4] and is also is employed in a modified form in DSM-IV, despite the fact that there is little evidence that it reflects a natural cleavage into discrete types of illness based on distinct pathophysiology or aetiology. In clinical practice, the major limitation of the classical sub-typing is the fact that many individual cases exhibit characteristics of several different subtypes.

Reactive vs process schizophrenia

While the classical subdivision is based predominantly on symptom type, an alternative approach is to divide the illness according to time-course. The simplest such classification divides the illness into reactive and process types [45]. Reactive schizophrenia is characterised by abrupt onset of episodes of florid symptoms, possibly related to a stressful event, with subsequent remission of symptoms and minimal residual disability. Process schizophrenia is characterised by gradual onset, with subsequent persistence of symptoms and disability. The major weakness of the reactive/process classification arises from the observation that there is a continuum of chronicity of illness, and it has proven impossible to identify a clear-cut boundary between reactive and process types. Nonetheless, a large body of evidence supports the conclusion that process schizophrenia is more strongly associated with indices of diffuse brain abnormality. For example, process schizophrenia is associated with more severe, wide-ranging cognitive deficits [46]. It appears that reactive and process schizophrenia lie on a continuum that reflects an increasing severity of diffuse brain abnormality towards the process end of the spectrum. In relation to the hypothesised continuum extending from bipolar disorder *via* schizoaffective disorder to schizophrenia, reactive schizophrenia lies adjacent to schizoaffective disorder while process schizophrenia lies at the far end of the continuum. While the reactive/process distinction is not currently employed in clinical practice, it has shaped several recent classification schemes that have sought to subdivide the illness on the basis of pathophysiology or aetiology, such as Crow's type 1/type 2 hypothesis [25, 27].

Type 1/type 2 schizophrenia

The type 1/type 2 hypothesis is based on the observation that negative symptoms tend to be chronic while positive symptoms tend to be acute and transient. Crow proposed that type 1 schizophrenia, which is manifest as positive symptoms, arises from biochemical imbalance, such as dopaminergic hyperactivity. He postulated that type 2 schizophrenia, which is manifest as negative symptoms and cognitive impairment, arises from structural abnormality of the brain, such as is reflected in increased size of the cerebral ventricles relative to the volume of brain tissue.

It should be noted that Crow did not actually propose that type 1 and type 2 schizophrenia were different illnesses, but rather two different processes that could occur within a single illness. Other investigators, such as Andreasen and Olsen [47], did attempt to define positive and negative schizophrenia as distinct conditions. However, approximately a third of their cases could not be assigned to either group because they exhibited an approximately equal mixture of the symptoms characteristic of both types, indicating that positive and negative schizophrenia are not separate illnesses.

Crow's type 1/type 2 distinction is broadly consistent with a substantial body of evidence [27, 48], and it provided a powerful stimulus to research into the mechanisms of schizophrenic symptoms in the 1980's. However, Crow did not address the question of whether it is symptom type or symptom chronicity that is the essential clinical attribute distinguishing the postulated type 1 and type 2 pathological processes. The observation that negative symptoms do respond at least partially to antipsychotic medication [23], while in a substantial proportion of cases positive symptoms persist despite adequate blockade of dopamine receptors [49], suggests that, on the one hand, biochemical imbalance plays a part in negative symptoms, while, on the other hand, factors other than dopamine overactivity are involved in producing positive symptoms. Furthermore, enlargement of cerebral ventricles is associated with poor response to treatment, irrespective of symptom type [50]. Therefore, it is plausible to propose that the relative contributions of biochemical imbalance and structural abnormality to the production of symptoms determines the tendency to chronicity of symptoms, rather than symptom type *per se*.

According to this perspective, episodic dopamine overactivity is responsible for acute exacerbations of symptoms, while an enduring cerebral structural abnormality is responsible for persistent symptoms and chronic disability. A large body of evidence indicates that the mechanism of the florid episodes involves dopaminergic over-activity. For example indirect dopamine agonists can promote an exacerbation of symptoms that are predominantly positive, although negative symptoms, such as flat affect and apathy, can also be induced [51]. Schizophrenic patients are prone to exhibit a greater release of endogenous dopamine than healthy subjects, and the amount of dopamine release is correlated with the severity of induced symptoms [52]. Plasma homovanillic acid increases during florid relapse [24], and the amplitude of this increase is correlated with the severity of both positive and negative symptoms.

Defect vs non-defect schizophrenia

Another recent attempt to describe the heterogeneity of schizophrenia that has its roots in both the reactive/process distinction and the positive/negative dichotomy is the defect/non-defect distinction proposed by Carpenter and colleagues [53]. Defect schizophrenia is characterised by chronic negative symptoms that have persisted for at least 1 year. Carpenter and colleagues have assembled a substantial body of evidence indicating that defect patients differ from non-defect patients in many respects that are potentially relevant to pathophysiology or aetiology. For example, they have found that defect patients are more likely to have enlarged cerebral ventricles. They emphasise that many of the pathological and/or etiological variables that are associated with the defect state are not significantly correlated with negative symptom score when transient negative symptoms are included. Whether or not defect schizophrenia is a distinct illness or merely the severe end of a continuum remains to be firmly established. It should be noted that only about 10–15% of patients with established schizophrenia satisfy rigorous criteria for the defect state.

Overall, there is only a small amount of evidence indicating that schizophrenia can be divided into discrete sub-types on the basis of type or time-course of symptoms. The relative lack of success of attempts at sub-typing schizophrenia after a century of clinical investigation points towards the possibility that most of the heterogeneity of clinical features reflects variations along several dimensions of pathophysiology within a single illness, albeit an illness that arises from a multitude of causal factors.

The pathophysiology of schizophrenia

The evidence discussed above supports the proposal that there is a subtle neurodevelopmental anomaly that produces relatively mild impairment of function in childhood, but predisposes to a florid crisis, mediated by dopaminergic hyperactivity, at time of stress in young adulthood. While treatment with dopamine blockers usually induces remission of the florid episode, the demonstration that even positive schizophrenic symptoms can persist despite adequate dopamine blockade [49] suggests that dopamine hyperactivity is merely a mechanism of symptom exacerbation, rather than the primary pathophysiological mechanism.

Studies of regional cerebral activity associated with persistent symptoms [14] indicate that each of the three syndromes of characteristic symptoms is associated with a specific pattern of aberrant activity in a distributed neural network embracing areas of association cortex and related subcortical nuclei (see Table 2). For each syndrome, the cerebral sites involved include those sites that are normally engaged during the type of mental processes implicated in that syndrome [11,14].

The nature of the enduring aberrant function in the relevant cerebral circuits is a matter for speculation. There is evidence for an overt structural abnormality, at least in the most persistent cases [54]. However the observation that the majority of cases exhibit a degree of recovery in late middle age [3] implies that whatever the nature of the neuronal abnormality, it can be overcome. This observation is reinforced by studies of regional cerebral activity during tasks such as word generation. Even in very severe persistent cases, the magnitude of cerebral activation in the left lateral frontal site that plays a cardinal role in word generation is normal, provided the rate of word generation is paced [55]. However the relationship of activation in frontal cortex to regional activity at other cerebral sites is abnormal. In particular, the reduction of activity in the superior temporal gyrus that accompanies the frontal activation in healthy subjects is less

Table 2. Cognitive deficits and patterns of aberrant regional cerebral activity associated with the characteristic syndromes of schizophrenia [14]

Syndrome	Cognitive deficit	Increased rCBF	Decreased rCBF
Reality distortion	Evaluation of mental activity	Medial temporal lobe L lateral frontal cortex Ventral striatum	Posterior cingulate L lateral temporal lobe
Disorganization	Selection of mental activity	R anterior cingulate Thalamus	R ventral frontal cortex R & L parietal cortex
Psychomotor poverty	Initiation of mental activity	Caudate nuclei	L lateral frontal cortex L parietal cortex

R = right, L = left, rCBF = regional cerebral blood flow.

marked, or absent, in schizophrenic patients [55–57], and the magnitude of thalamic activation is reduced [56]. This indicates impaired coordination of cerebral activity at diverse sites, and suggests that the essential pathophysiological process in schizophrenia might be a failure to develop efficient connections between cerebral sites.

References

1 Kraepelin E (1919) *Dementia praecox and paraphrenia*. (Trans. RM Barclay, 1919, facsimile edition, published 1971) Kreiger, New York

2 Bleuler E (1911) *Dementia praecox or the group of schizophrenias*. (Trans. J. Zinkin, 1950) International Universities Press, New York

3 Harding CM, Zubin J, Strauss JS (1992) Chronicity in schizophrenia: revisited. *Br J Psychiatry* 161 (suppl 18): 27–37

4 World Health Organization (1993) *The tenth revision of the international classification of diseases. (ICD10)*. WHO, Geneva

5 American Psychiatric Association (1994) *Diagnostic and statistical manual of mental disorders, fourth edition*. American Psychiatric Association, Washington DC

6 Liddle PF (1984) *Chronic schizophrenic symptoms, cognitive function and neurological impairment*. (Dissertation) Royal College of Psychiatrists, London

7 Liddle PF (1987) The symptoms of chronic schizophrenia: a re-examination of the positive-negative dichotomy. *Br J Psychiatry* 151: 145–151

8 Arndt S, Alliger RJ, Andreasen NC (1991) The distinction of positive and negative symptoms. The failure of a two-dimensional model. *Br J Psychiatry* 158: 317–322

9 Bilder RM, Mukherjee S, Reider RO, Pandurangi AK (1985) Symptomatic and neuropsychological components of defect states. *Schizophr Bull* 11: 409–419

10 Kulhara P, Kota SK and Joseph S (1986) Positive and negative subtypes of schizophrenia: a study from India. *Acta Psychiatr Scand* 74: 353–379

11 Malla AK, Norman RMG, Williamson P, Cortese L, Diaz F (1993) Three syndrome concept of schizophrenia, a factor analytic study. *Schizophr Res* 10: 143–150

12 Arndt S, Andreasen NC, Flaum M, Miller D, Nopoulos P (1995) A longitudinal study of symptom dimensions in schizophrenia. *Arch Gen Psychiatry* 52, 352–360

13 Liddle PF (1995) Inner connections within the domain of dementia praecox: the role of supervisory mental processes in schizophrenia. *Eur Arch Psychiatr Clin Neurosci* 245: 210–215

14 Liddle PF, Friston KJ, Frith CD, Jones T, Hirsch SR, Frackowiak RSJ (1992) Patterns of cerebral blood flow in schizophrenia. *Br J Psychiatry* 160: 179–186

15 Schneider K (1959) *Clinical Psychology*. (Trans. MW Hamilton) Grune Stratton, New York

16 O'Grady JC (1990) The prevalence and diagnostic significance of first-rank symptoms in a random sample of acute psychiatric in-patients. *Br J Psychiatry* 156: 496–500

17 Liddle PF, Morris DL (1991) Schizophrenic syndromes and frontal lobe performance. *Br J Psychiatry* 158: 340–345

18 McGrath JJ (1992) The neuropsychology of thought disorder. *Schizophr Res* 6: 157.

19 Baxter RD, Liddle PF (1998) Neuropsychological deficits associated with schizophrenic syndromes. *Schizophr Res* 30: 239–250

20 Spohn HE, Coyne L, Larson L (1986) Episodic and residual thought pathology in chronic schizophrenics. *Schizophr Bull* 12: 394–407

21 Allen HA, Frith CD, Liddle PF (1993) Negative features, retrieval processes and verbal fluency in schizophrenia. *Br J Psychiatry* 163: 769–775

22 Dollfus S, Petit M (1995) Negative symptoms in schizophrenia: their evolution during an acute phase. *Schizophr Res* 17: 187–194

23 Tollefson GD, Sanger TM (1997) Negative symptoms: a path analytic approach to a double-blind, placebo and haloperidol-controlled clinical trial with olanzapine. *Am J Psychiatry* 154: 466–476

24 Pickar D, Labarca R, Doran A, Wolkowicz OM, Roy A, Brier A, Linnoila M, Paul SM (1986) Longitudinal measurements of plasma homovanillic acid levels in schizophrenic patients. *Arch Gen Psychiatry* 43: 669–679
25 Crow TJ (1980) The molecular pathology of schizophrenia: more than one disease process. *BMJ* 280: 66-68
26 Johnstone EC, Crow TJ, Frith CD (1978) Mechanism of the antipsychotic effect in the treatment of acute schizophrenia. *Lancet* ii: 848–851
27 Crow TJ (1985) The two syndrome concept: origins and current status. *Schizophr Bull* 11: 471–486
28 Andreasen NC (1982) Negative symptoms in schizophrenia: definition and reliability *Arch Gen Psychiatry* 39: 784–788
29 Kay SR (1991) *Positive and negative syndromes in schizophrenia.* Brunner Mazel, New York
30 Overall JE, Gorham DR (1962) The brief psychiatric rating scale. *Psychological Reports* 10: 799–812
31 Leff J, Tress K, Edwards B (1988) The clinical course of depressive symptoms in schizophrenia. *Schizophr Res* 1: 25–30
32 Barnes TRE, Curson D, Liddle PF, Patel M (1989) The nature and prevalence of depression in chronic schizophrenic in-patients. *Br J Psychiatry* 154: 486–491
33 Tollefson GD, Sanger TM, Lu Y, Thieme ME (1998) Depressive signs and symptoms in schizophrenia: a prospective blinded trial of olanzapine and haloperidol. *Arch Gen Psychiatry* 55: 250-258
34 Goldberg TE, Ragland DR, Gold J, Bigelow LB, Torrey EF, Weinberger DR (1990) Neuropsychological assessment of monozygotic twins discordant for schizophrenia. *Arch Gen Psychiatry* 47: 1066–1072
35 Park S, Holzman PS, Goldman-Rakic PS (1995) Spatial working memory deficits in the relatives of schizophrenic patients. *Arch Gen Psychiatry* 52: 821–828
36 Jones P, Rodgers B, Murray R (1994) Child development risk factors for adult schizophrenia in the British 1946 birth cohort. *Lancet* 344: 1398–1402
37 Done DJ, Crow TJ, Johnstone EC, Sacker A (1994) Childhood antecedents of schizophrenia and affective illness: social adjustment at ages 7 and 11 *BMJ* 309: 699–703
38 Green MF, Marshall BD, Wirshing WC, Ames D, Marder SR, McGurk S, Kern RS, Mintz J (1997) Does risperidone improve working memory in treatment-resistant schizophrenia? *Am J Psychiatry* 154: 799–804
39 Walker E, Lewine RJ (1990) Prediction of adult-onset schizophrenia from childhood home videos of the patients *Am J Psychiatry* 89: 704–716
40 McNeil TF (1995) Perinatal risk factors and schizophrenia: selective review and methodological concerns. *Epidemiological Reviews* 17: 107–112
41 Mellor CS (1992) Dermatoglyphic evidence of fluctuating asymmetry in schizophrenia. *Br J Psychiatry* 160: 467–472
42 Akbarian S, Bunney WE jr, Potkin SG (1993) Altered distribution of nicotinamide-adenine dinucleotide phosphate diaphorase cells in frontal lobe of schizophrenics implies anomalous cortical development. *Arch Gen Psychiatry* 50: 178–187
43 Watt DC, Katz K, Shepherd M (1983) The natural history of schizophrenia: a 5 year prospective follow-up study of a representative sample of schizophrenics by means of a standardized clinical and social assessment. *Psychol Med* 13: 663–670
44 Crow TJ, MacMillan JF, Johnson AL, Johnstone EC (1986) The Northwick Park Study of first episodes of schizophrenia. I. A randomised controlled trial of prophylactic treatment. *Br J Psychiatry* 148:120–127
45 Garmezy N (1968) Process and reactive schizophrenia: some conceptions and issues. In: MM Katz, JO Cole, WE Barton (eds) *The role and methodology of classification in psychiatry and psychopathology (Publication No. 1584).* US Public Health Service, Washington DC
46 Heaton RK, Baade LE, Johnson KL (1978) Neuropsychological test results associated with psychiatric disorders in adults. *Psychol Bull* 85: 141–162
47 Andreasen NC, Olsen S (1982) Negative v. Positive schizophrenia: definition and validation. *Arch Gen Psychiatry* 39: 789–794
48 Liddle P, Carpenter WT, Crow T (1994) Syndromes of schizophrenia: the classic literature. *Br J Psychiatry* 165: 721–727

49 Wolkin A, Barouche F, Wolf AP (1989) Dopamine blockade and clinical response: evidence for two biological sub-groups of schizophrenia. *Am J Psychiatry* 146: 905–908
50 Lewis SW (1990) Computerised tomography in schizophrenia 15 years on. *Br J Psychiatry* 157 (suppl 9): 16–24
51 Fibiger HC (1991) The dopamine hypothesis of schizophrenia and mood disorders: contradictions and speculations. In: P Willner and J Scheel-Kruger (eds): *The mesolimbic dopamine system: from motivation to action.* John Wiley, Chichester, 615–637
52 Laruelle M, Abi-Dargham A, van Dyck CH, Gil R, D'Souza CD, Erdos J, McCance E, Rosenblatt W, Fingado C, Zoghbi S et al (1996) Single photon emission computerized tomography imaging of amphetamine-induced dopamine release in drug-free schizophrenic subjects. *Proc Nat Acad Sci USA* 93: 9235–9240
53 Carpenter WT jr, Heinrichs DW, Wagman AM (1988) Deficit and non-deficit forms of schizophrenia: the concept. *Am J Psychiatry* 145: 578–583
54 Chua SE, Wright IC, Poline J-B, Liddle PF, Murray RM, Frackowiak RSJ, Friston KJ, McGuire PK (1997) Grey matter correlates of syndromes in schizophrenia: a semi-automated analyses of structural magnetic resonance images. *Br J Psychiatry* 170: 406–410
55 Frith CD, Friston KJ, Herold S, Silbersweig D, Fletcher P, Cahill C, Dolan RJ, Frackowiak RSJ, Liddle PF (1995) Regional brain activity in chronic schizophrenic patients during the performance of a verbal fluency task. *Br J Psychiatry* 167: 343–349
56 Liddle PF, Passmore M, Friston KJ, Frith CD (1997) Functional connectivity during word generation in schizophrenia. *Schizophr Res* 24: 16
57 Fletcher PC, McKenna PJ, Frith CD, Grasby PM, Friston KJ, Dolan RJ (1998) Brain activations in schizophrenia during a graded memory task studied with functional neuroimaging. *Arch Gen Psychiatry* 55: 1001–1008

Atypical Antipsychotics
ed. by B.A. Ellenbroek and A.R. Cools

From first to second generation antipsychotics

John L. Waddington[1,2] and John F. Quinn[2,1]

[1] *Department of Clinical Pharmacology, Royal College of Surgeons in Ireland, St. Stephen's Green, Dublin 2, Ireland*
[2] *Stanley Foundation Research Unit, St. Davnet's Hospital, Monaghan, Ireland*

Introduction

As late as 1993, 85% of psychotic inpatients at a major university psychiatric referral centre in the United States were found to be receiving antipsychotic drugs that had been available for some three decades or more, most commonly perphenazine and haloperidol, with an additional 2% receiving loxapine and 13% receiving clozapine [1]. Since the identification in the 1950s of chlorpromazine as the archetype antipsychotic, a profound advance that has received personal, historical documentation by one of the principal innovators [2], their properties have been subject to extensive contemporary review [3–7]. Yet these reviews share at least one chastening theme: enduring uncertainty, in the face of extensive clinical use over four decades, as to a number of quite fundamental aspects of their antipsychotic actions, including such basic issues as diagnostic specificity, time-course of therapeutic effect, optimal dosage and most effective treatment strategy.

Diagnostic specificity

There is evidence from controlled clinical trials that treatment with a conventional first-generation (typical) antipsychotic appears effective in alleviating "positive" psychotic symptoms in patients with functional psychosis (including schizophrenia, schizoaffective disorder, schizophreniform disorder, bipolar disorder, depression with psychotic features, paranoid disorder and atypical psychosis) [8], and that this occurs in a manner unrelated to the presence or absence of elevated or depressed mood, each of which remained substantially unaltered by such treatment; conversely, lithium appeared to have little effect on such psychotic symptoms or depressed mood but reduced elevation in mood.

Time-course of therapeutic effect

Though it is widely held that the full antipsychotic effect of first-generation agents may not be manifested until 2–4 weeks following initiation of treatment, evidence for the proposition from controlled clinical trials is far from substantial [9]. These reviewers concluded that controlled studies of shorter duration (hours-days) observed moderate improvement, while those of longer duration (days-weeks) observed little improvement over the first few days and marked improvement only over weeks of treatment; they speculate that the early effects of such antipsychotics may be non-specific and might be largely the same as those of sedative agents or else reflective of hospitalisation or other non-pharmacological clinical interventions. More recent studies continue to suggest clinically meaningful, though not necessarily maximal improvement over 3–10 days of treatment with perphenazine or haloperidol [10–12]; this occurs in the face of essentially maximal (73–92%) occupancy of brain D_2-like dopamine receptors, the presumed primary common action of such agents, within a few hours of acute ingestion of modest doses (4–7.5 mg), of haloperidol, at least by normal, volunteer subjects studied using positron emission tomography (PET) [13].

Optimal dosage

It is of particular note that optimal dosage, even for extensively utilised agents such as haloperidol, has received little empirical study. A review in 1986 revealed a paucity of studies but suggested that moderate doses are adequate for most patients, with little evidence to support the usage of high doses which might actually be associated with reduced efficacy as well as more prominent adverse effects [14]. Subsequent studies have confirmed these suggestions and elaborated on the quantitative relationships. In particular, a series of studies now indicate that the effectiveness of haloperidol appears maximal at approximately ≤ 10 mg daily in most patients, with higher doses being of no greater efficacy and possibly of reduced efficacy though, unexpectedly, not always of greater adverse effect liability [15–18]; on the basis of studies with fluphenazine [19], it has been suggested that a relationship between dosage and effectiveness may be most evident when non-responding patients are excluded. Similarly, pharmacokinetic studies now indicate that optimal effectiveness of haloperidol is attained at plasma concentrations in the range of 5–12 ng/ml; no predictable additional benefit appears to derive from higher levels and, in some instances, reducing higher plasma concentrations towards this general range was associated with further improvement [20–23]. The pharmacokinetics of long-acting ("depot") injectable preparations of antipsychotic drugs are considerably more complex [24].

In accordance with such findings, occupancy of brain D_2-like receptors, as evaluated by PET, approached maximal values (70–89%) at daily doses of 4–6 mg haloperidol, 200 mg chlorpromazine, 300–400 mg thioridazine, 10 mg trifluoperazine and 6 mg flupenthixol [25]; occupancy of D_2-like receptors reaches such values at 5–15 ng/ml haloperidol [26], in accordance with clinical pharmacokinetic studies. Subsequent investigations have confirmed that modest doses of haloperidol [oral, 2–4 mg daily; decanoate, 30–50 mg monthly] can be effective therapeutically while occupying 53–82% of D_2-like receptors [27, 28]; these effects appear to endure for some months following discontinuation of haloperidol decanoate [29]. However, one recent study, while supporting the clinical effectiveness of modest haloperidol doses, suggests some incompatibility between an optimal plasma concentration of 8–12 ng/ml and occupancy of 60–80% of D_2-like receptors [30].

Treatment strategy

It has been considered whether targeted antipsychotic therapy, whereby medication is discontinued after a period of clinical stability and reinstituted only on prodromal signs of psychotic relapse/decompensation, might prove an effective treatment strategy which would decrease the amount of antipsychotic administered and perhaps reduce the long-term burden of adverse effects. However, studies of this strategy continue to indicate an increased rate of relapse/decompensation and rehospitalization relative to continuous treatment, with or without reduction in adverse effects [31–33]. Studies of the sequelae of antipsychotic withdrawal, with a view either to long-term discontinuation or to periodic "drug holidays", confirm the risk of relapse to be increased substantially relative to continuation of medication [34, 35].

Reappraisal of domains of antipsychotic activity

Enduring uncertainty as to optimal dosage and treatment strategy is accompanied by similar uncertainty as to what domains of psychopathology are ameliorated by antipsychotics. Psychopathology has been commonly dissociated into "positive" and "negative" symptoms [see Liddle chapter 1], with the former accepted to be more responsive and the latter posited to respond less readily or hardly at all to such medication [5,7, 36,37]. Paradoxically, it is the current wave of extensive, multicentre double-blind controlled trials in which second-generation ("atypical") antipsychotics are compared with placebo and a first-generation ("typical") reference agent, usually haloperidol, that has allowed the profiles of such first-generation agents to be re-evaluated from a contemporary perspective.

Effects on "positive" vs "negative" symptom scores

In trials establishing the clinical profiles of risperidone [38], olanzapine [39], sertindole [40] and quetiapine [41], reference-placebo comparisons consistently confirm haloperidol to reduce overall severity of illness, total psychopathology and "positive" symptom scores, but with more modest [40, 41] or minimal [38, 39] effects on "negative" symptom scores when given for 6–8 weeks; this profile was generally apparent using fixed doses of 4, 8, 12, 16 or 20 mg, or flexible dosage within the range of 10–20 mg haloperidol daily. Importantly, in the one study which included three fixed doses of haloperidol [4, 8 and 16 mg], the first such double-blind, placebo-controlled dosage comparison over four decades of availability, 8 mg haloperidol daily was found to be the most effective [40], in accordance with findings from studies that had adopted alternative or less rigorous approaches to the issue (see "*Optimal dosage*").

Nature of effects on "negative" symptom scores

When such effects are evident, a distinction between changes in *primary* (or *deficit*) and in *secondary* "negative" symptoms (i.e. apparent reductions in scores due indirectly to effects on "positive", depressive or extrapyramidal features) is now recognised to be important conceptually; it has been argued that at least first-generation antipsychotics have little or no activity against *primary/deficit* symptoms, with reductions in "negative" symptom scores reflecting effects on *secondary* features [42]. In this new wave of controlled clinical trials, "path analysis" has been offered as a statistical route to clarifying the extent to which drug-induced changes in total "negative" symptom scores reflect effects on *primary vs secondary* features [43]; this approach suggests the modest overall effect of 10–20 mg haloperidol daily on "negative" symptom scores to be attributable mainly to *secondary* effects on "positive" symptoms [44]. Evidence to indicate that reducing plasma levels of haloperidol after the first 3 weeks of treatment can decrease mild but not severe negative symptoms [45] may reflect plasma concentrations more optimal for reduction in "positive" symptoms or extrapyramidal features.

Alternative perspectives of effectiveness

It is increasingly recognised that evaluation of the effectiveness of antipsychotics should not be limited to quantification of symptom suppression but, rather, be related more holistically to each patient's individual impairments, functional status, perceptions and social capacity, in both the short- and long-term.

Quality-of-life

This concept is generic to all branches of medicine but has received only limited application in schizophrenia, where it seeks to access these aspects of individual patient well-being through integration of the multiplicity of impairments and consequences of the illness with beneficial and adverse effects (to be considered below) over the course of treatment [46]. Recently, among responders to acute haloperidol treatment who continued in a double-blind extension phase of a trial that included haloperidol as a reference agent [39], quality-of-life was assessed following 24 weeks of treatment. At this time, and in the face of enduring reduction in total psychopathology, but not in "negative" symptom or overall severity scores, haloperidol was not associated with any improvement in quality-of-life indices in terms of intrapsychic foundations (cognition, conation and affectivity), interpersonal relations (social relations and interpersonal experience), instrumental role category (functioning in one's social role) or common objects and activities (possession of objects indicative of community participation and engagement in regular activities). This complex area is in need of much further study.

Long-term outcome

Beyond acute symptom suppression, and in elaboration of quality-of-life estimates, long-term outcome in psychotic illness should include clinical, rehabilitative, humanitarian and public safety domains; the effectiveness of antipsychotic agents should involve proximal effects, not only on "positive" and "negative" symptoms but also on other aspects of psychopathology and on relational functions, followed by distal effects on functional status, individual quality-of-life and family well-being, and to ensure public safety [47]. It must be emphasised that the effects of first-generation antipsychotics on long-term outcome remain very poorly understood in these most important terms.

Treatment refractoriness

Despite overwhelming evidence that antipsychotic drugs exert a profound overall effect on psychotic symptoms, some 25% of patients do not respond adequately in one or more domains of psychopathology, or at all, to treatment with first-generation agents; these constitute a major therapeutic problem [48, 49]. In the course of ineffective treatment, such patients demonstrate by PET an occupancy of D_2-like receptors indistinguishable from those of responders, and hence they cannot be accounted for in terms of any failure to attain adequately, for either pharmacokinetic or pharmacodynamic reasons, the presumed primary mechanistic effect of these agents [50, 51]. There is no consistent body of evidence to indicate the effectiveness of unusually high doses of antipsychotics in such patients [48, 49]; rather, there is preliminary evidence that some may actually benefit from a gradual reduction in what is commonly a high but currently ineffective dose [52].

Reappraisal of adverse effect profiles for first-generation antipsychotics

These same decades of extensive clinical experience, over which several fundamental aspects of therapeutic efficacy have remained unclear, have generated what is often thought to be a better, though still incomplete, understanding of their adverse effects. Here, these effects are outlined, before considering further their consequences in the context of the need for improved, second generation antipsychotics and how such agents should be defined.

Neurological adverse effects

The classical "acute" extrapyramidal side-effects (EPS) of first-generation antipsychotics, primarily Parkinsonism, dystonia and akathisia, are well recognised and documented [7, 53, 54]. Their pathophysiological bases are at least partially understood or else the subject of heuristic hypotheses [55]. More specifically, there has been considerable interest in evidence from PET studies that such EPS become more likely at occupancies of D_2-like receptors above some threshold between 74% and 82%, and that occupancies between 70% and that threshold are less likely to be associated with EPS while antipsychotic efficacy is retained [25]. It should be noted that only recently has the prototypical agent chlorpromazine been examined in detail using PET for its relative occupancy of 5-HT_2-like *vis-à-vis* D_2-like receptors, a ratio thought to underlie propensity to induce EPS [56], and results direct attention back onto D_2-like receptor occupancy [57; see also 58].

This level of understanding does not extend to rarer EPS such as rabbit syndrome and for very rare but potentially life-threatening reactions characterised by more severe and generalised neurological dysfunction, such as neuroleptic malignant syndrome (NMS); similarly, the nature and pathophysiology of abnormal, involuntary movement disorder in patients receiving long-term exposure to first-generation antipsychotics (i.e. "tardive dyskinesia") continues to engender controversy [6, 53–55]. Furthermore, it is often overlooked that the spectrum of neurological adverse effects of such antipsychotics extends beyond EPS to encompass subjective dysphoria, unwanted sedation, lowering of seizure threshold and, controversially, cognitive dysfunction [54]; the extent to which antipsychotics impair cognitive function or alleviate illness-related cognitive impairment as an additional domain of antipsychotic efficacy is still widely debated [59–61].

Additional domains of adverse effect

Such an understandable emphasis on what can be highly visible and problematic EPS often results in insufficient attention being paid to an unfortunately broad range of other adverse effects of first-generation antipsychotics which, though often more subtle and covert in their presentation, can be a cause of serious debility [7, 54, 62, 63]: hyperprolactinemia, with associated endocrinological sequelae; sexual dysfunction, constituting a major impediment to holistic recovery; weight gain, presenting both medical and cosmetic-social problems; autonomic/cardiovascular effects, which engender particular concern in relation to sudden unexpected death, especially in association with high dose therapy and in a forensic setting [64–66].

There can also be adverse effects, of variable likelihood and significance, on diverse physiological systems: dermatological, ophthalmic, gastrointestinal, respiratory, hepatic, and haematological [7, 54]; this latter effect is highlighted by concern over the raised propensity of clozapine, the prototypical second-generation antipsychotic, to induce leucopenia-agranulocytosis when the reference rate thereof for first-generation agents is still uncertain. Such agents may be associated with increased morbidity and mortality in patients with Lewy body dementia [67] or asthma [68]; we have recently reported antipsychotic polypharmacy to be associated with reduced survival over 10-years among older inpatients [69], in the face of little or no systematic evidence to justify the administration of more than one antipsychotic concurrently [70].

Patient perception and compliance

Those recent double-blind, controlled clinical trials establishing the clinical profiles of several second-generation antipsychotics [38–41] have also allowed, *via* their reference-placebo comparisons, rigorous re-examination of the adverse effects of haloperidol from a contemporary perspective. While confirming its EPS liability, these trials indicate otherwise perhaps a somewhat more benign profile than might have been expected on the basis of the above analysis; this may reflect doses [4–20 mg daily] lower than those used previously both in research studies and in clinical practice.

However, this should engender no complacency. To consider such adverse effects at an empirical-mechanistic level fails to acknowledge their impact on patients" subjective sense of (lack of) well-being over the course of medication. Firstly, psychiatrists appear to evidence only limited understanding of which adverse effects are most likely to cause distress to patients [71]. Furthermore, while the role of such adverse effects, including but not confined to EPS in general and akathisia in particular, to the emergence of antipsychotic drug-associated dysphoria is not straightforward, the consequences thereof are more clear; it contributes materially to the multifaceted problem of non-compliance with prescribed medication and associated increase in risk for subsequent relapse [72, 73].

Expectations for and the definition of second-generation antipsychotics

It is self-evident that multiple problems associated with the use of conventional antipsychotic drugs constitute an imperative for seeking new, improved agents. However, the renaissance of clozapine and the introduction of remoxipride (now withdrawn), followed by the emergence of yet newer agents which include amisulpride, olanzapine, quetiapine, sertindole, ziprasidone and zotepine [74], are welcome advances which also challenge us as to what our expectations should be and how they should be classified. The term "atypical" conveys simplistically the sense of antipsychotics that are different in some advantageous manner from conventional or "typical" agents. However, despite such widespread usage, it is far from clear that this terminology evolved from clear theoretical underpinnings [62, 75, 76].

At the core of "atypicality" is a reduced liability to induce EPS, and this definition continues to enjoy broad acceptance; however, it appears to be incomplete: for example, as we have argued elsewhere, such a definition is satisfied by the 40-year-old agent thioridazine as well as by remoxipride, with clinical differences in favour of remoxipride being evident, rather, in terms of sedative, autonomic, sexual and other non-neurological adverse effects [78]. Furthermore, clozapine confirms that it is realistic to have yet higher expectations for new antipsychotics, to include also superior efficacy. Thus, the term "atypical" conveys little specific sense of what can be diverse advantages, beyond some generic (though no less welcome) reduction in liability to induce EPS; the term "EPS- sparing" [79] is more pragmatic, but similarly incomplete. It has been suggested that the term second-generation, as applied to advances in antimicrobial therapy is to be preferred as a general descriptor [80], and that broader domains of [dis]advantage beyond EPS liability should be specified for each agent to operationalise the similarities and differences between what are actually heterogeneous agents [62]. Yet the term "atypical" has over the past decade acquired considerable currency, often in association with commercial considerations, and may not be easily displaced; rather, our raised expectations for and classification of second-generation/"atypical" antipsychotics should focus not only on the core property of reduced liability for EPS but also on a broad concept of superior efficacy, an improved adverse effects profile beyond EPS, and pharmacoeconomic considerations [62], as outlined below.

Broader concepts of superior efficacy

New, second-generation antipsychotics and their third-generation successors should demonstrate (ideally superior) efficacy not only against all domains of "positive" symptoms (i.e. reality distortion and disorganisation; see Liddle, this volume) but also against "negative" symptoms (i.e. psychomotor poverty/deficit) domains. Furthermore, they should be effective in patients who are refractory to conventional agents. However, efficacy should extend beyond the domains of psychopathology to encompass alleviation of often disabling cognitive impairment and of co-morbid features such as affective symptoms, anxiety and aggression. These acute actions should endure over continuing therapy to maintain stability and to improve overall quality of life and long-term functional outcome.

Broader concepts of improved adverse effects beyond EPS

Critically, such agents should demonstrate reduced (ideally no) liability in relation to induction not only of EPS but also particularly of subjective dysphoria, unwanted sedation, autonomic/cardiac effects, prolactin elevation and weight gain. In the longer term, new antipsychotics should be associated even less commonly (ideally not at all) with the emergence of involuntary movements ("tardive dyskinesia") and of rare but potentially serious idiosyncratic reactions and unexpected sudden deaths that might otherwise become apparent over phase IV scrutiny.

Pharmacoeconomics

Health economics have moved on from a situation where antipsychotic drug costs could be tabulated on an average purchase price per month for an acute dosage schedule [81] to one which considers in an integrative manner the cost implications of psychotic illness itself *vis-à-vis* all aspects of its treatment in relation to resource allocation [82]. Antipsychotics are coming under increasing fiscal as well as clinical scrutiny, stimulated by the introduction of considerably more expensive second-generation agents with attendant cost-benefit implications [83, 84].

Requirements for future studies

To evaluate new antipsychotics fully in these regards will necessitate variants of contemporary, double-blind, placebo- and reference antipsychotic-controlled multicentre clinical trials over large numbers of patients. Studies will need to include assessment not only of acute efficacy/adverse effects in a much broader sense but also prolonged extension phases to establish these parameters and functional outcome on a long-term basis. It will be important to include in clinical development programmes not only comparisons with first-generation antipsychotics but also "head-to-head" comparisons with current second-generation agents, so that their relative (dis-)merits can be established. There endures the problem of generalising results from the rarefied atmosphere of the controlled clinical trial in carefully screened patients of demographic and diagnostic homogeneity, to those who will receive these agents in "front-line" clinical practice; hence the necessity for enhanced phase IV evaluation.

Early intervention

Over the past several years, there has emerged renewed evidence that the longer psychosis proceeds unchecked following onset, the longer is the latency to attain remission on antipsychotics, the poorer is the quality of that remission, the greater is the likelihood of subsequent relapse and, when initially untreated psychosis is particularly prolonged, the more severe are negative symptoms and cognitive impairment in the long-term; that is, initially untreated (and perhaps treated but non-responsive) psychosis may reflect an active, morbid process that is associated with increasingly poor long-term outcome unless ameliorated by antipsychotic drugs [85–89]. In our own studies, focusing on older inpatients admitted in the pre-neuroleptic era [88, 90], increasing duration of initially untreated illness was associated on regression analysis with increasing severity of current "negative" symptoms, essentially in the psychomotor poverty domain, and, to a lesser extent, of general cognitive impairment. Modest rates of change in outcome measures, together with relatively modest extents of variance therein accounted for [91], suggest that factor(s) additional to duration of initially untreated illness also appear to exert material influence(s) on these features. However, a corollary is that some improvement in long-term outcome may be obtained when intervention with antipsychotics is both as effective and as prompt as possible following the earliest signs of psychotic disturbance [74, 92, 93].

If intervention with medication at the earliest signs of psychotic disturbance can exert some advantageous effect on outcome, this is most likely to be attained using antipsychotics which combine high efficacy with minimal side-effects; given the limited efficacy of conventional agents and particularly their well recognised range of adverse effects, it is perhaps not surprising that physicians can sometimes be reluctant to prescribe such medication until the clinical picture "becomes more clear" and patients can be reluctant to take such medication in the face of subjective discomforture over the very phase of the illness when compliance may be of particular benefit [74]. The fundamental challenge is the extent to which new antipsychotics might shift this balance materially both towards reduced physician concerns over possible long-term consequences of early intervention, perhaps for a condition which may prove subsequently not to be schizophrenia, and towards improved patient compliance [62]. More provocatively, to what extent do the new antipsychotics impact on the practical and ethical debate [94] over intervention with medication at a yet earlier, prodromal phase of the illness; here, there are additional problems of definition and specificity, given that the likelihood of treating some behavioural states which are not the harbingers of a psychotic process is amplified considerably [74]. It will become increasingly important to evaluate new antipsychotics in first-episode populations [95].

Conclusions

It is sobering that reports from the schizophrenia Patient Outcomes Research Team (PORT), set up to develop and disseminate recommendations for the treatment of schizophrenia based on existing scientific evidence, mostly in relation to first-generation agents, re-emphasise the deficiencies in current knowledge; furthermore, PORT findings indicate that current usual treatment practices often fall substantially short of what would be recommended based on the best available evidence [96, 97]. "Evidence-based" practice should be a primary objective for second-generation antipsychotics.

Acknowledgements
The authors' studies are supported by the Stanley Foundation.

References

1 Baldessarini RJ, Kando JC, Centorrino F (1995) Hospital use of antipsychotic agents in 1989 and 1993. *Am J Psychiat* 152: 1038–1044
2 Deniker P (1983) Discovery of the clinical use of neuroleptics. In: MJ Parnham, J Bruinvels (eds): *Discoveries in pharmacology*, Vol 1: *Psycho- and Neuropharmacology*. Elsevier, Amsterdam, 163–180
3 Ellenbroek BA (1993) Treatment of schizophrenia: a clinical and preclinical evaluation of neuroleptic drugs. *Pharmacol Ther* 57: 1–78
4 Johnstone EC (1993) Schizophrenia: problems in clinical practice. Lancet 341: 536–538
5 Dixon LB, Lehman AF, Levine J (1995) Conventional antipsychotic medications for schizophrenia. *Schizophr Bull* 21: 567–577
6 Waddington JL (1995) The clinical psychopharmacology of antipsychotic drugs in schizophrenia. In: SR Hirsch, DR Weinberger (eds): *Schizophrenia*. Blackwell, Oxford, 341–357
7 Kane JM (1996) Drug therapy: Schizophrenia. *N Engl J Med* 334: 34–41
8 Johnstone EC, Crow TJ, Frith CD, Owens DGC (1988) The Northwick Park "functional" psychosis study: diagnosis and treatment response. *Lancet ii*: 119–125
9 Keck PE, Cohen BM, Baldessarini RJ, McElroy SL (1989) Time course of antipsychotic effects of neuroleptic drugs. *Am J Psychiat* 146: 1289–1292
10 Glovinsky D, Kirch DG, Wyatt RJ (1992) Early antipsychotic response to resumption of neuroleptics in drug-free chronic schizophrenic patients. *Biol Psychiat* 31: 968–970

11 Mazure CM, Nelson JC, Jatlow PI, Bowers MB (1992) Drug-response symptoms during early neuroleptic treatment. *Psychiat Res* 41: 147–154
12 Stern RG, Kahn RS, Harvey PD, Amin F, Apter SH, Hirschowitz J (1993) Early response to haloperidol treatment in chronic schizophrenia. *Schiz Res* 10: 165–171
13 Nordstrom AL, Farde L, Halldin C (1992) Time course of D_2-dopamine receptor occupancy examined by PET after single oral doses of haloperidol. *Psychopharmacology* 106: 433–438
14 Baldessarini RJ, Cohen B, Teicher MH (1988) Significance of neuroleptic dose and plasma level in the pharmacological treatment of psychoses. *Arch Gen Psychiat* 45: 79–91
15 Van Putten T, Marder SR, Mintz J (1990) A controlled dose comparison of haloperidol in newly admitted schizophrenic patients. *Arch Gen Psychiat* 47: 754–578
16 Rifkin A, Doddi S, Karajgi B, Borenstein M, Wachspress M (1991) Dosage of haloperidol for schizophrenia. *Arch Gen Psychiat* 48: 166–170
17 McEvoy JP, Hogarty GE, Steingard S (1991) Optimal dose of neuroleptic in acute schizophrenia. *Arch Gen Psychiat* 48: 739–745
18 Stone CK, Garver DL, Griffith J, Hirschowitz J, Bennett J (1995) Further evidence of a dose-response threshold for haloperidol in psychosis. *Am J Psychiat* 152: 1210–1212
19 Levinson DF, Simpson GM, Singh H, Yadalam K, Jain A, Stephanos MJ, Silver P (1990) Fluphenazine dose, clinical response, and extrapyramidal symptoms during acute treatment. *Arch Gen Psychiat* 47: 761–768
20 Van Putten T, Marder SR, Mintz J, Poland RE (1992) Haloperidol plasma levels and clinical response: a therapeutic window relationship. *Am J Psychiat* 149: 500–505
21 Volavka J, Cooper T, Czobor P, Bitter I, Meisner M, Laska E, Gastanaga P, Krakowski M, Chou J, Crowner M, Douyon R (1992) Haloperidol blood levels and clinical effects. *Arch Gen Psychiat* 49: 354–361
22 Volavka J, Cooper TB, Czobor P, Meisner M (1995) Plasma haloperidol levels and clinical effects in schizophrenia and schizoaffective disorder. *Arch Gen Psychiat* 52: 837–845
23 Coryell W, Miller DD, Perry PJ (1998) Haloperidol plasma levels and dose optimization. *Am J Psychiat* 155: 48–53
24 Marder SR, Hubbard JW, Van Putten T, Midha KK (1989) Pharmacokinetics of long-acting injectable neuroleptic drugs: clinical implications. *Psychopharmacology* 98: 433–439
25 Farde L, Nordstrom AL, Wiesel FA, Pauli S, Halldin C, Sedvall G (1992) Positron emission tomographic analysis of central D_1 and D_2 dopamine receptor occupancy in patients treated with classical neuroleptics and clozapine. *Arch Gen Psychiat* 49: 538–544
26 Wolkin A, Brodie JD, Barouche F, Rotrosen J, Wolf AP, Smith M, Fowler J, Cooper TB (1989) Dopamine receptor occupancy and plasma haloperidol levels. *Arch Gen Psychiat* 46: 482–483
27 Nyberg S, Farde L, Halldin C, Dahl ML, Bertilsson L (1995) D_2 dopamine receptor occupancy during low-dose treatment with haloperidol decanoate. *Am J Psychiat* 152: 173–178
28 Kapur S, Remington G, Jones C, Wilson A, DaSilva J, Houle S, Zipursky R (1996) High levels of dopamine D_2 receptor occupancy with low-dose haloperidol treatment: a PET study. *Am J Psychiat* 153: 948–950
29 Nyberg S, Farde L, Halldin C (1997) Delayed normalization of central D_2 dopamine receptor availability after discontinuation of haloperidol decanoate. *Arch Gen Psychiat* 54: 953–958
30 Kapur S, Zipursky R, Roy P, Jones C, Remington G, Reed K, Houle S (1997) The relationship between D_2 receptor occupancy and plasma levels on low dose oral haloperidol: a PET study. *Psychopharmacology* 131: 148–152
31 Carpenter WT, Hanlon TE, Heinrichs DW, Summerfelt AT, Kirkpatrick B, Levine J, Buchanan BW (1990) Continuous vs. targeted medications in schizophrenic outpatients: outcome results. *Am J Psychiat* 147: 1138–1148
32 Jolley AG, Hirsch SR, Morrison E, McRink A, Wilson L (1990) Trial of brief intermittent neuroleptic prophylaxis for selected schizophrenic outpatients: clinical and social outcome at two years. *Br Med J* 301: 837–842
33 Schooler NR, Keith SJ, Severe JB, Matthews SM, Bellack AS, Glick ID, Hargreaves WA, Kane JM, Ninan PT, Frances A et al (1997) Relapse and rehospitalization during maintenance treatment of schizophrenia. *Arch Gen Psychiat* 54: 453–463
34 Gilbert PL, Harris MJ, McAdams LA, Jeste DV (1995) Neuroleptic withdrawal in schizophrenic patients. *Arch Gen Psychiat* 52: 173–188

35 Viguera AC, Baldessarini RJ, Hegarty MD, van Kammen DP, Tohen M (1997) Clinical risk following abrupt and gradual withdrawal of maintenance neuroleptic treatment. *Arch Gen Psychiat* 54: 49–55
36 Moller HJ, van Praag HM, Aufdembrinke B, Bailey P, Barnes TRE, Beck J, Bentsen H, Eich FX, Farrow L, Fleishhacker WW et al (1994) Negative symptoms in schizophrenia: considerations for clinical trials. *Psychopharmacology* 115: 221–228
37 King DJ (1998) Drug treatment of the negative symptoms of schizophrenia. *Eur Neuropsychopharmacol* 8: 33–42
38 Marder SR, Meibach RC (1994) Risperidone in the treatment of schizophrenia. *Am J Psychiat* 151: 825–835
39 Hamilton SH, Revicki DA, Genduso LA, Beasley CM (1998) Olanzapine vs. placebo and haloperidol: quality of life and efficacy results of the North American double-blind trial. *Neuropsychopharmacol* 18: 41–49
40 Zimbroff DL, Kane JM, Tamminga CA, Daniel DG, Mack RJ, Wozniak PJ, Sebree TB, Wallin BA, Kashkin KB and the Sertindole Study Group (1997) Controlled, dose-response study of sertindole and haloperidol in the treatment of schizophrenia. *Am J Psychiat* 154: 782–791
41 Arvanitis LA, Miller BG and the Seroquel Trial 13 Study Group (1997) Multiple fixed doses of "Seroquel" (quetiapine) in patients with acute exacerbation of schizophrenia: a comparison with haloperidol and placebo. *Biol Psychiat* 42: 233–246
42 Kirkpatrick B, Carpenter WT (1995) Drug development and the deficit syndrome of schizophrenia. *Biol Psychiat* 38: 277–278
43 Moller HJ, Muller H (1997) Statistical differentiation between direct and indirect effects of neuroleptics on negative symptoms. *Eur Arch Psychiat Clin Neurosci* 247: 1–5
44 Tollefson GD, Sanger TM (1997) Negative symptoms: a path analytic approach to a double-blind, placebo- and haloperidol-controlled clinical trial with olanzapine. *Am J Psychiat* 154: 466–474
45 Volavka J, Cooper TB, Czobor P, Meisner M (1996) Effect of varying haloperidol plasma levels on negative symptoms in schizophrenia and schizoaffective disorder. *Psychopharmacol Bull* 32: 75–79
46 Voruganti L, Heslegrave R, Awad AG, Seeman MV (1998) Quality of life measurement in schizophrenia: reconciling the quest for subjectivity with the question of reliability. *Psychol Med* 28: 165–172
47 Lehman AF (1996) Evaluating outcomes of treatments for persons with psychotic disorders. *J Clin Psychiat* 57 (Suppl 11): 61–67
48 Kinon BJ, Kane JM, Johns C, Perovich R, Ismi M, Koreen AM, Weiden P (1993) Treatment of neuroleptic-resistant schizophrenic relapse. *Psychopharmacol Bull* 29: 309–314
49 Conley RR, Buchanan RW (1997) Evaluation of treatment-resistant schizophrenia. *Schizophr Bull* 23: 663–674
50 Wolkin A, Barouche F, Wolf AP, Rotrosen J, Fowler JS, Shiue CY, Cooper TB, Brodie JD (1989) Dopamine blockade and clinical response: evidence for two biological subgroups of schizophrenia. *Am J Psychiat* 146: 905–908
51 Coppens HJ, Slooff CJ, Paans AMJ, Wiegman T, Vaalburg W, Korf J (1991) High central D_2-dopamine receptor occupancy as assessed with positron emission tomography in medicated but therapy-resistant schizophrenic patients. *Biol Psychiat* 29: 629–634
52 Liberman RP, Van Putten T, Marshall BD, Mintz J, Bowen L, Kuehnel TG, Aravagiri M, Marder SR (1994) Optimal drug and behaviour therapy for treatment-refractory schizophrenic patients. *Am J Psychiat* 151: 756–759
53 Barnes TRE, McPhillips MA (1996) Antipsychotic-induced extrapyramidal symptoms: role of anticholinergic drugs in treatment. *CNS Drugs* 6: 315–330
54 Hansen TE, Casey DE, Hoffman WF (1997) Neuroleptic intolerance. *Schizophr Bull* 23: 567–582
55 Waddington JL (1992) Mechanisms of neuroleptic-induced extrapyramidal side effects. In: JM Kane, JA Lieberman (eds): *Adverse effects of psychotropic drugs*. Guilford Press, New York, 246–265
56 Meltzer HY (1995) Atypical antipsychotic drug therapy for treatment-resistant schizophrenia. In: SR Hirsch, DR Weinberger (eds): *Schizophrenia*, Blackwell, Oxford, 485–502

57 Trichard C, Paillere-Martinot ML, Attar-Levy D, Recassens C, Monnet F, Martinot JL (1998) Binding of antipsychotic drugs to cortical 5-HT_{2A} receptors: a PET study of chlorpromazine, clozapine, and amisulpride in schizophrenic patients. *Am J Psychiat* 155: 505–508
58 Kapur SJ, Zipursky R, Remington G, Jones C, McKay G, Houle S (1997) PET evidence that loxapine is an equipotent blocker of 5-HT_2 and D_2 receptors: implications for the therapeutics of schizophrenia. *Am J Psychiat* 154: 1525–1529
59 Bilder RM, Turkel E, Lipschutz-Broch L, Lieberman JA (1992) Antipsychotic medication effects on neuropsychological functions. Psychopharmacol Bull 28: 353–366
60 Green JF, King DJ (1996) Cognitive functioning in schizophrenia: effects of drug treatment. *CNS Drugs* 6: 382–398
61 Mortimer AM (1997) Cognitive function in schizophrenia – do neuroleptics make a difference? *Pharmacol Biochem Behav* 56: 789–795
62 Waddington JL, O'Callaghan E (1997) What makes an antipsychotic "atypical"? Conserving the definition. *CNS Drugs* 7: 341–346
63 Ackerman S, Nolan LJ (1998) Bodyweight gain induced by psychotropic drugs. *CNS Drugs* 9: 135–151
64 Jusic N, Lader M (1994) Post-mortem antipsychotic drug concentrations and unexplained deaths. *Br J Psychiat* 165: 787–791
65 Warner JP, Barnes TRE, Henry JA (1996) Electrocardiographic changes in patients receiving neuroleptic medication. *Acta Psychiat Scand* 93: 311–313
66 Working Group of the Royal College of Psychiatrists, Psychopharmacology Sub-Group (1997) The association between antipsychotic drugs and sudden death. *Council Report CR57*, Royal College of Psychiatrists, London
67 McKeith I, Fairbairn A, Perry R, Thompson P, Perry E (1992) Neuroleptic sensitivity in patients with senile dementia of Lewy body type. *Br Med J* 305: 673–678
68 Joseph KS, Blais L, Ernst P, Suissa S (1996) Increased morbidity and mortality related to asthma among asthmatic patients who use major tranquillisers. *Br Med J* 312: 79–83
69 Waddington JL, Youssef HA, Kinsella A (1998) Mortality in schizophrenia: antipsychotic polypharmacy and absence of adjuctive anticholinergics over the course of a 10-year prospective study. *Br J Psychiat* 173: 325–329
70 Kane JM (1995) Psychopharmacological approaches to schizophrenia: practical aspects. In: JA Den Boer, HGM Westenberg, HM Van Praag (eds): *Advances in the neurobiology of schizophrenia*. Wiley, Chichester, 245–263
71 Day JC, Kinderman P, Bentall R (1998) A comparison of patients' and prescribers' beliefs about neuroleptic side-effects: prevalence, distress and causation. *Acta Psychiat Scand* 97: 93–97
72 Awad AG (1993) Subjective response to neuroleptics in schizophrenia. *Schizophr Bull* 19: 609–616
73 Fenton WS, Blyler CR, Heinssen RK (1997) Determinants of medication compliance in schizophrenia: empirical and clinical findings. *Schizophr Bull* 23: 637–651
74 Waddington JL, Scully PJ, O'Callaghan E (1997) The new antipsychotics, and their potential for early intervention in schizophrenia. *Schizophr Res* 28: 207–222
75 Gerlach J, Casey DE (1994) Drug treatment of schizophrenia: myths and realities. *Curr Opinion Psychiat* 7: 65–70
76 Kinon BJ, Lieberman JA (1996) Mechanisms of action of atypical antipsychotic drugs: a critical analysis. *Psychopharmacology* 124: 2–34
77 Kerwin R, Taylor D (1996) New antipsychotics: a review of their current status and clinical potential. *CNS Drugs* 6: 71–82
78 Keks N, McGrath J, Lambert T, Catts S, Vaddadi K, Burrows G, Varghese F, George T, Hustig H, Burnett P et al (1994) The Australian multicentre double-blind comparative study of remoxipride and thioridazine in schizophrenia. *Acta Psychiat Scand* 90: 358–365
79 Copolov D (1997) New name for atypical antipsychotics? Am J Psychiat 154: 439
80 Kane JM (1997) Commentary on "What makes an antipsychotic atypical?" *CNS Drugs* 7: 347–348
81 Davis JM (1976) Comparative doses and costs of antipsychotic medication. *Arch Gen Psychiat* 33: 858–861
82 Bosanquet N (1995) Schizophrenia: developing new strategies for effective care. *Br J Med Econ* 8: 51–64

83 Knapp M (1997) Costs of schizophrenia. *Br J Psychiat* 171: 509–518
84 Robert G, Kennedy P (1997) Establishing cost-effectiveness of atypical neuroleptics. *Br J Psychiat* 171: 103–104
85 Wyatt RJ (1991) Neuroleptics and the natural course of schizophrenia. *Schizophr Bull* 17: 325–351
86 Loebel AD, Lieberman JA, Alvir JMJ, Mayerhoff DI, Geisler SH, Szymanski SR (1992) Duration of psychosis and outcome in first-episode schizophrenia. *Am J Psychiat* 149: 1183–1188
87 Szymanski SR, Cannon TD, Gallacher F, Erwin RJ, Gur RE (1996) Course of treatment response in first-episode and chronic schizophrenia. *Am J Psychiat* 153: 519–525
88 Scully PJ, Coakley G, Kinsella A, Waddington JL (1997) Psychopathology, executive (frontal) and general cognitive impairment in relation to duration of initially untreated vs. subsequently treated psychosis in chronic schizophrenia. *Psychol Med* 27: 1303–1310
89 Wyatt RJ, Green MF, Tuma AH (1997) Long-term morbidity associated with delayed treatment of first admission schizophrenic patients: a re-analysis of the Camarillo State Hospital data. *Psychol Med* 27: 261–268
90 Meagher D, Quinn J, Murphy P, Kinsella A, Mullaney J, Waddington JL (1998) Duration of initially untreated psychosis predicts selectively the "psychomotor poverty" factor in schizophrenia. *Schizophr Res* 29: 37
91 Waddington JL, Scully PJ (1998) Untreated psychosis and long-term outcome in schizophrenia. *Schizophr Bull* 24: 34–35
92 McGlashan TH, Johannessen JO (1996) Early detection and intervention with schizophrenia: rationale. *Schizophr Bull* 22: 201–222
93 Birchwood M, McGorry P, Jackson H (1997) Early intervention in schizophrenia. *Br J Psychiat* 170: 2–5
94 McGorry PD, Edwards J, Mihalopoulos C, Harrigan SM, Jackson HJ (1996) EPPIC: an evolving system of early detection and optimal management. Schizophr Bull 22: 305–326
95 Sheitman BB, Lee H, Strauss R, Lieberman JA (1997) The evaluation and treatment of first-episode psychosis. *Schizophr Bull* 23: 653–661
96 Lehman AF, Steinwachs DM, and the co-Investigators of the PORT project (1998) At issue: translating research into practice: The schizophrenia Patient Outcomes Research Team (PORT) treatment recommendations. *Schizophr Bull* 24: 1–10
97 Lehman AF, Steinwachs DM and the survey co-Investigators of the PORT project (1998) Patterns of usual care for schizophrenia: initial results from the schizophrenia Patient Outcomes Research Team (PORT) client survey. *Schizophr Bull* 24: 11–20

Atypical Antipsychotics
ed. by B.A. Ellenbroek and A.R. Cools

Animal models for schizophrenia: an introduction

Bart A. Ellenbroek and Alexander R. Cools

Department of Psychoneuropharmacology, University of Nijmegen, P.O. Box 9101, 6500 HB Nijmegen, The Netherlands

Introduction

Although both Kraepelin and Bleuler already recognised schizophrenia as a brain disease, the exact underlying brain disturbance(s) have so far not been identified. The main reason for this, apart from the difficulties in diagnosis (see Liddle, this volume), is the limited accessibility of the human brain. Until about 20 years ago, the investigation of the brains of patients was limited to *post mortem* analysis. This technique (with a high spatial resolution) has been very useful in studying the neuropathology of, for instance, Parkinson's, Huntington or Alzheimer's disease. However, very few anatomical abnormalities were observed in the brains of schizophrenic patients. Given the nature and course of the schizophrenic symptomatology, this is not surprising. Most symptoms, such as hallucinations and delusions wax and wane over time, suggesting a functional rather than a morphological brain disturbance. Moreover, most patients suffering from schizophrenia acquire the disease early in life (between 18 and 30 years) and may live well into their sixties or seventies. Even if, in *post mortem* studies, brain abnormalities are found, it is virtually impossible to determine whether these disturbances are related to the cause of the illness, or are a result of it, or due to the (many) treatments these patients usually undergo throughout life.

The study of the human brain has dramatically changed in the last few decades due to the introduction of new imaging techniques that make it possible to study the living brain. Techniques such as computer tomography (CT), Positron Emission Tomography (PET), Single Photon Emission Computer Tomography (SPECT) and Nuclear Magnetic Resonance Imaging (NMRI) have significantly improved our possibilities. These techniques differ in spatial and temporal resolution but also in type of information obtained. Thus CT and NMRI scanning primarily yields structural information, whereas PET and SPECT are used to obtain functional (dynamical) information on neurotransmitter receptor, blood flow or glucose utilisation. A very recent technique is the functional Magnetic Resonance Imaging (fMRI) technique, which offers a combination of structural and dynamical information. Although these techniques are widely used, they still have quite a number of limitations, most importantly the spatial and/or temporal resolution. Next to the limitations in resolution, the available techniques also do not (yet) allow us to study the activity of individual neurotransmitters in the brain. Although it is possible to study the density of neurotransmitter receptors, the techniques do not have the sensitivity and the temporal resolution to study changes in neurotransmitter activity.

Apart from the technical limitations, studying the human brain is also limited by more ethical considerations. Ideally, if one wants to study the involvement of a specific brain structure in a certain type of behaviour or symptom, one would activate or block the neurotransmission in that particular brain region and study the functional consequences. Thus if one is interested in the role of the amygdala in locomotor activity, one would inject a specific drug directly in the amygdala and investigate whether this manipulation alters the locomotor activity of the subject. Obviously, such experiments can not be performed in humans. Therefore, the study of brain functioning in humans is almost always limited to a correlative analysis. For instance Weinberger et al. [1] studying the function of the dorsolateral prefrontal cortex in the Wisconsin Card Sorting Test found that there was a negative correlation in schizophrenic patients between the number of errors made in the test and the activation of this particular brain region (using PET). These data strongly suggest that the cause of the poor performance of schizophrenic patients on this test is the inability of these patients to activate the dorsolateral prefrontal cortex. Alternatively, one might speculate that good performance induces activation of the dorsolateral prefrontal cortex, and thus the lack of activation of this area in schizophrenic patients would be the *result* of a poor performance. An experiment to resolve this question would be to deliberately reduce the activity in this area and study the performance.

Studying the function of the brain in animals has a number of clear advantages. First of all, the available techniques have high spatial and temporal resolution. Techniques such as *in vivo* voltammetry and *in vivo* microdialysis allow the registration of neurotransmitter changes in very small areas of the brain (~ 0.5 mm) in very short periods of time (< 10 min). Such techniques are sensitive enough to measure neurotransmitter concentrations in the range of 20–50 fmol per 20 min. Moreover, through the stereotactical implantation technique it is possible to locally inject drugs directly into the brain and study the resulting changes in freely moving animals. The use of experimental drugs is also much easier in animals than in humans. Thus drugs which have not (yet) been approved in man can already be used in rats. Likewise drugs which have been withdrawn from the human market due to unwanted side-effects can still be used in animals, mostly because they are only used once. Clozapine, for example, was withdrawn from most European countries and the United States in the late 1970s because of reports of agranulocytosis with repeated treatment [2]. However, it continued to be used in animal studies and the findings in these studies of the unique character of this drug (see Naber et al., this volume) have undoubtedly contributed to its reintroduction in clinical practice in the eighties. Likewise drugs such as remoxipride and raclopride are very selective dopamine D_2 receptor antagonists (see Den Boer and Korf, this volume). Due to side-effects these drugs have been withdrawn (remoxipride) or never reached (raclopride) clinical practice. Nevertheless they have been instrumental in furthering our knowledge of the functional role of dopamine D_2 receptors in behaviour.

Although animal models offer a great number of advantages over human studies, there are also a number of limitations to them. Obviously, the brain of an animal (especially the most commonly used species, the rat) is not identical with the human brain. Indeed in no other species has the cerebral cortex (especially the frontal parts) developed so extensively as in man. On the other hand, all neurotransmitters and neurotransmitter receptors known to occur in humans have also been found in rats and *vice versa*. One of the few possible exceptions is the 5-HT_{1B} receptor, which only occurs in rats. In humans two 5-HT_{1D} receptors have been identified, one of which only occurs in humans (the 5-$HT_{1D\alpha}$). Interestingly, the human 5-$HT_{1D\beta}$ shows a large structural similarity with the rat 5-HT_{1B} receptor ($>90\%$ amino acid homology). This structural homology is also seen with most other neurotransmitter receptors. The human and rat D_2 receptor, for instance, differ in only 17 out of 415 amino acids [3].

Another important similarity between the human and the rat brain is the projection of nerve cells. Not only do humans and rats share the same neurotransmitters and neurotransmitter receptors; they are also found in the same brain areas in both species. The dopaminergic cells, for instance, are localised within a number of very discrete cell groups (usually referred to as the A_8–A_{12} cell groups) in both species. The termination area of these cells is also the same in humans and rats. The A_9 cell group for instance predominantly terminates in circumscribed areas within the caudate putamen complex, whereas the A_{10} cell group projects to areas within the nucleus accumbens and the frontal cortex.

Despite these clear similarities in brain morphology, one essential difference between humans and rats (and monkeys) is the use of language. Humans can express their emotions and feelings whereas animals can not. This makes animal modelling (especially in the field of psychiatry) difficult. Whereas humans can indicate that they feel sad, that they hear voices or that they have delusional thoughts, the presence of such symptoms is impossible to ascertain in animals.

A classification of animal models

The inherent difficulty in modelling human ideas and thoughts in animals has led to a plethora of animal models in search of the ideal model for a specific disease. Since such ideal models have not yet been found, it is important to realise what goal one pursues with a specific model. As discussed by a number of authors [4, 5] it has proven useful to subdivide animal models in a number of general categories, not based on the specific type of technique, but rather on the general field of research. Thus Willner suggested a sub-division in three types of animal models: screening models, behavioural bioassays and simulations [4] (see Fig. 1). Screening models are developed for the sole purpose of identifying new drugs for clinical treatment. They represent pharmacology based models and as such are closely similar to what other authors have described as models with predictive validity [5] or models with pharmacological isomorphism [6]. Behavioural bioassays are used to investigate specific brain functions. For instance the study of the role of the nucleus accumbens in locomotor activity [7] or the role of the neostriatum in play behaviour [8] represent behavioural bioassays. Such models are therefore very brain-oriented, and thus represent models in the general field of neuroscience. Simulations are models in which one tries to analyse human mental processes. They represent models from a more psychological point of view, or (since most models investigate human disease states) from a clinical point of view. Simulations are closely similar to animal models with face and construct validity [5] and to animal models with symptom similarity and models with cross-species psychological processes [6].

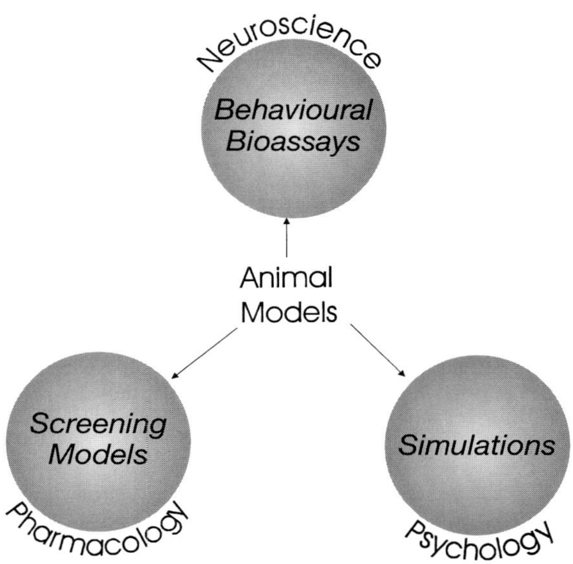

Figure 1. Based on the general aim and the principal discipline involved, animal models can be subdivided into three different classes: Behavioural Bioassays, Screening Models and Simulations.

When studying human diseases such as schizophrenia, most models fall within the categories of screening models or simulations. This does not imply that behavioural bioassays are not relevant for investigating specific aspects of diseases. In fact the border between these two animal models is often difficult to draw. For instance the prepulse inhibition of the acoustic startle response is generally considered to be a good simulation for (aspects of) schizophrenia [9] (see below). Studying the involvement of the prefrontal cortex in the mediation of prepulse inhibition [10], is a behavioural bioassay, yet may provide valid information on the neuronal structure of prepulse inhibition and possibly on the disease process underlying schizophrenia.

Screening models

Screening models are by far the largest group of animal models. They are developed in order to have a fast and valid method for determining the possible clinical applications of a new drug. In general these models are based on one (or more) standard drugs (Fig. 2). The model's starting point is a "*gold standard*" viz. a drug which has a very clear, unequivocal therapeutic action with respect to a specific clinical condition. Such drugs usually have a long history of clinical application. Examples are imipramine or amitriptyline (in screening models for depression) or diazepam or chlordiazepoxide (in models for anxiety). In the case of schizophrenia the gold standard is usually haloperidol or chlorpromazine. Although not absolutely necessary, an animal model would greatly benefit from a "*gold standard*" with few side-effects. As will be described below, this is beneficial in the validation procedure.

The next step in screening model building is to evaluate the effects of the gold standard in a specific behavioural model in animals. A number of aspects should be considered in selecting the appropriate animal model. First of all, virtually all screening models use rats (or mice) as animal species. The reason for selecting these species is based purely on financial and practical grounds. The second prerequisite for a useful screening model is that it should be simple and fast, in order to cope with the large number of new drugs, which need to be screened. This prerequisite seems to be somewhat paradoxical. Most of the psychotherapeutic drugs (especially antidepressants and antipsychotic drugs) need at least several weeks before the full therapeutic response is achieved. One should, however, keep in mind that screening models are only concerned with making accurate predictions with respect to the therapeutic efficacy, and not with modelling the therapeutic efficacy per se. A third requirement of a good screening model is that the parameter (or parameters) measured in the test can be unequivocally assessed. Although it is often advantageous to have an automatic detection system (for instance a video tracking device), this is not an

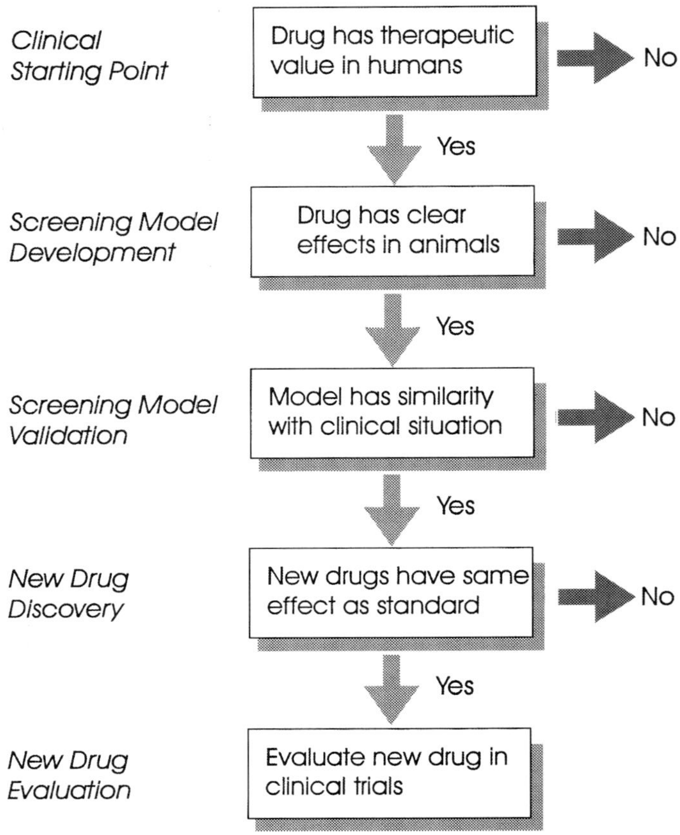

Figure 2. A flow diagram illustrating the most important steps in developing screening models.

absolute prerequisite. Moreover a parameter measured on a ratio or interval scale is preferred over a parameter on a nominal or ordinal level. Ratio and interval measures allow for more powerful statistics.

Taking all these requirement into consideration, a large number of screening models have been developed. In some cases the screening model may attempt to simulate a clinical condition (such as the elevated plus maze as a model for anxiety and the Porsolt swimming test as a model for depression) this is, however, not a requirement. In fact it may even be a disadvantage, since these similarities are often only assumed and may, upon further scrutiny of the testing condition, turn out to be incorrect. Since such models are often confused with simulation models (see below) this may negatively influence the general opinion of the test, irrespective of its usefulness as a screening model. A good example of this trap is the Porsolt Swimming test. In this test a rat is emersed in water from which he can not escape. Animals will fairly rapidly adopt a characteristic immobile posture and make no attempt to escape. It has been suggested [11] that this is due to a state of "*behavioural despair*" which suggests that it may be a simulation model for depression. However, as discussed by Willner [12] there is, in fact, very little evidence to support this assumption. Nevertheless, the model seems to be a fairly good screening test for antidepressant drugs [12, 13].

In the case of schizophrenia, a large variety of screening models have been described (see also Arnt, this volume). These models can be based on the effects of antipsychotic drugs on spontaneous behaviour, like feeding [14], catalepsy [15], the paw test [16] and spontaneous locomotor activity [14]. Alternatively, the effects of antipsychotics on learned behaviour, like conditioned avoidance response [15], intracranial self stimulation [17], or Morris water maze swimming [18] are used for screening purposes. Finally a large number of screening models are based on the effects of antipsychotics on drug induced behaviour. In this field, the effects of antipsychotic drugs on dopamine related behaviours have taken a prominent place, like apomorphine induced emesis in dogs [19], 6,7-ADTN induced locomotor activity [20], amphetamine induced locomotor activity [21], amphetamine induced drug discrimination [22] and methylphenidate induced behavioural activation [23]. Earlier research also concentrated on the effects of antipsychotics on noradrenaline and serotonin related behaviours [14, 24] and recently, the effects of antipsychotics on glutamate dependent behaviours has received particular attention [25, 26].

The third step (Fig. 2) is by far the most critical phase in screening model building, the validation step. Since psychotherapeutic drugs produce a large number of effects (both beneficial and unwanted), it is important to determine whether the effects observed in the screening model predict the therapeutic action of psychotherapeutic agents or one of the side-effects. For this purpose a number of criteria have been developed largely based on the clinical pharmacology of these drugs [5, 27]. The criteria for evaluating the validity of a screening model can be subdivided into two categories: general and specific. The general criteria are important for every screening model, independent of the type of drug one is screening for, whereas the specific criteria only apply to one type of screening model. Table 1 represents the general and specific criteria for screening models for antipsychotics.

The first general criterion states that drugs of different chemical classes must be active in the screening model. In the case of antipsychotic drugs, quite a large number of chemical classes have been developed such as phenothiazines (like chlorpromazine and thioridazine), butyrophenones (like haloperidol and benperidol), thioxanthenes (like thiothixene and flupenthixol), dibenzazepines (like clozapine and loxapine), benzamides (like sulpiride and amisulpiride) as well as a large number of other compounds. In a good screening model, compounds from all these classes should be effective. Criterion 2 is related to criterion 1. A false negative is a drug which is effective in clinical practice, but which does not show "*gold*

Table 1. The validation criteria for screening models for schizophrenia

General Criteria

1. Drugs of different chemical classes should be effective
2. No false positives should occur
3. No false negatives should occur
4. There should be a relationship between the potency of drugs in the clinical setting and potency of these drugs in the model

Specific Criteria

5. Anticholinergic drugs should not reduce the effects of antipsychotics in the model
6. Chronic treatment should not reduce the effects of antipsychotic drugs in the model
7. Benzodiazepines should enhance the effects of antipsychotic drugs

standard"-like results in the model. In screening models for antipsychotic drugs, a number of antipsychotics have often shown up as false negatives. Most prominent among them are clozapine and sulpiride. A false positive (criterion 3) is a drug which behaves like the "*gold standard*" in the model, yet appears to be ineffective in clinical practice. This is a difficult criterion for two reasons. First of all, it is often difficult to definitely conclude that a specific drug is not therapeutically effective. For instance the neuropeptide des-enkephaline-γ-endorphin has been reported to have antipsychotic activity by some [28], but not by others [29]. Likewise benzodiazepines have been found effective in some [30, 31], but not in other studies [32, 33]. Secondly, it is obviously impossible to test all potentially false negatives, so one has to make a decision, which drugs to test and which to leave out. Since the performance of rats in screening models almost always involves motor action (behaviour), drugs which influence the motor performance are potentially false negatives. Indeed, in a number of cases drugs like morphine (which reduce spontaneous movement and increase muscle tone) or diazepam (which reduce spontaneous movement and decrease muscle tone) represent false negatives. Other potentially false negatives are domperidon (a butyrophenone like haloperidol which does not cross the blood brain barrier), promethazine (a non antipsychotic phenothiazine) and trans-flupenthixol (the inactive enantiomer of the effective antipsychotic cis-flupenthixol). The fourth criterion (Table 1) should be considered with some caution. The potency of a drug strongly depends on its metabolism and bio-availability. Since these factors may (strongly) differ between rats and humans (which are also ill), this may lead to differences in potency between the two species, which are unrelated to the model. In general, rats tend to receive higher doses than humans. For instance haloperidol is usually given in doses around 0.5 mg/kg in rats, which would be equivalent to about 35 mg per day for humans. Thus, an absolute correlation between human and animal potency is not a necessary prerequisite, although in most models drugs like haloperidol and fluphenazine are much more potent than drugs like chlorpromazine and thioridazine [27].

The three specific criteria are derived from clinical pharmacological experience with antipsychotic drugs, and are intended to differentiate between the therapeutic effects of antipsychotics and the extrapyramidal side-effects. These side-effects occur with a large number of antipsychotics [27] (see also Waddington and Quinn, this volume), and represent the most cumbersome of side-effects. Moreover, since they occur with a large number of antipsychotics, it is possible that the screening model is more related to these side-effects than to the therapeutic efficacy. This is nicely illustrated with the catalepsy test, which was originally designed as a screening model for antipsychotics [14], but is now generally considered to be a model for the extrapyramidal side-effects [27]. Criterion 5 is based on the clinical finding that anticholinergics drugs reduce extrapyramidal side-effects without influencing the therapeutic efficacy to any great extent. Although there is some evidence that anticholinergics may affect the therapeutic efficacy of antipsychotics, this is likely due to high doses, or to the fact that some anticholinergics also inhibit dopamine re-uptake. Criterion 6 is based on clinical findings that the extrapyramidal side-effects are most prominent early during the treatment and usually wane with repeated application. Since the therapeutic effects seem to increase rather than decrease with repeated treatment, this represents another way of separating the therapeutic and the extrapyramidal side-effects. The final criterion is based on a number of publications which show that adjunctive treatment with benzodiazepines enhance the therapeutic effects of antipsychotic drugs, while at the same time reducing (at least some) extrapyramidal side-effects [27].

When this third step in the screening model building is (successfully) completed, we have a valid screening model and can proceed to the last step in the model, the evaluation of new chemical compounds. When one of these substances has been detected, the drug can be evaluated in clinical practice, after extensive pharmacological and toxicological evaluation of course.

Limitations and possibilities of screening models

Although screening models have been used extensively to detect new antipsychotics (see also Arnt, this volume), such models have some inherent limitations. The most important limitation is that it is highly unlikely that screening models can lead to novel pharmacotherapeutic approaches. Drugs with a completely new mode of action, like glutamate agonists, or selective serotonin antagonists are unlikely to show behavioural responses similar to the "*gold standard*". This is not surprisingly, since the principal objective of screening models is to compare new chemical substances with known drugs. Given this limitation, it is not surprising that only few breakthroughs have occurred in the pharmacotherapy of schizophrenia. The few exceptions (such as clozapine) have been found by serendipity, and usually show up as false negatives in most screening models [27]. Some authors have tried to circumvent this limitation by using two different "*gold standards*", like haloperidol and clozapine [16]. However, this does not eliminate the problem, it only leads to drugs with similarity to either haloperidol or clozapine.

In spite of this limitation, the screening models are important for two reasons, first to detect novel therapeutic drugs which may be more beneficial than current medication, and second to study the neuronal mechanism underlying the therapeutic action of antipsychotic drugs. With respect to the first reason, most research is now concentrated on finding substances with a mechanism of action similar to clozapine, but lacking the agranulocytosis side-effect. In this case, screening models may be very useful.

With respect to the second reason, good screening models can serve as behavioural bioassays of antipsychotic drug action. For instance, we have used the paw test to study the differences in neuronal mechanism between haloperidol and clozapine. The results show that whereas the actions of haloperidol can be reversed by dopamine D_2 agonists, the effects of clozapine can be reversed by dopamine D_1 agonists [34]. Likewise, whereas the 5-HT_2 antagonist ketanserin blocks the effects of haloperidol, the 5-HT_2 agonist DOI reverses the effects of clozapine [35]. These data strongly indicate that clozapine and haloperidol have different mechanisms of action. Since the paw test has been extensively validated as a screening model, these data may have implications for the therapeutic activity as well.

Simulations

Despite the above-mentioned limitations, screening models have been used extensively in preclinical research on schizophrenia. This is due to the fact that there are only very limited possibilities to develop simulation models for schizophrenia. As discussed above, simulation models try to mimic the disease under investigation, usually by trying to simulate one or more of the symptoms. In the case of schizophrenia, very few of the symptoms can be modelled in animals, since the assessment of these symptoms is dependent on an oral account by the patient. However, there are a few symptoms, which can be assessed with more objective methods, most notably stereotyped behaviour, social withdrawal and anhedonia.

During the last two decades, it has become increasingly recognised that simulation models not necessarily have to be limited to symptoms, but may also apply to cognitive processes. Using a variety of psychological and psychophysiological techniques, a number of these second-generation simulation models have been developed for schizophrenia.

Simulations of schizophrenic symptoms of schizophrenic symptoms

Stereotypy

Stereotypy (or stereotyped behaviour) refers to the repetition of well-defined behavioural acts, which seem to be repeated without any apparent adaptive function. Stereotyped behaviours can occur in a large number of different conditions. In animals, captivity is a strong inducer of stereotypy, as any casual visitor to a zoo can readily observe. In humans stereotypy can occur both in stressful and in very boring situations [36] as well as in a number of neurological and psychiatric conditions such as Parkinson's disease, Huntington's Chorea, autism, Gilles de la Tourette and of course schizophrenia [37–41].

In schizophrenic patients, stereotypy can take many different forms. Especially Kraepelin and Bleuler have give very precise examples of stereotyped (or perseverative) behaviour in schizophrenic patients [40, 41] such as stereotyped speech, hand movements, walking patterns and mannerisms. However, more complex behaviours, including polydipsia and boulimia, may also become stereotyped. According to Luchins and co-workers, stereotyped behaviour occurs in at least 21% of the acute and 47% of the chronic schizophrenic patients [42].

Although Bleuler has stressed the importance of stereotyped behaviour in schizophrenic patients, relatively little attention is paid to this phenomenon. This is probably due to the large individual difference in the expression of stereotypy, as described above. Frith and Done have used a two choice guessing task to specifically induce stereotyped responding. Subjects are positioned in front of a computer screen, which displays two squares [43]. The subjects have to guess behind which square a cross is hidden. The crosses are presented in a pseudo-random order. Faced with such a problem, healthy volunteers adopt a strategy which is guided by the results (win-stay, loose-shift). Schizophrenic patients, however, develop stereotyped responses, either alternating between left and right or favoring one side. Lyon and co-workers [44, 45] showed that stereotyped responding was observed in both schizophrenic patients and in bipolar patients. Patients with neurosis and with schizoid personality did not differ from normal controls. Although some authors have tried to adapt this strategy for animal research [46] so far few pharmacological studies have been performed [27].

Anhedonia

Anhedonia refers to the inability to experience pleasure or joy and was already recognised by Bleuler and Kraepelin as an important characteristic of schizophrenia, although it is also a core symptom of major depression

[47]. Rado [48] suggested that anhedonia plays a fundamental role in the development of schizophrenia. According to this author, anhedonia prevents the development of normal healthy sexual relationships, impairs the ability to form relationships with other people and weakens the feelings of joy, affection, love, pride and self-respect. In accordance with this, Andreasen and Olsen considered anhedonia one of the principal negative symptoms, closely related to social withdrawal or asociality [49].

In an attempt to quantify anhedonia, Chapman and colleagues [50] developed two anhedonia scales, the Physical and the Social Anhedonia Scales (PAS and SAS). The PAS consists of 40 and the SAS of 48 statements which have to be answered with true or false. Examples are "*I have always had a number of favourite foods*" (PAS) or "*I have often enjoyed long discussions with other people*" (SAS). The authors found that the scores of both anhedonia scales showed a large correlation suggesting that both forms are governed by the same underlying mechanisms (or that the questionnaires do not differentiate enough). The authors also found that schizophrenic patients were indeed more anhedonic than controls. In accordance with the hypothesis of Rado (see above), several authors have found that anhedonia is particularly high in subjects with an elevated risk for schizophrenia [51–53].

Social withdrawal

One of the most troublesome symptoms of schizophrenia is the lack of social contact. Schizophrenic patients often live alone, have very few social contacts and in many cases seem to actively avoid social behaviour. Reductions in social behaviour are already present in the premorbid stages of the illness [54], and it has even been shown that during very early childhood, pre-schizophrenic patients show significantly reduced playing behaviour. According to Bellack et al. [55] social withdrawal worsens during prodromal periods and during exacerbations of the illness, but it generally persists during periods of remission. These authors looked in detail into the origins of social withdrawal in schizophrenic patients. Their data clearly indicate that social withdrawal is not an epiphenomenon, secondary to other disturbances seen in schizophrenic patients, but rather results from a fundamental deficit in social skills [56, 57]. This deficit in social skills seems to be a very stable phenomenon in schizophrenic patients. In comparison to schizoaffective and affective patients, schizophrenic patients have the lowest premorbid adjustment and social skills and both were predictive of poor outcome [57]. Using a multiple choice questionnaire measuring social knowledge, it was found that schizophrenic patients score worse than manic and depressed patients on social competence [58].

Simulations of information processing abnormalities in schizophrenia

As described above, the symptoms of schizophrenia are difficult to model in schizophrenic patients. Moreover, even symptoms for which animal models have been developed (stereotypy, anhedonia and social withdrawal), are difficult to objectively quantify in humans. This lack of quantification makes it difficult to assess the effects of therapeutic drugs, which hampers validation studies in animals (see above). This has led investigators to look for more objectively measurable disturbances in schizophrenic patients.

As discussed in previous papers, schizophrenic patients are known to suffer from information processing deficits [5, 59, 60]. Information processing encompasses a large number of different processes [61, 62], involving, among others perception, selection and processing of stimuli. The deficits seen in schizophrenic patients are often considered to represent a general failure of inhibition [60] and can be seen at many different stages of information processing, most prominently at the level of stimulus perception and stimulus selection.

One of the first stages in information processing is the sensory gating phase, in which the total amount of information is quantitatively reduced to provide a functional barrier against incoming sensory information [62, 63]. It has long been recognised that schizophrenic patients suffer from deficits in this early, preconscious stage of information processing [64, 65]. Especially Venables has suggested that this failure leads to sensory "*flooding*" which eventually may culminate in cognitive disintegration [60, 64]. Such sensory gating mechanisms have traditionally been viewed as inhibitory mechanisms and can be measured with several paradigms. In schizophrenia research two paradigms have most often been used to study these inhibitory processes: the P_{50} gating [66] and the prepulse inhibition paradigm [67].

In the P_{50} gating paradigm, auditory stimuli are presented in pairs every 10 s and the resulting changes in the electrical currents are measured on the skull. It is hypothesised that the first stimulus conditions (activates) inhibitory neuronal gating mechanisms, the strength of which is tested by the second stimulus. When the interstimulus interval between the two clicks is 500 ms, schizophrenic patients fail to decrement P_{50} responses to the test stimulus [66]. This deficit appears to be relatively independent of the clinical state of the patient [68]. Interestingly, the deficit in gating can not be normalised by antipsychotics, with the exception of clozapine [69].

In the prepulse inhibition paradigm, inhibitory processes are assessed by studying the influence of prestimuli upon the startle response. Upon presentation of a very intense stimulus (usually an acoustic stimuli, although tactile stimuli are also effective) a subject will show a startle response. In humans this is usually quantified by measuring the eye blink response [67].

When this startle stimulus is preceded by a much weaker stimulus, which by itself does not induce a startle response, the startle response is significantly reduced. When the interval between the prepulse and the startle stimulus is 100 ms, schizophrenic patients show significantly less inhibition of the startle response.

Another important stage in information processing is Broadbent's selective attention filter. This filter refers to a psychological process, which operates as a qualitative filter, selecting sensory stimuli for further perceptual processing. It is important to realise that this filtering process does not completely eradicate unselected or irrelevant stimuli from awareness. It merely attenuates them in order to allocate more attentional capacity to the processing of the selected or relevant stimuli [59, 62]. The dichotic listening task [70] represents one of several paradigms in which selective attention can be assessed. In this task, subjects are asked to attend to a voice presented on one side of an earphone, while ignoring the voice from the other channel of the earphone. Schizophrenic patients show severe deficits in this task. Unfortunately, so far no animal analogue of this task has been developed.

Two psychological paradigms in which attentional deficits are probed, and which have been used in both humans and rats are latent inhibition and the Kamin blocking effect. Latent inhibition refers to the phenomenon that previous presentation of a stimulus retards the subsequent conditioning of that stimulus [71]. From this definition it is clear that latent inhibition involves two different groups (a preexposed and a nonpreexposed group) and, at least, two phases, a preexposure and a learning stage. In many occasions a third phase is necessary to test the strength of the learned association. Baruch and colleagues have studied latent inhibition in schizophrenic patients [72]. In the first phase subjects were asked to listen to a tape and to count one of several nonsense syllables that were presented. This was done for two reasons. First of all, since all nonsense syllables were presented five times the authors could check whether the subjects had paid attention to the audio tape. Second, in the preexposed group, the nonsense syllables were interspersed with a number of noise bursts, the actual stimulus, which later will be used in the conditioning paradigm. In humans latent inhibition can only be observed when this to be conditioned stimulus is masked [73]. In the learning stage, the subjects are given the same audio tape, but this time they are seated in front of a counter which increases every time the noise burst is presented on the tape. The subjects have to learn this rule. The study of Baruch and co-workers first of all showed that normal subjects preexposed to the noise bursts needed significantly more trials to learn the rule than subjects not preexposed, indicating that latent inhibition indeed occurs. More importantly, however, they also showed that schizophrenic patients showed significantly less latent inhibition than normal healthy volunteers. This is particularly important since this indicates that the preexposed schizophrenic patients learned the rule *faster* than the preexposed healthy volunteers, a rare finding in psychological research with schizophrenic patients. Unfortunately, the disturbance in latent inhibition seems to be rather transient, occurring only in the more acute phase of the disease [72, 74]. Moreover, some authors have been unable to replicate this disturbance in latent inhibition [75].

A phenomenon closely related to latent inhibition is the Kamin blocking effect. In this paradigm, subjects are again subdivided in two groups, a preexposed and a nonpreexposed group. The preexposed group is exposed to one stimulus (A), which they have to associate with a specific response. In the second phase, both groups are exposed to a combination of stimuli (AB) which they have to associate with a response. In the third phase the associative strength of stimulus B is tested. In normal healthy volunteers the associative strength of stimulus B is markedly reduced in the preexposed group. The theoretical explanation of this phenomenon is that due to the preexposure to stimulus A, this stimulus is much more important in the second phase and thus will divert attention away from stimulus B. Since schizophrenic patients have difficulty in selective attention, one would expect this blocking to be reduced. This has indeed been found, at least for the subgroups of paranoid schizophrenics [76].

Conclusion

Although simulation models for schizophrenia were rare in the past, the situation has clearly changed in the last couple of years. The recognition that apart from several symptoms, a number of psychophysiological and psychological deficits of schizophrenic patients can be used in simulation models has greatly improved our possibility to study aspects of schizophrenia in animals. However, all simulation models suffer from two major drawbacks. First of all, since we do not know the exact aetiology or the pathophysiology of schizophrenia, it is still unclear how a "schizophrenia-like" condition can be most optimally induced in rats. Several different methods have so far been used, which will be described in Ellenbroek et al., this volume. Secondly, neither the symptoms, nor the psychophysiological or psychological deficits appear to be selective for schizophrenia. Thus, stereotypy can also occur in for instance Huntington's chorea, Parkinson's disease, Gilles de la Tourette syndrome and autism [37, 48]. Anhedonia is one of the most prominent symptoms of depression, and social withdrawal is also often seen in patients with major depression. Likewise P_{50} gating appears to be reduced in manic patients [77], and prepulse inhibition is disturbed in patients with obsessive compulsive disorders, Gilles de La Tourette syndrome, autism and Huntington's chorea [78]. Relatively little research has so far been done on latent inhibition and blocking, but both phenomena appear to be disturbed in psychotic prone subjects, and, as discussed above, appear only in a subgroup of schizophrenic patients, and only for a short period of time. At this moment, it is completely unknown whether the disturbances seen in, for instance prepulse inhibition seen in schizophrenia are similar, or even identical to those observed in any of the other diseases. Much more clinical research will be necessary in order to investigate this problem, which will be important for developing validation criteria for simulation models.

References

1 Weinberger DR, Berman KF, Zec RF (1986) Physiological dysfunction of dorsolateral prefrontal cortex in schizophrenia. *Arch Gen Psychiatry* 43: 114–124
2 Idänpäan-Heikkilä, Alhave E, Olkinuora M, Palva I (1977) Agranulocytosis during treatment with clozapine. *Eur J Clin Pharmacol* 11:193–198
3 Dal Toso R, Sommer B, Ewert M, Herb A, Pritchert DB, Bach A, Ahivers BD, Seeberg PH (1989) The dopamine D_2 receptor: Two molecular form generated by alternative splicing. *EMBO J* 8: 4025–4034
4 Willner P (1991) Behavioural models in psychopharmacology. In: P Willner (ed): *Behavioural models in psychopharmacology: Theoretical, industrial and clinical perspectives.* Cambridge Univ. Press, Cambridge, 3–18
5 Ellenbroek BA, Cools AR (1990) Animal models with construct validity for schizophrenia. *Behav Pharmacol* 1: 469–490
6 Matthysse S (1986) Animal models in psychiatric research. *Prog Brain Res* 65: 259–270
7 Pijnenburg AJJ, Honig WMM, vanderHeyden JAM, van Rossum JM (1976) Effects of chemical stimulation of the mesolimbic dopamine system in the rat. *Eur J Pharmacol* 35: 45–58
8 Pellis SM, Casteneda E, McKenna MM, Tran-Nguyen LTL, Whishaw IQ (1993) The role of the striatum in organizing sequences of play fighting in neonatally dopamine depleted rats. *Neurosci Lett* 158: 13–15
9 Swerdlow NR, Braff DL, Taaid N, Geyer MA (1994) Assessing the validity of an animal model of deficient sensorimotor gating in schizophrenic patients. *Arch Gen Psychiatry* 51: 139–154
10 Ellenbroek BA, Budde S, Cools AR (1996) Prepulse inhibition and latent inhibition: The role of dopamine in the medial prefrontal cortex. *Neuroscience* 75: 535–542
11 Porsolt RD, Bertin A, Jalfre M (1977) Behavioural despair in mice: A primary screening test for antidepressants. *Arch Int Pharmacodyn Ther* 229: 327–336
12 Willner P (1984) The validity of animal models of depression. *Psychopharmacology* 83: 1–16
13 Porsolt RD, Lenègre A, McArthur RA (1991) Pharmacological models of depression. In: B Olivier, J Mos, JJ Slangen (eds): *Animal models in psychopharmacology.* Birkhäuser, Basel, 137–159
14 Janssen PAJ, Niemegeers CJE, Schellekens KHL (1965) Is it possible to predict the clinical effects of neuroleptic drugs (major tranquilizers) from animal data? Part I. "Neuroleptic activity spectra" for rats. *Arzneim Forsch* 15: 104–117
15 Arnt J (1982) Pharmacological specificity of conditioned avoidance response inhibition in rats: Inhibition by neuroleptics and correlation to dopamine receptor blockade. *Acta Pharmacol Toxicol* 51: 321–329
16 Ellenbroek BA, Peeters B,W, Honig WM, Cools AR (1987) The paw test: A behavioural paradigm for differentiating between classical and atypical neuroleptic drugs. *Psychopharmacology* 93: 343–348.
17 Wauquier A (1979) Neuroleptics and brain self-stimulation. *Int Rev Neurobiol* 21: 335–403
18 Skarsfeldt T (1996) Differential effect of antipsychotics on place navigation of rats in the Morris water maze. A comparative study between novel and reference antipsychotics. *Psychopharmacology* 124: 126–133
19 Niemegeers CJE (1982) Antiemetic specificity of dopamine antagonists. *Psychopharmacology* 78: 21–213

20 Arnt J (1983) Neuroleptic inhibition of 6,7-ADTN induced hyperactivity after injection into the nucleus accumbens. Specificity and comparison with other models. *Europ J Pharmacol* 90: 47–55
21 Arnt J (1995) Differential effects of classical and newer antipsychotics on the hypermotility induced by two dose levels of d-amphetamine. *Europ J Pharmacol* 283: 55–62
22 Arnt J (1996) Inhibitory effects on the discriminative stimulus properties of d-amphetamine by classical and newer antipsychotics do not correlate with antipsychotic activity. Relation to effects on the reward system? *Psychopharmacology* 124: 117–125
23 Koek W, Colpaert FC (1993) Inhibition of methylphenidate-induced behaviors in rats: Differences among neuroleptics. *J Pharmacol Exp Ther* 267: 181–191
24 Niemegeers CJE, Lenaerts FM, Artois KSK, Janssen PAJ (1977) Interaction of drugs with apomorphine, tryptamine and norepinephrine. A new "*in vivo*" approach: the ATN test in rats. *Arch Int Pharmacodyn* 227: 238–253
25 Hoffman DC (1992) Typical and atypical neuroleptics antagonize MK-801 induced locomotion and stereotypy in rats. *J Neural Trans* 89: 1–10
26 Gleason SD, Shannon HE (1997) Blockade of phencyclidine-induced hyperlocomotion by olanzapine, clozapine and serotonin receptor subtype selective antagonists in mice. *Psychopharmacology* 129: 79–74
27 Ellenbroek BA (1993) Treatment of schizophrenia: A clinical and preclinical evaluation of neuroleptic drugs. *Pharmacol Ther* 57: 1–78
28 Verhoeven WMA, van Praag HM, van Ree JM, de Wied D (1979) Improvement of schizophenic patients by treatment with des-tyr-γ-endorphin. *Arch Gen Psychiatry* 36: 294–302
29 Manchanda R, Hirsch SR, Barnes TRE (1988) Criteria for evaluating improvement in schizophrenia in psychopharmacological research (with special reference to gamma endorphin fragments). *Br J Psychiatry* 153: 354–358
30 Maculans GA (1964) Comparison of diazepam chlorprothixene and chlorpromazine in chronic schizophrenic patients. *Dis Nerv Syst* 25: 164–168
31 Rao AV (1964) A controlled trial with "valium" in some psychiatric disorders. *Indian J Psychiatry* 4: 188–192
32 Stonehill E, Lee H, Ban TA (1966) A comparative study of benzodiazepines in chronic psychotic patients. *Dis Nerv System* 27: 411–413
33 Merlis S, Turner WJ, Krumholz W (1964) A double-blind comparison of diazepam, chlordiazepoxide and chlorpromazine in psychotic patients. *J Neuropsychiatry* 3 (Suppl 1): S133–S138
34 Ellenbroek BA, Artz M, Cools AR (1991) The involvement of dopamine D_1 and D_2 receptors in the effects of the classical neuroleptic haloperidol and the atypical neuroleptic clozapine. *Europ J Pharmacology* 196: 103–108
35 Ellenbroek BA, Prinssen EPM, Cools AR (1994) The role of serotonin receptor subtypes in the behavioural effects of neuroleptic drugs. A paw test study in rats. *Europ J Neuroscience* 6: 1–8
36 Asendorpf J (1980) Nichtreaktive Stressmessung: Bewegungsstereotypien als Aktivierungsindikatoren. *Z Exp Ang Psychol* 27: 44–58
37 Stoessl AJ (1990) Sterotyped motor phenomena in neurological disease. In: SJ Cooper, CT Dourish (eds): *Neurobiology of stereotypeed behaviour*. Clarendon Press, Oxford, 260–292
38 Frith CD, Done DJ (1990) Stereotyped behaviour in madness and in health. In: SJ Cooper, CT Dourish (eds): *Neurobiology of stereotypeed behaviour*. Clarendon Press, Oxford, 232–259
39 Ellenbroek BA, Cools AR (1993) Stereotyped behaviour. In: F van Haren (ed): *Methods in behavioral pharmacology*, Elsevier, Amsterdam, pp 519–538
40 Ridley RM (1994) The psychology of perseverative and stereotyped behaviour. *Prog Neurobiol* 44: 221–231
41 Crider A (1997) Perseveration in schizophrenia. *Schizoph Bull* 23: 63–74
42 Luchins DJ, Goldman MB, Lieb M, Hanrahan P (1992) Repetitive behaviorus in chronically institutionalized schizophrenic patients. *Schizophr Res* 8: 119–123
43 Frith CD Done DJ (1983) Stereotyped responding by chronic schizophrenic patients on a two-choice guessing task. *Psychol Med* 13: 779–786
44 Lyon N, Mejsholm B, Lyon M (1986) Stereotyped responding by schizophrenic outpatients: crosscultural confirmation of perseverative switching on a two-choice guessing task. *J Psychiat Res* 20: 137–150

45 Lyon N, Gerlach J (1988) Perseverative switching of responses by schizophrenic and affective disorder patients. *J Psychiatr Res* 22: 261–277
46 Evenden JL, Robbins TW (1983) Increased response swtiching, perseveration and perseverative switching following *d*-amphetamine in the rat. *Psychopharmacology* 80: 67–77.
47 American Psychiatric Association (1994) *Diagnostic and statistical manual of mental disorders*, 4th edition, American Psychiatric Press, Washington DC
48 Rado S (1962) *Psychoanalysis of behavior: Collected papers (vol. 2)*. Grune and Stratton, New York
49 Andreasen NC, Olsen S (1902) Negative vs positive schizophrenia: definition and validation. *Arch. Gen. Psychiatry* 39: 789–794
50 Chapman LJ, Chapman JP, Raulin ML (1976) Scales for physical and social anhedonia. *J Abn Psychol* 85: 374–382
51 Clementz BA, Grove WM, Katsanis J, Iacono WG (1991) Psychometric detection of schizotypy: perceptual aberration and physical anhedonia in relatives of schizophrenics. *J Abn Psychol* 100: 607–612
52 Erlenmeyer-Kimling L, Cornblatt BA, Rock D, Roberts S, Bell M, West A (1993) The New York high-risk project: Anhedonia, attentional deviance and psychopathology. *Schizophr Bull* 19: 141–153
53 Franke P, Maier W, Hardt J, Hain C (1993) Cognitive functioning and anhedonia in subjects at risk for schizophrenia. *Schizophr Res* 10: 77–84
54 Strauss JS, Kokes RF, Klorman R, Sacksteder JL (1977) Premorbid adjustment in schizophrenia: Concepts, measures, and implications. I. The concept of premorbid adjustment. *Schizophrenia Bull* 3: 182–185
55 Bellack AS, Morrison RL, Wixted JT, Mueser KT (1990) An analysis of social competence in schizophrenia. *Br J Psychiatry* 156: 809–818
56 Bellack AS, Morrison RL, Mueser KT, Wade JH, Sayers SL (1990) Role playing for assessing the social competence of psychiatric patients. *Psychol Assessm* 2: 248–255
57 Mueser KT, Bellack AS, Morrison RL, Wixted JT (1990) Social competence in schizophrenia: Premorbid adjustment, social skill, and domains of functioning. *J Psychiat Res* 24: 51–63
58 Cutting J, Murphy D (1990) Impaired ability of schizophrenics, relative to manics or depressives, to appreciate social knowledge about their culture. *Br J Psychiatr* 157: 355–358
59 Ellenbroek BA and Cools AR (1994) Animal models of psychotic disturbances. In: JA Den Boer, HGM Westenberg, HM van Praag (eds): *Advances in the neurobiology of schizophrenia*. John Wiley & Sons, Chichester, (1995), 89–109
60 Braff DL (1993) Information processing and attention dysfunctions in schizophrenia. *Schizophr Bull* 19: 233–260
61 Broadbent DE (1971) *Decision and stress*. Academic Press, London
62 Carr V, Wale J (1986) Schizophrenia: An information processing model. *Austr N Zealand J Psychiatry* 20: 136–155
63 Shagass C (1976) An electrophysiological view of schizophrenia. *Biol Psychiatry* 11: 3–30
64 Venables PH (1964) Input dysfunction in schizophrenia. *Prog Exp Pers Res* 1: 1–47
65 McGhie A, Chapman J (1961) Disorders of attention and perception in early schizophrenia. *Br J Med Psychol* 34: 103–116
66 Adler LE, Pachtman E, Franks RD, Pecevich M, Waldo MC, Freedman, R (1982) Neurophysiological evidence for a defect in neuronal mechanisms involved in sensory gating in schizophrenia. *Biol Psychiatry* 17: 639–654
67 Braff DL, Stone C, Callaway E, Geyer MA, Glick ID, Bali L (1978) Prestimulus effects on human startle reflex in normals and schizophrenics. *Psychophysiology* 14: 339–343
68 Freedman R, Adler LE, Waldo MC, Pachtman E, Franks RD (1903) Neurophysiological evidence for a defect in inhibitory pathways in schizophrenia: Comparison of medicated and drug-free patients. *Biol Psychiatr* 18: 537–551
69 Nagamoto HT, Adler LE, Hea RA, Griffith JM, McRae KA, Freedman R (1996) Gating of auditory P_{50} in schizophrenics: Unique effects of clozapine. *Biol Psychiatr* 40: 181–188
70 Spring B, Weinstein L, Freeman R, Thompson S (1991) Selective attention in schizophrenia. In: SR Steinhauer, JH Gruzelier, J Zubin (eds): *Handbook of schizophrenia, vol 5, Neuropsychology, psychophysiology and information processing*. Elsevier, Amsterdam, 371–396
71 Lubow RE (1973) Latent inhibition. *Psychol Bull* 79: 398–407

72 Baruch I, Hemsley DR, Gray JA (1988) Differential performance of acute and chronic schizophrenics in a latent inhibition task. *J Nerv Ment Dis* 176: 598–606
73 Lubow RE (1989) *Latent inhibition and conditioned attention theory*. Cambridge Univ Press, Cambridge.
74 Gray NS, Pilowsky LS, Gray JA, Kerwin RW (1995) Latent inhibition in drug naïve schizophrenics: Relationship to duration of illness and dopamine D_2 binding using SPET. *Schizophr Res* 17: 95–107
75 Swerdlow NR, Braff DL, Hartston H, Perry W, Geyer MA (1996) Latent inhibition in schizophrenia. *Schizophr Res*, 20: 91–103
76 Jones SH, Gray JA, Hemsley DR (19923) Loss of Kamin blocking effect in acute but not chronic schizophrenics. *Biol Psychiat* 32: 739–755
77 Adler LE, Gerhardt GA, Franks RD, Baker N, Nagamoto H, Drebing C, Freedman R (1990) Sensory physiology and catecholamines in schizophrenia and mania. *Psychiatr Res* 31: 297–309
78 Swerdlow NS, Geyer MA (1998) Using an animal model of deficient sensorimotor gating to study the pathophysiology and new treatments of schizophrenia. *Schizophr Bull* 24: 285–301

The preclinical evaluation of atypical antipsychotics

Atypical Antipsychotics
ed. by B.A. Ellenbroek and A.R. Cools

Receptor profile of antipsychotics

Josée E. Leysen

Department of Biochemical Pharmacology, Janssen Research Foundation, Turnhoutseweg 30, B-2340 Beerse, Belgium

Introduction

The aetiology of schizophrenia is still unknown, but aberrant neurotransmitter actions have been hypothesised to underlie symptoms of schizophrenia. The most considered are the dopaminergic [1], the serotonergic (5-hydroxytryptamine, 5-HT) [2, 3] and the glutamatergic systems [4]. The hypotheses essentially emerged from clinical observations with drugs, whose properties became well-documented in pharmacological and biochemical studies. Today's knowledge of neurotransmitter receptors is greatly evolved and a broad range of symptoms of schizophrenia has been described. Besides the positive symptoms, negative symptoms and impairment of cognition receive increasing attention [5, 6]. It is clear that a single neurotransmitter system, let alone a particular neurotransmitter receptor subtype, cannot account for the complicated picture of the disease. Today, a vague hypothesis could be that excessive stimulation of dopamine D_2-type receptors plays a role in the positive symptoms of schizophrenia whereas imbalance in the stimulation of excitatory 5-HT_{2A} receptors may be involved in the expression of some of the negative symptoms of schizophrenia, and defective signalling of N-methyl-D-aspartate (NMDA)-type glutamate receptors may underlie the deregulation of the other neurotransmitter systems.

The first-generation neuroleptics, developed between the early 1950s and mid-1980s, were designed to be dopamine antagonists. The butyrophenone, haloperidol, is the prototype for a more selective dopamine antagonist. Over 70 neuroleptics, belonging to several different chemical classes were brought to the European market [7]. All these compounds appeared to block dopamine D_2-type receptors in the brain and a correlation was demonstrated between their affinity for D_2 receptors and dosages used for treating schizophrenia [8]. However, blockade of D_2 receptors also induces extrapyramidal symptoms (EPS).

Pharmacological and receptor studies revealed that neuroleptics could interact with several neurotransmitter systems [2, 7]. The identification, in 1978, of 5-HT_2-type receptors in the brain and the finding that certain neuroleptics had high affinity for these receptors [9] initiated the development of a second generation of antipsychotics with predominant 5-HT_2 and some D_2 antagonism. In the pioneer study, the possible benefits of 5-HT_2 antagonism were suggested from the exceptional pharmacological and clinical properties of pipamperone. In contrast to other neuroleptics, this butyrophenone was found to be primarily a 5-HT_2 and only a weak D_2 antagonist. In clinical studies it was reported to have particular anti-agitation properties, to normalise disturbed sleep rhythms in psychiatric patients and to improve social interaction [9]. Later studies with the potent and selective 5-HT_2 antagonist, ritanserin, demonstrated the beneficial effects of central 5-HT_2 antagonism on dysthymia and on negative symptoms of schizophrenia. Furthermore it appeared that ritanserin could attenuate neuroleptic-induced EPS [10–13]. Clozapine too showed more potent 5-HT_2 than D_2 antagonism [9]. In spite of serious risks for fatal haematological complications, special attention was paid to this compound (see [14–16]). Based on clinical observations, clozapine was designated as an "atypical antipsychotic" because of its therapeutic efficacy in treatment-resistant patients with schizophrenia-like symptoms, the low incidence of inducing EPS and the absence of elevated prolactin levels. Meltzer and Nash [17] suggested that, in order to be classified as an "atypical antipsychotic" a compound should have at least 10 times higher affinity for 5-HT_2 than for D_2 receptors. For the second generation of antipsychotics, for which risperidone became the prototype, the term "balanced 5-$HT_{2/D2}$ antagonist" is preferred [18–23]. Compounds entering the market are olanzapine [24–26], quetiapine [27, 28], zotepine [29], sertindole [30] ziprasidone [31]. The clinical properties of these drugs were recently reviewed by King [6].

At present, discovery research pays attention to drugs tackling the glutamatergic system. This may yield future antipsychotics but the therapeutic value of such agents (and side-effects) remains to be demonstrated [4].

The explosive development of receptor research has revealed a host of neurotransmitter (mono-amine and amino acid) receptor subtypes. According to their protein structure, neurotransmitter receptors belong to two large receptor families: the super-family of G-protein coupled receptors (sometimes called metabotropic receptors) and the ligand-gated ion channel receptors. G-protein coupled receptors are protein monomers with seven trans-membrane domains. These receptors couple to a G-protein (a trimeric protein, $\alpha\beta\gamma$, of which the α subunit has guanosine triphosphate [GTP]-ase activity), which mediates signal transduction. Agonist binding activates the G-protein, upon which GTP is bound, the G-protein α and $\beta\gamma$ subunits dissociate from the receptor and activate an effector protein in the cell. The effector protein can be an enzyme which produces an intracellular second messenger (e.g. cyclic adenosine monophosphate [cAMP], inositol triphosphate [IP3], arachidonic acid), or an ion channel which allows ion fluxes. The second messengers further stimulate the responding mechanism within the cell. Agonists and antagonists can bind to distinct, mutually exclusive sites at the receptor protein and produce either activation or blockade of the receptor. Ligand-gated ion channels consist of several protein subunits which can associate as homomers or heteromers to form pores in cell membranes. They may have several co-operatively linked binding sites for endogenous and exogenous compounds.

The following numbers of neurotransmitter receptors have been identified to date: five muscarinic acetylcholine G-protein coupled receptors and multiple isoforms of alpha and beta subunits of the ionotropic nicotine receptors; nine G-protein coupled adrenoceptors; five G-protein coupled dopamine receptors; three histamine G-protein coupled receptors; 13 5-hydroxytryptamine receptors (12 G-protein coupled, one ionotropic); several subunits of ionotropic glutamate receptors: NMDA- receptors (five subunits), AMPA receptors (four subunits), kainate receptors (five subunits) and eight metabotropic glutamate receptors; several subunits of the chloride channel forming GABA-A receptor and the metabotropic GABA-B receptor. To complicate the picture even more, it appears that a drug can interact with many different receptor subtypes. The role of several new receptors, as identified by gene cloning, is still unclear. Yet, the availability of cloned receptors (mostly human genes) expressed in cell lines and of techniques for measuring drug affinities in competition binding experiments with radioligands, allows assessment of the receptor profiles of drugs. Receptors expressed in cells also facilitate the measurement of specific signal transduction events, giving information on agonist, partial agonist, antagonist or inverse agonist activity of drugs.

In this chapter, we will discuss the mono-amine receptor profile of the antipsychotics: haloperidol, pipamperone, risperidone, 9-hydroxyrisperidone, sertindole, ziprasidone clozapine, olanzapine, quetiapine and zotepine (chemical structures in Fig. 1). We report the binding affinities *in vitro* for 22 neurotransmitter receptor subtypes: four dopamine, 12 serotonin, four adrenoceptors, the histamine H_1 and the brain muscarinic acetylcholine receptor. We mostly used cloned human receptors expressed in cells. We report data from our own studies in which all the compounds were measured in parallel in a uniform way [3, 32]. Indeed, depending on assay conditions and applied radioligands, receptor binding affinities of compounds may vary between studies (see reviews [33, 34]), confounding valid comparison of data from different studies. Before discussing the *in vitro* receptor profiles of the drugs, we will briefly review the properties of the receptors which are targets for the antipsychotics and discuss the possible clinical consequences of the drug receptor interaction. We will further show data from *ex vivo* measurements of brain receptor occupancy by drugs administered to animals and we will relate the receptor occupancy to dopamine mediated behaviours observed in the animals.

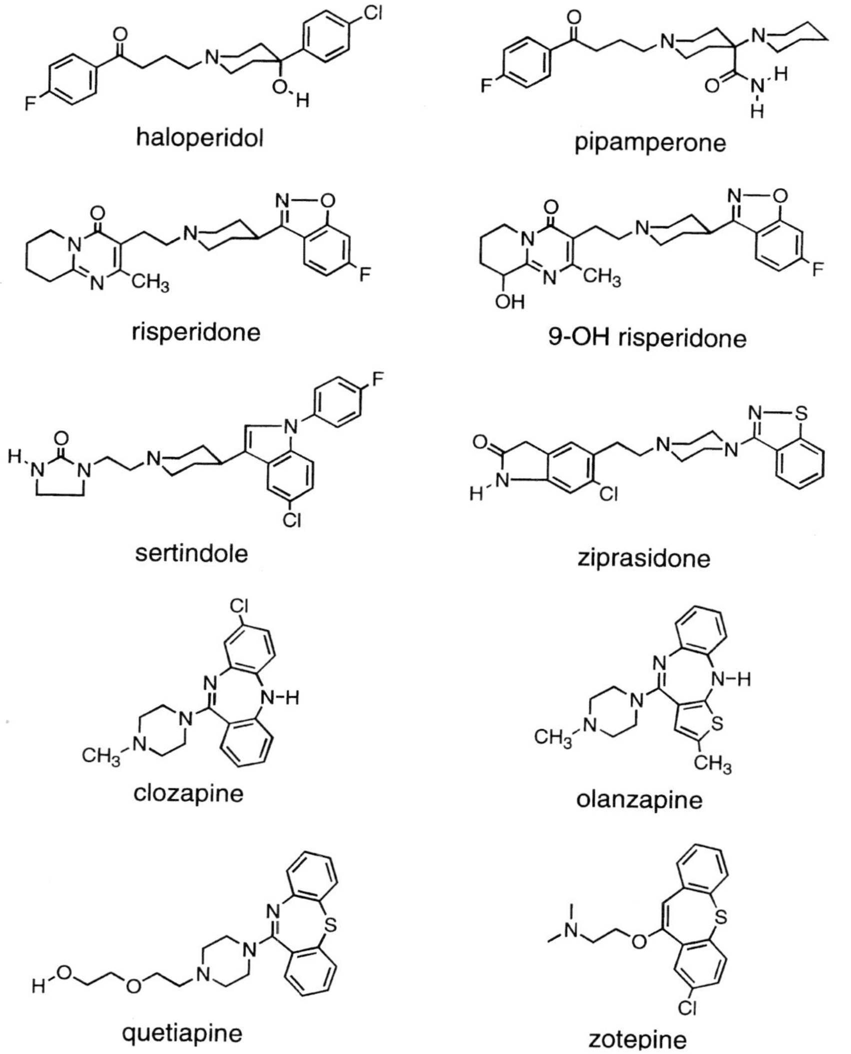

Figure 1. Chemical structure of antipsychotics.

Dopamine receptors

Dopamine receptors have been grouped into two main classes: D_1-like (D_1 and D_5) and D_2-like receptors (D_2, D_3, D_4). D_1-like receptors are positively coupled to adenylyl cyclase: activation of the receptor by an agonist produces an increase in cAMP. D_2-like receptors are negatively coupled to adenylyl cyclase: agonist stimulation produces a decrease in cAMP (for review see [35, 36]).

D_1 and D_5 receptors

D_1-like receptors occur in the caudate putamen, the nucleus accumbens and the frontal cortex. No drugs, neither agonists nor antagonists, are known yet which can differentiate between D_1 and D_5 receptors. D_1 receptors are more abundant in the brain and they appear to have a role in actions of dopamine to control motor, cognitive and cardiovascular functions [37]. Recent studies using D_5 receptor antisense, revealed a D_5 receptor role in the regulation by dopamine of progestin-dependent reproductive behaviour [38].

No linkage was found between D_1 and D_5 receptor genes and schizophrenia (see [35]). In primates, prefrontal cortical D_1 receptors seem to play a subtle role in regulating memory functions. A low occupation of these receptors by a D_1 antagonist can enhance neuronal activity in the memory field, whereas excessive D_1 receptor blockade induces hypofrontality and impairs cognitive function [39, 40]. Amongst the antipsychotics discussed in this review, clozapine and olanzapine show relatively potent D_1 receptor interaction (Tables 1 and 2).

A clinical study with the D_1 antagonist, SCH39166, could not demonstrate antipsychotic activity, on the contrary, a worsening of symptoms occurred [41]. For a more extensive discussion on the clinical effects of D_1 antagonists the reader is referred to Naber et al., this volume.

D_2 receptors

D_2 receptors are found at high density in caudate putamen, nucleus accumbens, tuberculum olfactorium and substantia nigra. Antagonism at central D_2 receptors is generally accepted to play a key role in the treatment of positive symptoms of schizophrenia. All presently known antipsychotics are D_2 antagonists and occupy these receptors to a certain extent at therapeutic dosages (with the exception of the obsolete mono-amine depleting agent, reserpine). Studies of receptor occupancy by positron emission tomography (PET), using tracer amounts of radioactive D_2 ligands in patients under antipsychotic treatment, have revealed that moderate blockade of central D_2 receptors can be adequate for the treatment of positive symptoms, whereas a high degree of D_2 receptor occupancy gives rise to EPS [42]. Prolonged, excessive blockade of central D_2 receptors may increase the risk for development of tardive dyskinesia. Antagonism at D_2 receptors in the anterior pituitary causes elevation of blood prolactin levels.

In brains of patients with schizophrenia, elevated levels of striatal D_2 receptors have been found in *post mortem* studies and in PET studies *in vivo*. However, it is still not entirely clear whether these increases in D_2 receptors are due to treatment with antipsychotic drugs or are related to the disease process [43].

Table 1. Receptor binding profiles of antipsychotics: pK_i-values ± SD (n), −log M

Receptor	Radioligand	Tissue	Temp.	Haloperidol	Pipamperone	Risperidone	9-OH-risperidone	Ziprasidone
dopamine								
rD_1	[^{3}H]SCH23390	rat striatum	37	6.56 ± 0.08 (3)	5.61 ± 0.03 (3)	6.21 ± 0.08 (3)	6.19 ± 0.11 (5)	6.47 ± 0.13 (3)
hD_{2L}	[^{3}H]spiperone	human D_{2L}-CHO	37	8.69 ± 0.09 (4)	6.71 ± 0.23 (5)	8.39 ± 0.23 (11)	8.37 ± 0.08 (3)	8.17 ± 0.10 (3)
hD_3	[^{125}I]iodosulpride	human D_3-CHO	37	8.25 ± 0.19 (3)	6.58 ± 0.17 (3)	7.85 ± 0.12 (11)	8.15 ± 0.10 (4)	7.61 ± 0.12 (2)
hD_4	[^{3}H]spiperone	human $D_{4.2}$-L929	37	7.93 ± 0.18 (5)	7.95 ± 0.37 (5)	7.82 ± 0.11 (5)	7.55 ± 0.09 (3)	6.98 ± 0.02 (2)
serotonin								
h5-HT$_{1A}$	[^{3}H]8OHDPAT	human 5-HT$_{1A}$-Hela	37	5.79 ± 0.13 (3)	5.46 ± 0.30 (3)	6.37 ± 0.13 (3)	6.23 ± 0.04 (5)	8.26 ± 0.18 (2)
h5-HT$_{1B}$	[^{3}H]alniditan	human 5-HT$_{1B}$-HEK293	37	< 5 (3)	5.54 + 0.15 (2)	6.84 ± 0.04 (2)	6.82 ± 0.24 (3)	8.06 ± 0.03 (2)
h5-HT$_{1D}$	[^{3}H]alniditan	human 5-HT$_{1D}$-C6 glioma	37	6.35 ± 0.23 (3)	6.14 ± 0.45 (5)	7.80 ± 0.38 (5)	7.98 ± 0.10 (4)	8.50 ± 0.11 (4)
h5-HT$_{1E}$	[^{3}H]5-HT	human 5-HT$_{1E}$-CHO	37	< 5 (3)	5.44 ± 0.01 (3)	5.68 ± 0.08 (3)	5.80 ± 0.04 (4)	6.12 ± 0.21 (3)
h5-HT$_{1F}$	[^{3}H]5-HT	human 5-HT$_{1F}$-COS7	37	< 5 (1)	< 5 (1)	< 5 (1)	< 5 (1)	6.86 ± 0.21 (2)
h5-HT$_{2A}$	[^{125}I]R093274	human 5-HT$_{2A}$-L929	37	6.52 ± 0.10 (3)	8.19 ± 0.08 (3)	9.39 ± 0.26 (6)	9.10 ± 0.22 (3)	8.68 ± 0.09 (5)
p5-HT$_{2C}$	[^{3}H]mesulergine	pig choroid plexus	37	< 5 (2)	6.92 ± 0.09 (5)	7.12 ± 0.15 (5)	7.16 ± 0.11 (7)	8.19 ± 0.23 (4)
m5-HT$_3$	[^{3}H]GR65630	NXG108CC15 cells	37	< 5 (3)	< 5 (2)	< 5 (5)	< 5 (1)	5.88 ± 0.31 (3)
h5-HT$_{4L}$	[^{3}H]R116712	human 5-HT$_4$-COS7	37	< 5 (3)	< 5 (3)	< 5 (3)	< 5 (2)	< 5 (1)
h5-HT$_5$	[^{3}H]5-carboxamido tryptamine	human 5-HT$_5$-HEK293	37	< 5 (1)	5.35 (1)	6.49 ± 0.06 (2)	6.44 ± 0.17 (2)	6.23 ± 0.25 (2)
h5-HT$_6$	[^{3}H]LSD	human 5-HT$_6$-HEK293	37	< 5 (1)	6.22 ± 0.03 (2)	5.53 ± 0.18 (3)	5.68 ± 0.15 (2)	7.43 ± 0.11 (4)
r5-HT$_7$	[^{3}H]LSD	rat 5-HT$_7$-HEK293	37	5.35 ± 0.02 (2)	6.26 ± 0.01 (2)	9.01 ± 0.05 (3)	8.86 ± 0.21 (2)	8.93 ± 0.03 (3)
adrenaline								
rα_1	[^{3}H]prazosin	rat cortex	25	7.58 ± 0.12 (4)	7.23 ± 0.14 (4)	8.61 ± 0.35 (4)	8.41 ± 0.09 (4)	7.88 ± 0.23 (3)
hα_{2A}	[^{3}H]rauwolscine	human α_{2A} -CHO	25	5.98 ± 0.08 (4)	6.15 ± 0.13 (4)	7.66 ± 0.10 (5)	7.55 ± 0.07 (4)	6.73 ± 0.13 (4)
hα_{2B}	[^{3}H]rauwolscine	human α_{2B} -CHO	25	6.29 ± 0.12 (4)	7.08 ± 0.05 (2)	8.06 ± 0.06 (5)	8.04 ± 0.12 (3)	7.08 ± 0.22 (3)
hα_{2C}	[^{3}H]rauwolscine	human α_{2C} -CHO	25	6.36 ± 0.10 (3)	6.25 ± 0.12 (4)	8.08 ± 0.22 (4)	8.02 ± 0.11 (4)	7.10 ± 0.12 (3)
histamine								
hH_1	[^{3}H]pyrilamine	human H_1-CHO	25	5.92 ± 0.10 (3)	5.74 ± 0.06 (2)	7.48 ± 0.56 (5)	7.47 ± 0.10 (4)	7.19 ± 0.05 (2)
acetylcholine								
muscarinic	[^{3}H]dexetimide	rat striatum	37	5.46 ± 0.38 (4)	5.23 ± 0.52 (5)	< 5 (4)	5.46 ± 0.12 (4)	5.61 ± 0.01 (2)

Table 1 (continued)

Receptor	Radioligand	Tissue	Temp.	Sertindole	Zotepine	Olanzapine	Clozapine	Quetiapine
dopamine								
rD_1	[^{3}H]SCH23390	rat striatum	37	6.89 ± 0.83 (4)	6.99 ± 0.16 (3)	6.93 ± 0.32 (3)	6.27 ± 0.04 (3)	5.35 ± 0.18 (3)
hD_{2L}	[^{3}H]spiperone	human D_{2L}-CHO	37	7.94 ± 0.19 (3)	7.90 ± 0.47 (4)	7.20 ± 0.52 (3)	6.75 ± 0.06 (4)	6.14 ± 0.05 (3)
hD_3	[^{125}I]iodosulpride	human D_3-CHO	37	8.00 ± 0.05 (3)	8.29 ± 0.14 (3)	7.30 ± 0.24 (3)	6.62 ± 0.14 (3)	6.03 ± 0.15 (5)
hD_4	[^{3}H]spiperone	human $D_{4.2}$-L929	37	7.62 ± 0.11 (54)	7.56 ± 0.28 (4)	7.53 ± 0.10 (4)	7.26 ± 0.14 (7)	5.65 ± 0.13 (5)
serotonin								
h5-HT_{1A}	[^{3}H]8OHDPAT	human 5-HT_{1A}-Hela	37	6.46 ± 0.10 (3)	6.50 ± 0.07 (3)	5.49 ± 0.06 (3)	6.72 ± 0.19 (3)	6.38 ± 0.21 (3)
h5-HT_{1B}	[^{3}H]alniditan	human 5-HT_{1B}-HEK293	37	6.60 ± 0.10 (3)	6.56 ± 0.05 (3)	5.56 ± 0.07 (3)	5.53 ± 0.07 (3)	5.34 ± 0.01 (4)
h5-HT_{1D}	[^{3}H]alniditan	human 5-HT_{1D}-C6 glioma	37	7.21 ± 0.30 (3)	6.93 ± 0.33 (4)	5.73 ± 0.24 (4)	5.96 ± 0.19 (6)	< 5 (3)
h5-HT_{1E}	[^{3}H]5-HT	human 5-HT_{1E}-CHO	37	6.38 ± 0.05 (3)	6.24 ± 0.12 (5)	5.59 (1)	6.06 ± 0.02 (3)	5.80 ± 0.04 (6)
h5-HT_{1F}	[^{3}H]5-HT	human 5-HT_{1F}-COS7	37	5.67 ± 0.18 (2)	5.93 ± 0.06 (2)	6.21 ± 0.24 (2)	6.76 ± 0.64 (2)	5.82 ± 0.25 (4)
h5-HT_{2A}	[^{125}I]R093274	human 5-HT_{2A}-L929	37	9.97 ± 0.04 (3)	8.58 ± 0.15 (3)	8.63 ± 0.09 (7)	8.20 ± 0.13 (4)	6.56 ± 0.49 (2)
p5-HT_{2C}	[^{3}H]mesulergine	pig choroid plexus	37	8.84 ± 0.03 (4)	8.68 ± 0.25 (3)	7.74 ± 0.58 (2)	7.90 ± 0.12 (3)	5.61 ± 0.23 (4)
m5-HT_3	[^{3}H]GR65630	NXG108CC15 cells	37	5.50 ± 0.01 (2)	6.62 ± 0.05 (3)	6.87 ± 0.19 (3)	7.00 ± 0.23 (3)	5.58 ± 0.38 (4)
h5-HT_{4L}	[^{3}H]R116712	human 5-HT_4-COS7	37	< 5 (3)	5.94 ± 0.06 (3)	< 5 (3)	< 5 (2)	< 5 (4)
h5-HT_5	[^{3}H]5-carboxamido tryptamine	human 5-HT_5-HEK293	37	6.50 ± 0.01 (2)	7.17 ± 0.23 (2)	5.86 ± 0.01 (2)	5.75 ± 0.54 (2)	5.40 ± 0.07 (2)
h5-HT_6	[^{3}H]LSD	human 5-HT_6-HEK293	37	9.13 ± 0.26 (4)	8.09 ± 0.01 (2)	8.25 ± 0.30 (4)	8.04 ± 0.22 (3)	5.86 ± 0.46 (2)
r5-HT_7	[^{3}H]LSD	rat 5-HT_7-HEK293	37	7.97 ± 0.22 (3)	7.86 ± 0.12 (3)	7.27 ± 0.26 (3)	7.80 ± 0.10 (3)	6.24 ± 0.01 (3)
adrenaline								
$r\alpha_1$	[^{3}H]prazosin	rat cortex	25	8.71 ± 0.17 (4)	8.48 ± 0.04 (3)	7.24 ± 0.18 (2)	7.65 ± 0.10 (4)	7.28 ± 0.16 (2)
$h\alpha_{2A}$	[^{3}H]rauwolscine	human α_{2A} -CHO	25	6.45 ± 0.27 (4)	6.81 ± 0.14 (5)	6.37 ± 0.12 (3)	7.27 ± 0.13 (4)	5.75 ± 0.08 (4)
$h\alpha_{2B}$	[^{3}H]rauwolscine	human α_{2B} -CHO	25	6.48 ± 0.23 (4)	8.28 ± 0.05 (3)	6.78 ± 0.13 (3)	7.65 ± 0.10 (4)	7.05 ± 0.06 (4)
$h\alpha_{2C}$	[^{3}H]rauwolscine	human α_{2C} -CHO	25	6.54 ± 0.19 (4)	6.89 ± 0.04 (3)	6.67 ± 0.40 (3)	8.11 ± 0.10 (4)	6.54 ± 0.13 (4)
histamine								
hH_1	[^{3}H]pyrilamine	human H_1-CHO	25	6.31 ± 0.21 (4)	9.25 ± 0.70 (3)	8.92 ± 0.08 (2)	8.97 ± 0.09 (3)	8.08 ± 0.27 (4)
acetylcholine								
muscarinic	[^{3}H]dexetimide	rat striatum	37	5.61 ± 0.01 (4)	6.03 ± 0.36 (3)	7.26 ± 0.40 (4)	7.48 ± 0.06 (3)	5.97 ± 0.07 (3)

Up to a concentration of 10 µM the compounds did not bind to β_1, β_2, β_3 adrenoceptors, neuropeptide receptors (cholecystokinin CCKA, CCKB, neurokinin NK1, NK2, bradykinin BK_2), NMDA receptors (MK801 site, glycine site), AMPA receptors.
Some compounds bound at µM concentrations to opiate receptors (μ, δ, κ), dihydropyridine labelled Ca^{++} channel sites, batrachotoxin labelled Na^+ channels sites, DA, 5-HT, NE transporter. Zotepine showed $pK_i = 8.3$ on the rat NE transporter.
Haloperidol had nM affinity for haloperidol labelled σ sites, the other compounds had µM affinity.

Gene cloning techniques, have uncovered two splice variants of D_2 receptors; a short form, D_{2S}, and a long form, D_{2L}. The long form has a 29 amino acid repeat segment in the third cytoplasmic loop of the receptor protein. D_{2S} and D_{2L} receptors, reportedly, are unevenly distributed in the brain and may show differences in functional coupling to G-proteins. However, no relevant differences in the pharmacology of the receptor variants with regard to antipsychotic drug binding have been found thus far [32, 44].

No linkage between the D_2 receptor gene and schizophrenia has been demonstrated. Pharmacological effects of D_2 receptor blockade in animal behavioural models are: antagonism of effects induced by direct or indirect D_2 agonists (e.g. apomorphine- or amphetamine-induced agitation and stereotypy in rats, apomorphine-induced disruption of sound and light prepulse inhibition in rats, apomorphine-induced vomiting in dogs); inhibition of learned and conditioned behaviour in laboratory animals and suppression of motility and induction of catalepsy. D_2 receptor blockade increases dopamine turnover in the brain and increases cholinergic transmission. Chronic D_2 receptor blockade causes up-regulation of brain D_2 receptors and development of dopaminergic supersensitivity (for further review see [34]).

D_3 receptors

D_3 receptors occur at highest density in the Islands of Calleja. They are also observed in the nucleus accumbens and the cerebellum. D_3 receptors were discovered by gene cloning. In transfected cells, they display only weak signalling and in some studies agonist-induced inhibition of cAMP formation is found. Only few relatively selective D_3 agonists and antagonists are known. Current antipsychotics poorly differentiate between D_2 and D_3 receptors [2, 32]. Brain D_3 receptors may be strongly occupied by endogenous dopamine [45]. The physiological, pharmacological and pathological role of D_3 receptors is not understood.

A presumed linkage between the D_3 receptor gene and schizophrenia is controversial. A limited clinical study in schizophrenic patients with the D_3 antagonist, UH232, at the University of Maryland failed to demonstrate antipsychotic activity [46]. Possible clinical effects of D_3 antagonists are discussed in Naber et al., this volume.

D_4 receptors

D_4 receptors were also discovered by gene cloning. They have attracted special interest because clozapine was initially found to have over 20-fold higher affinity for D_4 than for D_2 receptors, although, the difference was

Table 2. Receptor profile and D_2 affinity potency ranking of antipsychotics

	Clinical dose range mg/day	D_2 affinity ratio K_i drug/K_i haloperidol	Rank order of receptors for which the drug has higher (> 3 x) or equal (≤ 3 x) affinity compared to its D_2 affinity
Haloperidol	5–20	1	$D_2 \sim D_3$*
Risperidone	4–6	2	$5HT_{2A} > 5HT_7 > \alpha_1 > D_2 \sim \alpha_{2C} \sim \alpha_{2B}$
9-OH-risperidone		2	$5HT_{2A} > 5HT_7 > \alpha_1 > D_2 \sim D_3 \sim \alpha_{2C} \sim \alpha_{2B}$
Ziprasidone	80–160	3.3	$5HT_7 > 5HT_{2A} \sim 5HT_{1D} > 5HT_{1A} \sim 5HT_{2C} \sim D_2 \sim 5HT_{1B} \sim \alpha_1$
Sertindole	16–24	5.6	$5HT_{2A} > 5HT_6 > 5HT_{2C} \sim \alpha_1 > D_3 \sim 5HT_7 \sim D_2 \sim D_4$
Zotepine	150–340	6.2	$H_1 > 5HT_{2C} \sim 5HT_{2A} > \alpha_1 \sim D_3 \sim \alpha_{2B} > 5HT_6 \sim D_2 \sim 5HT_7 \sim D_4$
Olanzapine	12.5–17.5	30	$H_1 > 5HT_{2A} > 5HT_6 > 5HT_{2C} > D_4 \sim D_3 \sim 5HT_7 \sim mACh \sim \alpha_1 \sim D_2 \sim D_1$
Clozapine	300–600	87	$H_1 > 5HT_{2A} \sim \alpha_{2C} \sim 5HT_6 \sim 5HT_{2C} > 5HT_7 \sim \alpha_{2B} \sim \alpha_1 \sim mACh >$ $\alpha_{2A} \sim D_4 \sim 5HT_3 > D_2 \sim 5HT_{1F} \sim 5HT_{1A} \sim D_3 \sim D_1$
Pipamperone	80–360	95	$5HT_{2A} > D_4 > \alpha_1 \sim \alpha_{2B} \sim 5HT_{2C} > D_2 \sim D_3$
Quetiapine	250–750	355	$H_1 \gg \alpha_1 > \alpha_{2B} > 5HT_{2A} \sim \alpha_{2C} \sim 5HT_{1A} >$ $5HT_7 \sim D_2 \sim D_3 \sim mACh \sim 5HT_6 \sim 5HT_{1F} \sim 5HT_{1E}$

* Haloperidol has equally high affinity for σ-sites, recently reported to be related to enzymes of the cholesterol synthase pathway.

much less in later studies [32, 47–49]. Few antipsychotics differentiate markedly between D_2 and D_4 receptors. Exceptions are pipamperone with a 15-fold higher D_4 than D_2 affinity (see Table 1) and raclopride, which is devoid of D_4-receptor binding affinity. Selective D_4-ligands, L745870, NGD94, have been described [50]. Although mRNA for D_4 receptors has been demonstrated in the brain and in the heart, radioligand binding to D_4 receptors in animal and human brain tissue is difficult to detect reliably. Initial claims of D_4 receptor labelling with non-specific radioligands ([^{3}H]nemonapride, [^{3}H]spiperone) could not be confirmed; the measurements seemed to be artefactual [51]. In addition, application of the recently available high affinity and selective D_4 ligand, [^{125}I]L-750667 [52], did not yield D_4 receptor positive autoradiograms on animal or human brain sections (unpublished observation). Only the use of [^{3}H]NGD-94-1 yielded positive findings. Highest levels were found in the hippocampus, temporal and entorhinal cortex and insula and elevated levels in brains (particularly substantia nigra) of patients with schizophrenia were noted [53]. D_4 receptor-like immunoreactivity with a reportedly specific D_4 receptor antibody was detected in monkey brain. Immunoreactivity was demonstrated in cortical pyramidal and non-pyramidal neuronal cells, in the hippocampus, the thalamic reticular nucleus, the globus pallidus and the substantia nigra. In many areas, D_4 receptor-like immunoreactivity coincided with GABA-ergic cells, hence the suggestion that D_4 receptors play a role in the modulation by dopamine of GABA-ergic neuronal activity [54].

By means of gene cloning, several splice variants of human D_4 receptors were detected and repeat segment in the third cytoplasmic loop was found to occur up to 11 times. Moreover, several amino acid point mutations can occur in these segments, leading to a great number of D_4 receptor variants [35]. A possible link between a D_4 receptor gene variant and novelty seeking was reported.

A recent clinical study in acutely psychotic schizophrenic patients with a potent and selective D_4 antagonist, L-745870, did not reveal antipsychotic activity [50]. Effects of D_4 antagonists on various symptoms in schizophrenia are to be explored further.

5-Hydroxytryptamine receptors

The 13 5-HT receptors comprise the 5-HT_1-class of receptors (5-HT_{1A}, 5-HT_{1B}, 5-HT_{1D}, 5-HT_{1E}, 5-HT_{1F}) which are inhibitory receptors negatively coupled to adenylate cyclase, the 5-HT_2-class receptors (5HT_{2A}, 5-HT_{2B}, 5-HT_{2C}) which are excitatory receptors and stimulate phospholipase C (inositol phosphate and diacylglycerol formation, Ca^{++} mobilisation) and phospholipase A_2 (arachidonic acid formation). The 5-HT_3 receptor is a cation channel, the 5-HT_4, the 5-HT_6 and 5-HT_7 receptors are positively coupled to adenylate cyclase, the 5-HT_5 receptor was recently found to inhibit adenylate cyclase [55].

For all of them the human genes were cloned and for several subtypes, variants and splice variants have been reported (for review see [3, 56, 57]). The 5-HT_{2A} receptor appears to be the most important of the 5-HT receptor subtypes with regard to the action of current antipsychotics (balanced 5-$HT_{2A/D2}$ antagonist) [2, 17, 32, 58]. Further, 5-HT receptors for which several (but not all) antipsychotics show relatively high binding affinity are the 5-HT_{2C}, the 5-HT_6 and the 5-HT_7 receptors (see Table 1). We do not report data on the 5-HT_{2B} receptor since its role in the brain is uncertain. Binding of some antipsychotics to the 5-HT_{2B} receptor has been reported [59]. Properties of 5-HT receptors hit by antipsychotics are discussed below.

5-HT_{2A} receptors

5-HT_{2A} receptor localisation in mammalian brain has been extensively studied by means of radioligand autoradiography [60], *in situ* hybridisation of mRNA [61, 62] and immunocytochemistry [63–66]. 5-HT_{2A} receptors mainly occur in the telencephalon and much less in the midbrain and hindbrain. Highest densities are found in the olfactory nucleus, -bulbus and -tuberculum, the cerebral cortex (layers II–VI), claustrum, mammilary body, hippocampus, nucleus accumbens, ventral pallidum, neostriatum, pedunculopontine nucleus, latero-dorsal tegmental nucleus, red nucleus and cranial motor nucleus. Literature reports are not unanimous with regard to the cellular localisation of 5-HT_{2A} receptors [63–66]. The most recent immunocytochemical studies [65, 66] in rat and monkey brain report extensive presence of 5-HT_{2A} receptors on apical dendrites of cortical pyramidal cells which use glutamate as neurotransmitter. Stimulation of 5-HT_{2A} receptors on these neurones enhances asynchronous excitatory transmission [67]. 5-HT_{2A} receptors are also detected on cortical GABA-ergic interneurons [63, 68]. In the neostriatum, the pedunculopontine nucleus and latero-dorsal tegmental nucleus they were found in cholinergic cells [64].

The most selective 5-HT_{2A} antagonist known is MDL100907 [69]. All the new antipsychotics show a relatively high affinity for 5-HT_{2A} receptors.

The pharmacological effects of 5-HT_{2A} antagonists are well documented. In mice, rats and guinea pigs they antagonise head twitches elicited by 5-HT_2 agonists (e.g. mescaline, dimethoxyphenylisopropylamines (DOM, DOB, DOI), 5-hydroxytryptophan). They antagonise discriminative stimulus effects induced by 5-HT_2 agonists (quipazine, LSD, DOM) and they antagonise 5-HT_2-agonist disruption of sound and light prepulse inhibition (role of 5-HT in the modulation of auditory and visual sensorimotor gating). 5-HT_{2A} antagonists can also attenuate effects induced by NMDA antagonists (phencyclidine, dizocilpine, AP-5) and by low dose amphetamine (see [34]).

In humans, 5-HT_{2A} antagonists attenuate hallucinations elicited by LSD, mescaline, DOM, DOB, DOI [70].

Central pharmacological activities of 5-HT_{2A} antagonists point to potential anxiolytic or thymostenic action, as demonstrated by anxiolytic activity in rats in an elevated plus maze paradigm or an antidepressant-like activity in a test of learned helplessness in rats (for review see [71]). In animals and in man 5-HT_{2A} antagonists increase the amount of slow wave sleep and decrease paradoxical sleep [72]. Slow wave or deep sleep is considered to be the restorative phase of sleep; improvement of the quality of sleep may contribute to the therapeutic effects of the compounds in dysthymia.

Important clinical findings attributed to 5-HT_{2A} antagonism are an improvement of negative symptoms in patients with schizophrenia [6, 13, 22], an enhancement of cognition [73] and an attenuation of EPS induced by dopamine D_2 antagonism [12]. A possible explanation of the beneficial effects of 5-HT_{2A} antagonism in schizophrenia can be derived from electrophysiological and neurochemical studies. 5-HT_{2A} antagonists were found to decrease GABA-ergic activity. They block the 5-HT-induced excitation of GABA-ergic cells in the periform and the frontal cortex, in the diagonal band of Broca and in the medial septum. By reducing the inhibitory GABA-ergic transmission in certain areas, 5-HT_{2A} antagonists may disinhibit glutamatergic transmission. Otherwise, 5-HT_{2A} antagonist may modulate apical dendritic gating mechanisms of the pyramidal cells [66]. Regulation of glutamatergic action is probably implicated in the therapeutic action of 5-HT_{2A} antagonists [74].

5-HT_{2A} antagonism can also potentiate and prolong inhibition of prefrontal cortex neurons by the 5-HT_{1A}-agonist, 8-OHDPAT. Indeed, electrophysiological studies have shown that excitatory 5-HT_{2A} receptors and inhibitory 5-HT_{1A} receptors co-exist on cortical cells [75].

Svensson and colleagues showed that systemic administration of 5-HT_{2A} antagonists can restore the burst firing pattern of mid-brain dopaminergic neurons (increase in burst firing and reduction of tonic activity), when the neuronal activity is impaired for example by local cooling of the frontal cortex (experimental hypofrontality) or by administration of low dose D_2 antagonist (causing increased tonic activity) [76–79]. 5-HT_{2A} antagonists were shown to enhance the dopamine efflux in the frontal cortex and the nucleus accumbens [80]. It is therefore suggested that a potent, predominant 5-HT_{2A} antagonism which restores dopaminergic neuron burst firing activity with a particular facilitation of cortical neurons, accounts for the beneficial effects on negative symptoms in schizophrenia and for the reduction in dopamine-antagonist-induced EPS.

5-HT_{2C} receptors

5-HT_{2C} receptors have a very widespread distribution in the CNS. They are abundant in the telencephalon, the midbrain, the hindbrain, the cerebellum and the spinal cord. The most dense occurrence of radioligand binding sites is in the choroid plexus [81].

Several compounds reveal relatively strong 5-HT_{2C} antagonistic activity (e.g. the antipsychotics: sertindole, zotepine, ziprasidone, clozapine, olanzapine and some antidepressants: mianserin, mirtazapine, certain tricyclic antidepressants) but a selective antagonist has only recently been described (SB-242084) [82]. No agonists can adequately distinguish between 5-HT_{2A} and 5-HT_{2C} receptors.

Animal and human pharmacological studies point to a possible role of 5-HT_{2C} receptors in anxiety. The 5-HT agonist, m-chlorophenyl piperazine (mCPP) induces anxiety in rats and mice and elicits panic attacks in humans. These effects are antagonised by 5-HT_{2C} antagonists with potencies which correlate with their 5-HT_{2C} receptor affinity. 5-HT_{2C} receptors also have a role in the regulation of food-intake. A reduction in food intake induced by mCPP or flenfluramine is reversed by 5-HT_{2C} antagonists. Dieting, together with low tryptophan intake, causes 5-HT_{2C} receptor supersensitivity. Finally, 5-HT_{2C} receptor knock-out mice grow to twice the weight of their normal littermates [83]. Hence 5-HT_{2C} receptor blockade may lead to substantial weight increase.

5-HT_{2C} receptors also have a role in development, in cell growth and differentiation and they modulate endocrine functions. 5-HT_{2C} receptor blockade can attenuate prolactin release [84]. In view of the widespread distribution throughout the brain and spinal cord other roles are expected to emerge.

5-HT_6 receptors

5-HT_6 receptors were discovered by gene cloning. Immunocytochemical studies [62, 85] have revealed that the density of these receptors is highest in the olfactory tubercle, nucleus accumbens, striatum, frontal and entorhinal cortex, the hippocampus (CA1 area, dentate gyrus) and the molecular layer of the cerebellum. They occur at moderate density in the thalamus, substantia nigra reticulata, superior colliculus, the motor trigeminal nucleus, and the facial nucleus. Immunoreactivity of the protein matches the mRNA distribution, suggesting localisation on dendritic processes. Selective 5-HT_6 antagonists, Ro 04-6790 and Ro 63-0563 were recently described [86]. LSD and some antipsychotics (sertindole, olanzapine, zotepine, clozapine, ziprasidone) show high affinity for 5-HT_6 receptors. 5-HT_6 receptor antisense oligonucleotide injection into rat brain caused yawning, stretching and chewing but had no effect on locomotor activity, body weight, food intake, body temperature, or nociception [87]. Similar effects were reported for the selective 5-HT_6 antagonists. Studies with these compounds revealed that 5-HT_6 antagonists enhance cholinergic transmission which can be blocked by muscarinic antagonists [86].

5-HT$_7$ receptor

5-HT$_7$ receptors were also originally detected by gene cloning. They are abundant in the medial thalamic nuclei, the molecular layer of the dentate gyrus, in the entorhinal cortex and cortical layers II-IV and in the amygdala. They occur at moderate density in the hippocampus (CA1, CA2, CA3), septum, hypothalamic nuclei, claustrum, ventral pallidum, globus pallidus, superior collicus, substantia nigra reticulata, dorsal raphe nucleus and locus coeruleus [88].

Some antipsychotics have high affinity for 5-HT$_7$ receptors: risperidone, 9-OH-risperidone, ziprasidone, or moderate affinity: sertindole, zotepine, clozapine, olanzapine. More selective 5-HT$_7$ antagonists are getting under way [89].

5-HT$_7$ receptors appear to be prone to downregulation: hypothalamic 5-HT$_7$ receptor binding sites are reduced following 21 days treatment with the 5-HT reuptake blocker, fluoxetine.

5-HT$_7$ receptors probably mediate 5-HT induced phase shifting in the circadian rhythm of melatonin secretion (a 5-HT agonist effect mimicking the effect of light).

The significance of 5-HT$_7$ receptor blockade with regard to antipsychotic drug action remains to be elucidated (for review see [90, 91]).

Neurotransmitter receptor binding profile *in vitro* of antipsychotics

Chemical structures of the antipsychotics discussed in this paper are shown in Figure 1: haloperidol and pipamperone are butyrophenones; risperidone and 9-OH-risperidone are benzisoxazoles; sertindole is an indole and ziprasidone a benzthiazole; clozapine, olanzapine, quetiapine and zotepine are tricyclic agents (6,7,6 or 6,7,5-membered rings).

The receptor binding affinity of the compounds for neurotransmitter receptor subtypes was assessed in competition binding assays with radioligands. The receptors, employed tissues and radioligands are listed in Table 1. Further details on methodology and assay conditions are reported in Schotte et al. [32] and Leysen et al. [92]. The binding affinities of the drugs in Table 3 are expressed as pK_i-values ($-\log K_i$, the K_i-value, apparent equilibrium dissociation constant, reflects the concentration of the drug which produces half maximal receptor occupancy).

To facilitate a comparison between the drugs, we show in Table 2 a ranking of the compounds according to decreasing binding affinity for D_2 receptors and for each drug we have ranked the receptors for which the drug shows higher or equal affinity as compared to its D_2 affinity. The table also contains the dose range at which the drugs were reported to be efficacious for treating symptoms of schizophrenia including positive and negative ones in case of the new compounds (see [6]).

Table 3. Binding affinity (K_i, nM) of compounds for cloned human muscarinic receptor subtypes expressed in cells. Data from Bolden [93] and Bymaster [25]

	m_1		m_2		m_3		m_4*		m_5
	ref Bo [93]	ref By [25]	ref Bo [93]	ref By [25]	ref Bo [93]	ref By [25]	ref Bo [93]	ref By [25]	ref Bo [93]
Clozapine	3.1	1.4	48	7	20	6	11	5	11.2
Olanzapine		2.5		13		10		6	
Zotepine	18		140		73		77		260
Quetiapine		135		705		225		2990	
Risperidone	⋙	⋙	⋙	⋙	⋙	⋙	⋙	⋙	⋙

⋙ No or very weak interaction.
* Agonistic activity at m_4 receptors was reported for clozapine EC_{50} 60 nM and olanzapine EC_{50} 1900 nM [94].

Although occupancy at a certain degree of D_2 receptors is thought to underlie the treatment of positive symptoms, for this series of compounds, the ratios in clinical dosages do not match the ratios in D_2 receptor affinity. The most conspicuous exceptions are zotepine and ziprasidone, which are used at very high dose. An explanation could be sought in unfavourable pharmacokinetics and metabolism but there may also be other reasons (see below). Tables 1 and 2 clearly illustrate the potency and selectivity of haloperidol for the D_2 receptor. In spite of its structural resemblance to haloperidol, pipamperone reveals an opposite profile. Risperidone, 9-OH-risperidone, ziprasidone, sertindole and zotepine bind quite potently to D_2-receptors. Quetiapine, appearing at the bottom of Table 2, is a very weak D_2 antagonist. All the new compounds show a higher $5\text{-}HT_{2A}$ than D_2 receptor affinity but the criterion of a ratio >10 is not met for zotepine, ziprasidone and quetiapine. Only risperidone, 9-OH-risperidone, sertindole and pipamperone bind primarily to $5\text{-}HT_{2A}$ receptors. As explained above, potent and primary $5\text{-}HT_{2A}$ receptor blockade probably confers the beneficial clinical properties to the drugs (treatment of negative symptoms, reduced risk to induce EPS).

All compounds, except haloperidol, bind to α_1 adrenoceptors with higher or equal potency as to D_2 receptors. It has been discussed that central α_1 receptor blockade may contribute to the antipsychotic activity and even may result in a more pronounced so-called limbic selectivity (see [34]). However α_1 receptor blockade also causes sedation, orthostatic hypotension, and reflex tachycardia. Another common property of all the new drugs (i.e. except haloperidol and pipamperone) is $5\text{-}HT_7$ receptor binding. One will have to await clinical studies with the upcoming selective agents [89] to unravel the significance of this property.

Risperidone and 9-OH-risperidone have almost the same receptor profile. All other compounds show different profiles. Clozapine remains the compound which hits most receptors (17) with more or equal potency compared to D_2 receptor binding. It is followed by quetiapine which binds to 13 receptors.

Olanzapine (hitting 11 receptors), although showing high structural resemblance to clozapine, differs from clozapine with regard to binding to particular receptors.

The tricyclics (zotepine, olanzapine, clozapine and quetiapine) have in common a primary H_1 receptor affinity. This may account for their severe sedative properties and for causing substantial weight gain. The potent $5\text{-}HT_{2C}$ receptor binding of zotepine, olanzapine and clozapine may in addition contribute to the weight gain. However $5\text{-}HT_{2C}$ receptor blockade (also a property of sertindole) may confer anxiolytic properties and may mitigate the rise in prolactin blood levels induced by D_2 blockade.

A further property of clozapine, olanzapine, zotepine and quetiapine is interaction with muscarinic acetylcholine receptors. Table 3 shows data reported in the literature for interaction with the cloned human m_1, m_2, m_3,

m_4 and m_5 receptor subtypes expressed in cells [25, 93]. Clozapine and olanzapine interact quite potently (nM affinity) with all subtypes. However, a marked difference between the compounds was reported for their action at m_4 receptors. In signal transduction assays clozapine was shown to be a strong agonist (inhibition of cAMP formation, EC_{50} 60 nM) whereas olanzapine was a weak agonist (EC_{50} 1900 nM) [94].

The agonistic effect of clozapine at m_4 receptors has been related to its strong hypersalivation effect, although other studies indicate that m_3 receptors mediate glandular secretion. The compounds are antagonists at m_1 receptors which are prevalent in the brain. This may counteract EPS but may impair cognition and cause confusion and pharmacogenic delirium. Also urinary incontinence, constipation and dry mouth are known side effects of muscarinic acetylcholine receptor blockade.

Further, exceptional properties of clozapine are 5-HT_3 receptor and histamine H_3 receptor blockade ($pK_i = 6.15$, [95]).

It is worth noting that risperidone, 9-OH-risperidone and clozapine bind with relatively high affinity to α_2-adrenoceptor subtypes. Blockade of the α_{2A}-subtype presumably will disinhibit adrenergic transmission and enhance release of various other neurotransmitters which may contribute to enhanced cognition and antidepressant effects. Peripheral α_2-adrenoceptor blockade can increase cardiac output.

In vivo receptor occupancy and pharmacological effects

In rats, antipsychotics produce various effects related to their dopamine antagonist property. In Figure 2, doses of the compounds are indicated which produce inhibition and complete blockade of amphetamine-induced agitation and which produce catalepsy. Haloperidol is the most potent compound, producing inhibition of amphetamine agitation at 0.018 mg/kg s.c. Risperidone is three times less potent, zotepine 16 times less, olanzapine 19 times less, sertindole 28 times less, and clozapine and quetiapine are 120 times less potent than haloperidol. The ratio between dosages for inhibition and blockade of amphetamine effects differ amongst the compounds. For example the dose ratio for haloperidol and zotepine is 2, for olanzapine it is 3, for risperidone, clozapine and quetiapine 5, and for sertindole 10. At high dose, the compounds produce catalepsy. The ratio between the dose to elicit the mild dopamine antagonistic effect (inhibition of amphetamine effects) and the dose for producing catalepsy, is again different for the compounds respectively. The ratio for haloperidol is 7, for clozapine 13, for olanzapine 31, for risperidone and zotepine 50, for sertindole and quetiapine it is 80. A relatively low potency for inducing catalepsy, may be predictive for a low propensity to induce EPS.

Using *ex vivo* quantitative receptor autoradiography in brain slices of rats treated with increasing dosages of antipsychotics, we investigated the

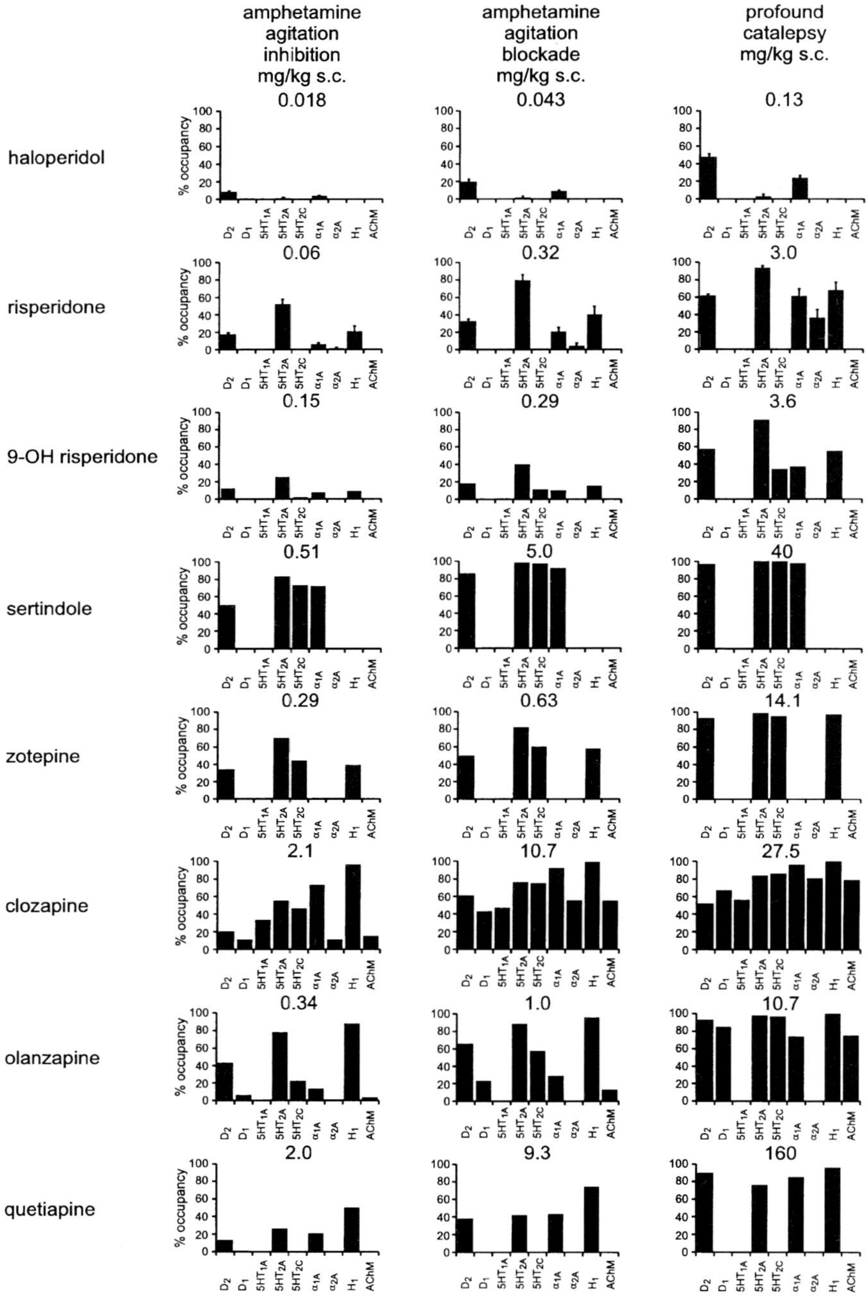
amphetamine agitation inhibition mg/kg s.c.
amphetamine agitation blockade mg/kg s.c.
profound catalepsy mg/kg s.c.
haloperidol
0.018
0.043
0.13
risperidone
0.06
0.32
3.0
9-OH risperidone
0.15
0.29
3.6
sertindole
0.51
5.0
40
zotepine
0.29
0.63
14.1
clozapine
2.1
10.7
27.5
olanzapine
0.34
1.0
10.7
quetiapine
2.0
9.3
160
% occupancy
0
20
40
60
80
100
D2
D1
5HT1A
5HT2A
5HT2C
α1A
α2A
H1
AChM

occupancy by the compounds of various receptors in various brain areas [2, 32]. The degree of occupancy of various receptors hit by the drugs, at dosages at which dopamine antagonistic behaviour was seen, was analysed [2, 3]. The profiles of receptor occupancy, taken from these studies, are shown in Figure 2. The dopamine receptor occupancy, at inhibition and blockade of amphetamine effects, was for haloperidol only 8 and 20%, for risperidone it was 16 and 32%, for clozapine 20 and 61%, for olanzapine 43 and 66% and for sertindole 50 and 86%, respectively. At the dose for producing catalepsy, D_2 receptor occupancy exceeded 50% and reached 100% for certain drugs (see Fig. 2). These pharmacological data illustrate that a particular dopamine antagonistic effect can be obtained at a particular degree of receptor occupancy and that this differs amongst the drugs. For example, for haloperidol effects are seen at very low D_2 receptor occupancy – hence careful dosing is mandatory. For sertindole a very high D_2 receptor occupancy is required to obtain similar behavioural effects. Sertindole binds relatively potently to D_2 receptors (see Table 1), but seems not to block the receptor effectively. We could recently corroborate this in *in vitro* studies measuring D_2 receptor mediated inhibition of cAMP production. Here also sertindole was a 130 times less potent antagonist as compared to its D_2 receptor binding affinity (Vanhauwe, unpublished observations).

The study illustrated in Figure 2 shows that at the dose for producing mild dopamine antagonistic effects, various other receptors are occupied to different degrees by the different compounds. Considering that a particular degree of D_2 receptor occupancy is required for treating positive symptoms, the degree of occupancy of other receptors will contribute to further therapeutic effects or may cause side-effects. Haloperidol, at low dose, occupies a minor part of D_2 receptors only. Risperidone, at the dose for amphetamine inhibition, produces a three times higher $5\text{-}HT_{2A}$ than D_2 receptor occupancy – other receptors are less occupied than the D_2 receptor. The high $5\text{-}HT_{2A}$ receptor occupancy at relatively low D_2 receptor occupancy, is beneficial for treating negative symptoms. At higher dosages, risperidone also occupies central α_1-and α_2-adrenoceptors and H_1 recep-

Figure 2. Brain receptor occupancy at doses producing behavioural effects in rats related to dopamine antagonism: inhibition of amphetamine agitation, complete suppression (blockade) of amphetamine agitation, profound catalepsy. Amphetamine (2.5 mg/kg, s.c.)-induced agitation was scored each quarter of an hour, starting 15 min after challenge. Scores were cumulated over the 1 h time interval. Criterion for inhibition: score < 11; for blockade: score < 5. Catalepsy was scored (0, 1, 2, 3) each hour of an 8 h observation by two independent trained observers. Criterion for catalepsy: total score of 6. Receptor occupancy was measured *ex vivo* in rat brain slices using quantitative receptor autoradiography [2, 32]. The respective receptors were measured in the following brain areas: D_2 and D_1: nucleus caudatus/putamen; $5\text{-}HT_{1A}$: hippocampus; $5\text{-}HT_{2A}$: frontal cortex; $5\text{-}HT_{2C}$: choroid plexus; α_1-adrenergic: thalamus; α_2-adrenergic: entorhinal cortex; acetylcholine muscarinic (AChM): nucleus caudatus/putamen; H_1: guinea pig cerebellum.

tors, although it should be noted that the affinity of risperidone for animal H_1 receptors is 10 times higher than its affinity for cloned human H_1 receptors [32], indicating species differences in H_1 receptor pharmacology.

Clozapine, at the dose for amphetamine inhibition produces complete H_1 receptor occupancy (tricyclics show similar affinity for human and animal H_1 receptors) and very high occupancy of α_1-adrenoceptors, 5-HT_{2A}, 5-HT_{2C} and 5-HT_{1A} receptors. Clozapine occupies muscarinic acetylcholine receptors to the same extent as D_2 receptors. At higher dosages, it also occupies D_1 receptors and α_2-adrenoceptors. Olanzapine produces high degrees of H_1, 5-HT_{2A} and 5-HT_{2C} receptor occupancy, and at higher dosages it occupies α_1-adrenoceptors, D_1 and muscarinic acetylcholine receptors. Sertindole, requiring high D_2 receptor occupancy for behavioural effects, occupies similarly high proportions of 5-HT_{2A}, 5-HT_{2C} and α_1-adrenoceptors.

Figure 2 also shows the receptor occupancy profile of 9-OH-risperidone (which is very similar to that of risperidone) and of zotepine and quetiapine. Ziprasidone and pipamperone are both very short acting compounds in the rat, which hampers the *ex vivo* study of receptor occupancy.

Conclusions

The most important message which can be inferred from the data reviewed is that the profiles and potencies of all the antipsychotics are different. Risperidone, ziprasidone and sertindole bind with relatively high potency to six to eight neurotransmitter receptors, the tricyclic compounds bind to 10 to 17 (clozapine) receptors. The ideal receptor occupancy profile is not known. However, it would seem clear that predominant 5-HT_{2A} antagonism and weaker D_2 antagonism is highly desirable for the simultaneous treatment of negative and positive symptoms with reduced EPS liability.

Risperidone and 9-OH-risperidone and sertindole score favourably in this respect. Sertindole is unusual because of its apparent ineffectiveness at D_2 receptor blockade. All compounds block α_1 adrenoceptors with relatively high potency, probably contributing to the antipsychotic activity, but also producing central and peripheral side-effects. Primary blockade of H_1 receptors will often be a drawback because of risk of sedation and weight increase. The tricyclics clozapine, olanzapine, zotepine and quetiapine score unfavourably in this respect. Muscarinic acetylcholine receptor blockade, which can become prominent for clozapine, olanzapine and quetiapine is highly unwanted in view of detrimental side-effects. Several of the compounds interact with 5-HT_{2C} receptors, which may confer anxiolytic activity, and reduce prolactin elevation but contribute to weight gain. All the new compounds interact with 5-HT_7 receptors and several bind to 5-HT_6 receptors but the roles of these and several other receptors remain to be elucidated.

References

1 Davis KL, Kahn RS, Ko G, Davidson M (1991) Dopamine in schizophrenia: a review and reconceptualization. *Am J Psychiatry* 148: 1474–1486

2 Leysen JE, Janssen PMF, Schotte A, Luyten WHML, Megens AAHP (1993) Interaction of antipsychotic drugs with neurotransmitter receptor sites *in vitro* and *in vivo* in relation to pharmacological and clinical effects: role of $5HT_2$ receptors. *Psychopharmacology* 112: S40–S54

3 Leysen JE, Janssen PMF, Heylen L, Gommeren W, Van Gompel P, Lesage AS, Megens AAHP, Schotte A (1998) Receptor interactions of new antipsychotics: relation to pharmacodynamic and clinical effects. *Int J Psychiatry Clin Pract* 2: S3–S18

4 Carlsson A, Hansson LO, Waters N, Carlsson ML (1997) Neurotransmitter aberrations in schizophrenia: new perspectives and therapeutic implications. *Life Sci* 61: 75–94

5 Carpenter WT (1995) Serotonin-dopamine antagonists and treatment of negative symptoms. *Clin Psychopharmacol* 16 (suppl 1): 30S–35S

6 King DJ (1998) Drug treatment of the negative symptoms of schizophrenia. *Eur Neuropsychopharmacol* 8: 33–42

7 Leysen JE, Niemegeers (1985) Neuroleptics. In: A Lajtha (ed): *Handbook of neurochemistry*, Plenum Publishing Corporation 9: 331–361

8 Seeman P, Lee T (1975) Antipsychotic drugs: direct correlation between clinical potency and presynaptic action on dopamine neurons. *Sci* 188: 1217–1219

9 Leysen JE, Niemegeers CJE, Tollenaere JP, Laduron PM (1978) Serotonergic component of neuroleptic receptors. *Nature* 272: 168–171

10 Leysen JE, Gommeren W, Van Gompel P, Wynants J, Janssen PFM, Laduron PM (1985) Receptor binding properties *in vitro* and *in vivo* of ritanserin: A very potent and long acting serotonin-S_2 antagonist. *Mol Pharmacol* 27: 600–611

11 Reyntjens A, Gelders YG, Hoppenbrouwers M-LJA, Vanden Bussche G (1986) Thymostenic effects of ritanserin (R55667), a centrally acting serotonin-S_2 receptor blocker. *Drug Dev Res* 8: 205–211

12 Bersani G, Grispini A, Marini S, Pasini A, Valducci M, Ciani N (1990) $5HT_2$ antagonist ritanserin in neuroleptic-induced Parkinsonism: a double-blind comparison with orphenadrine and placebo. *Clin Neuropharmacol* 13: 500–506

13 Duinkerke SJ, Botter PA, Jansen AAI, Van Dongen PA, Van Haaften AJ, Boom AJ, Van Laarhoven JH, Busard HL (1993) Ritanserin, a selective 5-$HT_{2A/2C}$ antagonist, and negative symptoms in schizophrenia: a placebo-controlled double-blind trial. *Br J Psychiatry* 163: 451–455

14 Coward DM, Imperato A, Urwyler S, White TG (1989) Biochemical and behavioural properties of clozapine. *Psychopharmacology* 99 (suppl): 6–12

15 Fitton A, Heel RC (1990) Clozapine. A review of its pharmacological properties, and therapeutic use in schizophrenia. *Drugs* 40: 722–747

16 Lindstrom LH (1989) A retrospective study on the long-term efficacy of clozapine in 96 schizophrenic and schizoaffective patients during a 13-year period. *Psychopharmacology* 99 (suppl): 84–86

17 Melzer HY, Nash JF (1991) Effects of antipsychotic drugs on serotonin receptors. *Pharmacol Rev* 43: 587–604

18 Janssen PAJ, Niemegeers CJE, Awouters F, Schellekens KH, Megens AA, Meert TF (1988) Pharmacology of risperidone (R64766), a new antipsychotic with serotonin-S_2 and dopamine-D_2 antagonistic properties. *J Pharmacol Exp Ther* 244: 685–693

19 Leysen JE, Gommeren W, Eens A, De Chaffoy de Courcelles D, Stoof JC, Janssen PAJ (1988) The biochemical profile of risperidone, a new antipsychotic. *J Pharmacol Exp Ther* 247: 661–670

20 Leysen JE, Janssen PMF, Gommeren W, Wynants J, Pauwels PJ, Janssen PAJ (1991) *In vitro* and *in vivo* receptor binding and effects on monoamine turnover in rat brain regions of the novel antipsychotics, risperidone and ocaperidone. *Mol Pharmacol* 41: 494–508

21 Megens AAHP, Awouters FHL, Schotte A, Meert TF, Dugovic C, Niemegeers CJE, Leysen JE (1994) Survey on the pharmacodynamics of the new antipsychotic risperidone. *Psychopharmacology* 114: 9–23

22 Davis JM, Janicak PG. (1996) Risperidone: a new, novel (and better?) antipsychotic. *Psychiatr Ann* 26: 78–87

23 Jones H (1997) Risperidone: A review of its pharmacology and use in the treatment of schizophrenia. *J Serotonin Res* 4: 17–28
24 Moore NA, Tye NC, Axton MS, Risius FC (1992) The behavioral pharmacology of olanzapine, a novel "atypical" antipsychotic agent. *J Pharmacol Exp Ther* 262: 545–551
25 Bymaster FP, Calligaro DO, Falcone JF, Marsh RD, Moore NA, Tye NC, Seeman P, Wong DT (1996) Radioreceptor binding profile of the atypical antipsychotic olanzapine. *Neuropsychopharmacol* 14: 87–96
26 Fulton B, Goa KL (1997) Olanzapine. A review of its pharmacological properties and therapeutic efficacy in the management of schizophrenia and related psychoses. *Drugs* 53: 281–298
27 Saller CF, Salama AI (1993) Seroquel: biochemical profile of a potential atypical antipsychotic. *Psychopharmacology* 112: 285–292
28 Migler BM, Warawa EJ, Malick JB (1993) Seroquel: behavioral effects in conventional and novel tests for atypical antipsychotic drug. *Psychopharmacology* 112: 299–307
29 Needham PL, Atkinson J, Skill MJ, Heal DJ (1996) Zotepine: preclinical tests predict antipsychotic efficacy and an atypical profile. *Psychopharmacol Bull* 32: 123–128
30 Hyttel J, Arnt J, Costall B, Domeney A, Dragsted N, Lembol HL, Meier E, Naylor RJ, Nowak G, Sanchez C et al. (1992) Pharmacological profile of the atypical neuroleptic sertindole. *Clin Neuropharmacol* 15 (suppl 1 Pt A): 267A–268A
31 Seeger TF, Seymour PA, Schmidt AW, Zorn SH, Schulz DW, Lebel LA, McLean S, Guanowsky V, Howard HR, Lowe JA 3rd et al. (1995) Ziprasidone (CP-88,059): a new antipsychotic with combined dopamine and serotonin receptor antagonist activity. *J Pharmacol Exp Ther* 275: 101–113
32 Schotte A, Janssen PFM, Gommeren W, Luyten WH, Van Gompel P, Lesage AS, De Loore K, Leysen JE (1996) Risperidone compared with new and reference antipsychotic drugs: *in vitro* and *in vivo* receptor binding. *Psychopharmacology* 124: 57–73
33 Richelson E (1996) Preclinical pharmacology of neuroleptics: focus on new generation compounds. *J Clin Psychiatry* 57 (suppl 11): 4–11
34 Arnt J, Skarsfeldt T (1998) Do novel antipsychotics have similar pharmacological characteristics ? A review of the evidence. *Neuropsychopharmacol* 18: 63–101
35 Seeman P (1995) Dopamine receptors and psychosis. *Sci Am* 273: 28–37
36 Baldessarini RJ, Tarazi FI (1996) Brain dopamine receptors: a primer on their current status, basic and clinical. *Harvard Rev Psychiatry* 3: 301–325
37 Bergson C, Mrzljak L, Smiley JF, Pappy M, Levenson R, Goldman-Rakic PS (1995) Regional, cellular and subcellular variations in the distribution of D_1 and D_5 dopamine receptors in primate brain. *J Neurosci* 15: 7821–7836
38 Apostolakis EM, Garai J, Fox C, Smith CL, Watson SJ, Clark JH, O'Malley BW (1996) Dopaminergic regulation of progesterone receptors: brain D_5 dopamine receptors mediate induction of lordosis by D_1-like agonists in rats. *J Neurosci* 16: 4823–4834
39 Goldman-Rakic PS (1995) Psychopathology and neuropathology of prefrontal cortex in schizophrenia. In: Fog R, Gerlach J, Hemmingsen R (eds): *Alfred Benzon Symposium 38: Schizophrenia, an integrated view*. Munksgaard, Copenhagen, 126–136
40 Williams GV, Goldman-Rakic PS (1995) Modulation of memory fields by dopamine D_1 receptors in prefrontal cortex. *Nature* 376: 572–575
41 Karlsson P, Smith L, Farde L, Harwyd C, Sedvall G, Wiesel FA (1995) Lack of apparent antipsychotic effect of the D_1-dopamine receptor antagonist SCH39166 in acutely ill schizophrenic patients. *Psychopharmacology* 121: 309–316
42 Nyberg S, Nakashima Y, Nordström AL, Halldin C, Farde L (1996) Positron emission tomography of *in-vivo* binding characteristics of atypical antipsychotic drugs. Review of D_2 and 5-HT_2 receptor occupancy studies and clinical response. *Br J Psychiatry* 168 (suppl 29): 40–44
43 Farde L, Halldin C (1995) D_2-dopamine receptors in schizophrenia. In: Fog R, Gerlach J, Hemmingsen R (eds): *Alfred Benzon Symposium 38: Schizophrenia, an integrated view.* Munksgaard, Copenhagen, 190–199
44 Leysen JE, Gommeren W, Mertens J, Luyten WHML, Pauwels PJ, Ewert M, Seeburg P (1993) Comparison of *in vitro* binding properties of a series of dopamine antagonists and agonists for cloned human dopamine D_{2S} and D_{2L} receptors and for D_2 receptors in rat striatal and mesolimbic tissues, using $[^{125}I]2'$-iodospiperone. *Psychopharmacology* 110: 27–36

45 Schotte A, Janssen PFM, Bonaventure P, Leysen JE (1996) Endogenous dopamine limits the binding of anti-psychotic drugs to D_3 receptors in the rat brain – A quantitative autoradiographic study. *Histochem J* 28: 791–799
46 Lahti AC, Albert PK, Warfel DT, Lahti RA, Tamminga CA (1995) Novel antidopaminergic strategies for the treatment of schizophrenia. *Schizophr Res* 15: 157
47 Lathi RA, Evans DL, Stratman NC, Figur LM (1993) Dopamine D_4 versus D_2 receptor selectivity of dopamine receptor antagonists: possible therapeutic implications. *Eur J Pharmacol* 236: 483–486
48 Roth BL, Tandra S, Burgess LH, Sibley DR, Meltzer HY (1995) D-4 Dopamine receptor binding affinity does not distinguish between typical and atypical antipsychotic drugs. *Psychopharmacology* 120: 365–368
49 Sanyal S, Van Tol HH (1997) Review the role of dopamine D_4 receptors in schizophrenia and antipsychotic action. *J Psychiatr Res* 31: 219–232
50 Bristow LJ, Kramer MS, Kulagowski J, Patel S, Ragan CI, Seabrook GR (1997) Schizophrenia and L-745,870, a novel dopamine D_4 receptor antagonist. *Trends Pharmacol Sci* 18: 186–188
51 Reynolds GP (1996) The importance of dopamine D_4 receptors in the action and development of antipsychotic agents. *Drugs* 51: 7–11
52 Patel S, Patel S, Marwood R, Emms F, Marston D, Leeson PD, Curtis NR, Kulagowski JJ, Freedman SB (1996) Identification and pharmacological characterization of [^{125}I]L-750, 667, a novel radioligand for the dopamine D_4 receptor. *Mol Pharmacol* 50: 1658–1664
53 Lahti RA, Roberts RC, Cochrane EV, Primus RJ, Gallager DW, Tamminga CA (1998) Dopamine D_4 receptors in human postmortem brain tissue of normal and schizophrenic subjects. An [^{3}] NGD-94-1 study. *Schizophr Res* 29: 93
54 Mrzljak L, Bergson C, Pappy M, Huff R, Levenson R, Goldman-Rakic PS (1996) Localization of dopamine D_4 receptors in GABAergic neurons of the primate brain. *Nature* 381: 245–248
55 Francken BJB, Jurzak M, Vanhauwe JFM, Luyten WHML, Leysen JE (1998) The human 5-HT_{5A} receptor couples to G_i/g_o proteins and inhibits adenylate cyclase in HEK 293 cells. *Europ J Pharmacol* 361: 299–309
56 Hoyer D, Clarke DE, Fozard JR, Hartig PR, Martin GR, Mylecharane EJ, Saxena PR, Humphrey PP (1994) International Union of Pharmacology classification of receptors for 5-hydroxytryptamine (serotonin). *Pharmacol Rev* 46: 157–203
57 Hoyer D, Martin GR (1996) Classification and nomenclature of 5-HT receptors: a comment on current issues. *Behav Brain Res* 73: 263–268
58 Schmidt CJ, Sorensen SM, Kehne JH, Carr AA, Palfreyman MG (1995) The role of 5-HT_{2A} receptors in antipsychotic activity. *Life Sci* 56: 2209–2222
59 Wainscott DB, Lucaites VL, Kursar JD, Baez M, Nelson DL (1996) Pharmacologic characterization of the human 5-hydroxytryptamine$_{2B}$ receptor: evidence for species differences. *J Pharmacol Exp Ther* 276: 720–727
60 Pazos A, Cortés R, Palacios JM (1985) Quantitative autoradiographic mapping of serotonin receptors in the rat brain. II. Serotonin-2 receptors. *Brain Res* 346: 231–249
61 Mengod G, Pompeiano M, Martínez-Mir MI, Palacios JM (1990) Localization of the mRNA for the 5-HT_2 receptor by *in situ* hybridization histochemistry. Correlation with the distribution of receptor sites. *Brain Res* 524: 139–143
62 Ward RP, Dorsa DM (1996) Colocalization of serotonin receptor subtypes 5-HT_{2A}, 5-HT_{2C}, and 5-HT_6 with neuropeptides in rat striatum. *J Comp Neurol* 370: 405–414
63 Morilak DA, Garlow SJ, Ciaranello RD (1993) Immunocytochemical localization and description of neurons expressing serotonin$_2$ receptors in the rat brain. *Neuroscience* 54: 701–717
64 Morilak DA, Ciaranello RD (1993) 5-HT_2 receptor immunoreactivity on cholinergic neurons of the pontomesencephalic tegmentum shown by double immunofluorescence. *Brain Res* 627: 49–54
65 Hamada S, Senzaki K, Hamaguchi-Hamada K, Tabuchi K, Yamamoto H, Yamamoto T, Yoshikawa S, Okano H, Okado N (1998) Localization of 5-HT_{2A} receptor in rat cerebral cortex and olfactory system revealed by immunohistochemistry using two antibodies raised in rabbit and chicken. *Mol Brain Res* 54: 199–211
66 Jakab RL, Goldman-Rakic P (1998) 5-hydroxyhyptamine 2A serotonin receptors in the primate cerebral cortex: possible site of action of hallucinogenic and antipsychotic drugs in pyramidal cell apical dentrites. *Proc Natl Acad Science USA* 95: 735–740

67 Aghajanian G, Marek GJ (1997) Serotonin induces excitatory postsynaptic potentials in apical dentrites of neocortical pyramidal cells. *Neuropharmacology* 36: 589–599
68 Marek GJ, Aghajanian GK (1996) LSD and the phenethylamine hallucinogen DOI are potent partial agonists at 5-HT_{2A} receptors on interneurons in rat piriform cortex. *J Pharmacol Exp Ther* 278: 1373–1382
69 Sorensen SM, Kehne JH, Fadayel GM, Humphreys TM, Ketteler HJ, Sullivan CK, Taylor VL, Schmidt CJ (1993) Characterization of the 5-HT_2 receptor antagonist MDL 100907 as a putative atypical antipsychotic: behavioral, electrophysiological and neurochemical studies. *J Pharmacol Exp Ther* 266: 684–691
70 Fiorella D, Rabin RA, Winter JC (1995) The role of the 5-HT_{2A} and 5-HT_{2C} receptors in the stimulus effects of hallucinogenic drugs. I: Antagonist correlation analysis. *Psychopharmacology* 121: 347–356
71 Stefanski R, Goldberg SR (1997) Serotonin 5-HT_2 receptor antagonists. Potential in the treatment of psychiatric disorders. *CNS Drugs* 7: 388–409
72 Dugovic C, Wauquier A, Janssen PA (1989) Differential effects of the new antipsychotic risperidone on sleep and wakefulness in the rat. *Neuropharmacology* 28: 1431–1433
73 Gallhofer B, Bauer U, Lis S, Krieger S, Gruppe H (1996) Cognitive dysfunction in schizophrenia: comparison of treatment with atypical antipsychotic agents and conventional neuroleptic drugs. *Eur Neuropsychopharmacol* 6: S2-13–S2-20
74 Gellman RL, Aghajanian GK (1994) Serotonin2 receptor-mediated excitation of interneurons in piriform cortex: antagonism by atypical antipsychotic drugs. *Neuroscience* 58: 515–525
75 Ashby CR Jr, Edwards E, Wang RY (1994) Electrophysiological evidence for a functional interaction between 5-HT_{1A} and 5-HT_{2A} receptors in the rat medial prefrontal cortex: an iontophoretic study. *Synapse* 17: 173–181
76 Svensson TH, Nomikos GG, Andersson JL (1993) Modulation of dopaminergic neurotransmission by 5HT_2 antagonism. In: Vanhoutte PM, Saxena PR, Paoletti R, Brunello N (eds): *Serotonin, from cell biology to pharmacology and therapeutics.* Kluwer, Dordrecht, The Netherlands, 263–270
77 Svensson TH, Tung CS (1989) Local cooling of prefrontal cortex induces pacemaker-like firing of dopamine neurons in rat ventral tegmental area *in vivo*. *Acta Physiol Scand* 136: 135–136
78 Ugedo L, Grenhoff J, Svensson TM (1989) Ritanserin, a 5HT_2 antagonist, activates midbrain dopamine neurons by blocking serotonergic inhibition. *Psychopharmacology* 98: 45–50
79 Svensson TH, Mathé JM, Andersson JL, Nomikos GG, Hildebrand BE, Marcus M (1995) Mode of action of atypical neuroleptics in relation to the phencyclidine model of schizophrenia: role of 5-HT_2 receptor and α_1-adrenoreceptor antagonism. *J Clin Psychopharmacol* 15: 11S–18S
80 Pehek EA (1996) Local infusion of the serotonin antagonist ritanserin or ICS205930 increases *in vivo* dopamine release in the rat medial prefrontal cortex. *Synapse* 24: 12–19
81 Abramowski D, Rigo M, Duc D, Hoyer D, Staufenbiel M (1995) Localization of the 5-hydroxytryptamine 2C receptor protein in human and rat brain using specific antisera. *Neuropharmacology* 34: 1635–1645
82 Bromidge SM, Duckworth M, Forbes IT, Ham P, King FD, Thewlis KM, Blaney FE, Naylor CB, Blackburn TP, Kennett GA et al. (1997) 6-Chloro-5-methyl-1-[[2-[(2-methyl-3-pyridyl)-oxy]-5-pyridyl]carbamoyl]-indoline (SB-242084): the first selective and brain penetrant 5-HT_{2C} receptor antagonist. *J Med Chem* 40: 3494–3496
83 Tecott LH, Sun LM, Akana SF, Strack AM, Lowenstein DH, Dallman MF, Julius D (1996) Eating disorder and epilepsy in mice lacking 5-HT_{2C} serotonin receptors. *Nature* 374: 542–546
84 Coccaro EF, Kavoussi RJ, Oakes M, Cooper TB, Hauger R (1996) 5-$HT_{2A/2C}$ receptor blockade by amesergide fully attenuates prolactin response to *d*-fenfluramine challenge in physically healthy human subjects. *Psychopharmacology* 126: 24–30
85 Gerard C, Martres MP, Lefevre K, Miquel MC, Verge D, Lanfumey L, Doucet E, Hamon M, El Mestikawy S (1997) Immuno-localization of serotonin 5-HT_6 receptor-like material in the rat central nervous system. *Brain Res* 746: 207–219
86 Sleight AJ, Boess FG, Bos M, Levettrafit B, Riemer C, Bourson A (1998) Characterization of Ro 04-6790 and Ro 63-0563 – potent and selective antagonists at human and rat 5-HT_6 receptors. *Br J Pharmacol* 124 (3): 556–562

87 Bourson A, Borroni E, Austin RH, Monsma FJ Jr, Sleight AJ (1995) Determination of the role of the 5-HT_6 receptor in the rat brain: a study using antisense oligonucleotides. *J Pharmacol Exp Ther* 274: 173–180

88 To ZP, Bonhaus DW, Eglen RM, Jakeman LB (1995) Characterization and distribution of putative 5-HT_7 receptors in guinea-pig brain. *Br J Pharmacol* 115: 107–116

89 Forbes IT, Dabbs S, Duckworth DM, Jennings AJ, King FD, Lovell PJ, Brown AM, Collin L, Hagan JJ, Middlemiss DN, et al. (1998) (R1-3,N-dimethyl-N-[1-methyl-piperidinin-1-yl)propyl] benzene sulfonamide: the first selective 5-HT_7 receptor antagonist. *J Med Chem* 41: 655–657

90 Sleight AJ, Boess FG, Bourson A, Sibley DR, Monsma FJ Jr (1997) 5-HT_6 and 5-HT_7 receptors: molecular biology, functional correlates and possible therapeutic indications. *DN and P* 10: 214–224

91 Eglen RM, Jasper JR, Chang DJ, Martin GR (1997) The 5-HT_7 receptor: orphan found. *Trends Pharmacol Sci* 18: 104–107

92 Leysen JE, Gommeren W, Heylen L, Luyten WHML, Van de Weyer I, Vanhoenacker P, Haegeman G, Schotte A, Van Gompel P, Wouters R et al. (1996) Alniditan, a new 5-hydroxytryptamine$_{1D}$ agonist and migraine-abortive agent: ligand-binding properties of human 5-hydroxytryptamine$_{1D\alpha}$, human 5-hydroxytryptamine$_{1D\beta}$, and calf 5-hydroxytryptamine$_{1D}$ receptors investigated with [^{3}H]5-hydroxytryptamine and [^{3}H]alniditan. *Mol Pharmacol* 50: 1567–1580

93 Bolden C, Cusack B, Richelson E (1991) Antagonism by antimuscarinic and neuroleptic compounds at the five cloned human muscarinic cholinergic receptors expressed in Chinese hamster ovary cells. *J Pharmacol Exp Ther* 260: 576–580

94 Zeng XP, Le F, Richelson E (1997) Muscarinic m4 receptor activation by some atypical antipsychotic drugs. *Eur J Pharmacol* 321: 349–354

95 Schlicker E, Marr I (1996) The moderate affinity of clozapine at H_3 receptors is not shared by its two major metabolites and by structurally related and unrelated atypical neuroleptics. *Naunyn Schmiedebergs Arch Pharmacol* 353: 290–294

Atypical Antipsychotics
ed. by B.A. Ellenbroek and A.R. Cools

Regional selectivity of antipsychotic drugs

Bart A. Ellenbroek and Alexander R. Cools

Department of Psychoneuropharmacology, University of Nijmegen, P.O. Box 9101, 6500 HB Nijmegen, The Netherlands

Introduction

Antipsychotic drugs have been in clinical practice for more than 40 years, and it is now well established that at comparable levels of antipsychotic efficacy, the incidence of side-effects (especially the extrapyramidal side-effects) differs between individual drugs. This has already been known for a long time, but the earlier studies were largely overlooked. Among the earlier papers were a number of clinical studies comparing several phenothiazine antipsychotics, such as the large multicentre double blind study conducted by the National Institute of Mental Health in 1964 [1]. This study showed that in therapeutically equivalent doses, thioridazine produced significantly less rigidity and dystonia than chlorpromazine and fluphenazine. Comparable findings were also reported by other groups [2–4]. After the introduction of clozapine, it became even more apparent that antipsychotic drugs not necessarily had to induce extrapyramidal side-effects [5–8], see also Naber et al., this volume. This drugs seems to be almost completely free of extrapyramidal side-effects, including tardive dyskinesia.

Since the introduction of clozapine a large number of drugs have been reported (or claimed) to induce less extrapyramidal side-effects than conventional antipsychotics (see Meltzer; Stahl and Shayegan, this volume). These drugs have been generally referred to as atypical antipsychotics, as opposed to the classical antipsychotics. A closer look at these drugs shows, however, that there is not a clear division in two groups. For instance risperidone induces less extrapyramidal side-effects at doses ranging from 4–8 mg/day. If, however, the dose is increased to about 12–16 mg/day, the extrapyramidal side-effects profile is similar to that seen for haloperidol. On the other hand, quetiapine, like clozapine, seems to induce very little side-effects, even at very high doses (see Meltzer, this volume). It seems therefore more logical to regards the antipsychotics not as subdivided in two groups, but rather as one group on a large scale of extrapyramidal side-effects, ranging from severe (in the case of fluphenazine and haloperidol) through moderate (i.e. thioridazine and risperidone) to very little (i.e. clozapine and quetiapine).

Even if one accepts that atypical antipsychotics do not form one specific group, the question remains why some antipsychotics induced less extrapyramidal side-effects than others. Generally, two different groups of theories have been proposed to explain this: (1) *The receptor diversity theories*; (2) *The regional selectivity theories* [8]. The receptor diversity theories generally explains the differential extrapyramidal side-effects liability on the basis of differences in receptor binding profiles, whereas the regional selectivity theories explain the differences on the basis of differences in the neuronal substrates affected by antipsychotic drugs.

Two important points have to be made here. First, it seems impossible that one common mechanism can be deduced from the binding profile of antipsychotic drugs (see also Leysen, this volume). For instance, when looking at the binding profile of drugs such as remoxipride, amisulpiride or pimozide, it is clear that these drugs are highly selective for the dopamine receptor [9–11]. However, compared to pimozide, remoxipride and amisulpiride appear to induce significantly less extrapyramidal side-effects (see Den Boer and Korf, this volume).

Another important point to make is that both groups of theories are not mutually exclusive (see also [8]). Thus it may very well be that the differences in binding profile may determine differences in regional selectivity. In fact, it was suggested [9] that clozapine, through its muscarinic antagonistic properties might have less influence in the neostriatum, and therefore induce less extrapyramidal side-effects. The same reasoning has also been used to explain why antipsychotics with a strong serotonergic component produce less extrapyramidal side-effects than antipsychotics with a stronger dopaminergic component [13].

This offers the perspective that due to specific (but different) receptor interactions certain antipsychotics may influence certain brain structures more than others, and therefore induce more or less extrapyramidal side-effects. There is indeed a large body of evidence from electrophysiological, biochemical and functional studies which show that differences exist between different antipsychotic drugs. Moreover, some studies have pointed to regional differences in binding capacity. The remainder of this chapter will deal with these differences.

Binding studies

LeFur and his colleagues were probably the first to point to regional differences in binding of different antipsychotic drugs [14]. These authors compared the binding of chlorpromazine and clozapine to dopamine receptors in the neostriatum and the olfactory tubercle, using [^{3}H]-haloperidol and found that clozapine had a much stronger affinity for the receptors in the olfactory tubercle (K_i ratio of 5.3) whereas the reverse was true for chlorpromazine (K_i ratio of 0.3). This selectivity for dopamine receptors in the olfactory tubercle has since been replicated by two independent groups [15, 16].

A somewhat different approach was taken by Bischoff and his co-workers [17]. These authors studied the *in vivo* displacement of [^{3}H]spiperone binding to neostriatal and hippocampal tissue. They found that certain neuroleptics, like clozapine, fluperlapine, sulpiride and a new substance called savoxepine showed a considerably higher affinity for displacing spiperone from the hippocampus. They proposed that this might be a good model for differentiating classical from atypical neuroleptic drugs. However, thioridazine showed only a very weak preference (ratio of 4.5), whereas several other non atypical neuroleptics also had a preference for displacing spiperone from the hippocampus (ratios: butaclamol 7.1; domperidon 8.7). Moreover, it has been found that savoxepine induces extrapyramidal side-effects comparable to haloperidol [18].

Electrophysiological studies

In 1983, two independent publications appeared [19, 20] describing the effects of acute and subchronic administration of antipsychotic drugs on the neural activity of the dopaminergic cells within the substantia nigra pars compacta (the so-called A_9 cell group) and the ventral tegmental area (the so-called A_{10} cell group). Both groups found that subchronic (3 weeks) treatment with haloperidol or chlorpromazine reduced cell firing in both the A_9 and the A_{10} cell groups, whereas clozapine and thioridazine only reduce cell firing in the A_{10} cell group. These results have been replicated by a number of others [21, 22] and has led to a general hypothesis on the mechanism of action of antipsychotic drugs. [23]. According to this general theory, all antipsychotic drugs block dopamine receptors, which results in a feedback excitation of the dopaminergic A_{10} cells. In the case of classical antipsychotics this excitation is also seen in A_9 cells. This feedback excitation produces an increase in dopamine release, which successfully competes with the antipsychotic drugs for the dopamine receptor. Therefore, according to the theory, there is no effect of acute antipsychotic treatment. Upon repeated treatment, however, the cells in both A_9 and A_{10} are "*over-excited*" which leads to a phenomenon known as depolarisation inactivation. This is a poorly understood phenomenon of dopaminergic cells, whereby the resting potential is above the threshold for action potentials, but due to some unknown factor, the spike generation capacity is disturbed. Decreasing the resting membrane potential by, for instance, apomorphine or GABA, will paradoxically activate the cells. All antipsychotics induce depolarisation inactivation in the A_{10}, but only the classical antipsychotics lead to depolarisation inactivation in A_9. This has led to the speculation that the A_{10} cells (and their output stations) are responsible for the therapeutic effect, whereas the A_9 cells (and their output stations) are responsible for the extrapyramidal side-effects.

There are, however, a number of problems with this general hypothesis. First of all, a number of extrapyramidal side-effects, most notably dystonia and akathisia, can occur already after the first administration of an antipsychotic drug. Moreover, it has been found that only a few of the novel antipsychotics, with fewer extrapyramidal side-effects, indeed show a selectivity for reducing cell activity in the A_{10} [24], most notably sertindole (see Arnt, this volume). On the other hand, olanzapine, ziprasidone and quetiapine do not show a clear preference for the A_{10} cell group, although a recent paper did find a A_{10} selectivity for olanzapine [25]. Moreover, morphine, which has no antipsychotic potential, also induces depolarisation inactivation of the A_{10} cell group [26]. There is also a large body of biochemical data not supporting a regional selectivity (see below). This has led some authors to speculate that the observed depolarisation inactivation may be an artefact induced by the general anaesthetic [27]. It has been shown that the firing properties of dopaminergic cells are influenced by general anaesthetics [28]. Such anaesthesia may reduce the amount of burst-firing, which may affect overall dopaminergic cell activity, and in turn alter the effects of antipsychotics on cell firing. Indeed, Zhang et al. [29] found that chloral hydrate decreased basal dopamine release as well as that haloperidol induced increase in firing. Likewise, Mereu et al. [30] found that haloperidol failed to reduce basal firing in either A_9 or A_{10} cells in unanaesthetised rats. Whether the anaesthesia is able to completely explain the differences between the biochemical and electrophysiological results is unclear. However, a recent study provided further support for this idea [31]. The authors investigated the effects of haloperidol in chloral hydrate anaesthetised rats and in rats immobilised with either d-tubocurarine, gallamine or succinylcholine. The authors found that subchronic treatment with haloperidol indeed reduced the number of active cells within the A_{10} cell group, but failed to do so in any of the immobilised groups, thus providing strong support for the idea that depolarisation inactivation may be an artefact. In a follow-up paper it was found that clozapine increased the firing rate of the A_9 cells in the dorsal striatum in immobilised animals, but not in anaesthetised rats [32].

There is also evidence that other brain structures may be selectively influenced by clozapine (as the prototypical antipsychotic with low extrapyramidal side-effects liability). Thus Rebec and colleagues [33] found that clozapine significantly increased cell firing in the amygdala (predominantly within the central nucleus), whereas haloperidol had no effect. Likewise, clozapine could reverse the increase in amygdala firing after local infusion of amphetamine, whereas haloperidol was without effect [34]. Although this points to an involvement of the amygdala in the actions of clozapine, it is unclear whether this structure also plays a role on other novel antipsychotics.

Another structure which has received some attention recently is the substantia nigra pars reticulata (SNR), one of the major output stations of the dorsal striatum and critically involved in muscular rigidity and catalepsy [35, 36]. It was found that acute or chronic administration of the atypical antipsychotics risperidone, clozapine and olanzapine decreased activity in the SNR, whereas the conventional antipsychotic haloperidol did not [37, 38].

Biochemical studies

A very large number of studies have focused on the potential difference between conventional and novel antipsychotics in activation specific neurochemical processes. Given the important role of dopamine, most of these studies have focussed on possible regional differences in this neurotransmitter. However, studies investigating other neurotransmitters and neuropeptides have also been reported. Recently, a more functional approach to regional selectivity has been introduced through the fos technique. Fos is a so-called immediate early gene, which is synthesised when neuronal cells are activated. It therefore allows a very precise mapping of brain regions, and even individual cells activated by antipsychotic drugs. Although the fos technique is rapidly becoming an important tool for studying functional activation of brain areas, there are also limitations to this technique which will be described below.

Regional differences in the dopaminergic system

Since dopamine has been implicated in the mechanism of action of antipsychotic drugs for a long time [39], it is not surprising that most studies on regional selectivity have focussed on this neurotransmitter system. Given the above discussion on the differential activation of nigrostriatal (A_9) vs. mesolimbic (A_{10}) dopamine cell groups, it is equally logical that most emphasis has been on the regional differences between different antipsychotics on the neostriatum (principal output station of the A_9 cells) and the nucleus accumbens (principal output station of the A_{10} cells).

Westerink and Korf [40] were probably one of the first to point to a difference between antipsychotic on dopamine metabolism. These authors compared the accumulation of homovanillic acid (HVA) the principal metabolite of dopamine within the neostriatum after the administration of different antipsychotic. As discussed above, acute administration of antipsychotic increases cell firing of dopaminergic cells, and thus increases the release of dopamine and its metabolites. However, the authors found that haloperidol and pimozide induced a much stronger increase in HVA accumulation than clozapine and thioridazine. Bürki et al., however, were unable to replicate these findings, and found clear enhancement of both DOPAC (3,4-dihydroxyphenylacetic acid) and HVA after administration of haloperidol, perlapine, thioridazine and clozapine [41]. Likewise, both conventional and atypical antipsychotics increase 3-methoxytyramine (3-MT, another important dopamine metabolite) within the neostriatum [42].

A distinct disadvantage of these earlier studies was that only the neostriatum was analysed, and not the nucleus accumbens. Since the cornerstone of the A_9/A_{10} hypothesis is not a general difference in potency between antipsychotic drugs, but a relatively selective action on one specific subgroup of cells, the dopamine release (or metabolite accumulation) should be measured in both the nucleus accumbens and the neostriatum. Moreover, the studies were usually done *in vitro*. The introduction of more sensitive techniques, such as microdialysis and voltammetry allow the direct *in vivo* registration of dopamine and/or its metabolites in different brain regions and can therefore be more helpful in elucidating the mechanisms underlying the action of conventional and atypical antipsychotics. Unfortunately, the data obtained with these techniques are not unequivocal. Thus, using *in vivo* voltammetry Lane and Blaha [43] found that conventional antipsychotics such as haloperidol and chlorpromazine increased dopamine release in both the neostriatum and the nucleus accumbens, whereas clozapine only increased dopamine release in the nucleus accumbens. Essentially the same regional selectivity was found after chronic administration [44]. Studies using the *in vivo* microdialysis technique also showed that chronic clozapine led to a reduction in dopamine release in the nucleus accumbens, but not in the neostriatum [45]. On the other hand, other studies have failed to find a regional selectivity for antipsychotics such as clozapine, using *in vivo* voltammetry [46, 47], microdialysis [48–50] or standard *ex vivo* voltammetry [51]. Likewise, olanzapine also increases dopamine release in both the nucleus accumbens and the neostriatum [52].

It is at present unclear why these studies gave such different results. One possible explanation may be that neither the neostriatum, nor the nucleus accumbens is a homogenous structure. Thus, within the neostriatum, specific patches (or striosomes) can be identified from the surrounding matrix using certain staining methods [53]. Within the nucleus accumbens the situation is even more complex; apart from a patch/matrix compartmentalisation, there is also a shell/core subdivision [54], the shell representing the more medial and ventral parts. Since the patch/matrix and the shell/core subregions each receive inputs from different structures and send its output to different target nuclei, it is quite conceivable that these structures are involved in different functions. For instance, it is the shell region of the nucleus accumbens which receives the strongest input from the hippocampus and the amygdala, and which projects to the ventral tegmental area. The core region, on the other hand, receives more input from thalamic regions and project to the substantia nigra pars reticulata [55]. This has led to the idea that the shell region may be more related to limbic functions and the core region more to motor functions. In agreement with this, it has been shown that after mild stress, dopamine is released from the shell but not the core region of the nucleus accumbens [56]. If this hypothesis is true, one would expect atypical antipsychotics to have less influence on the core region of the accumbens than conventional antipsychotics. This has indeed been shown by several authors [56, 57].

Apart from a nucleus accumbens/neostriatum or a core/shell differentiation, there is also evidence that conventional and novel antipsychotics differ in the degree in which they activate cortical *vs* subcortical dopaminergic projection. It was known for some time already that virtually all antipsychotics increase HVA levels in the prefrontal cortex [51]. Moreover, using microdialysis, both conventional and novel antipsychotics increase dopamine release in this structure [49, 58]. There have now been several reports that show that antipsychotics like haloperidol have a stronger influence on striatal dopamine than on prefrontal dopamine, whereas the reverse is true for clozapine and other novel antipsychotics [59, 60].

Overall, the data on dopamine release now show a relatively clear picture, with conventional antipsychotics influencing virtually all dopaminergic systems, whereas atypical antipsychotics having more effect on mesolimbic and mesocortical dopaminergic systems, innervation of the shell of the nucleus accumbens and the medial prefrontal cortex.

Regional selectivity in other neurotransmitters

The (hypothesised) differential involvement of the neostriatum and the nucleus accumbens in the extrapyramidal side-effects, respectively the therapeutic effects of antipsychotic drugs has led to a large number of studies investigating other aspects of these neuronal circuitries. Most of these studies compared only haloperidol with clozapine, thereby excluding a generalisation to all conventional or novel antipsychotics. Nylander and Terrenius [61], for instance, found that chronic administration of clozapine significantly increase substantia nigra levels of dynorphin and substance P, whereas chronic treatment with haloperidol decrease substantia nigra levels of substance P. From this one might conclude that classical and atypical antipsychotics show a differential regulation of neuropeptides in the substantia nigra. However, Angulo et al. [62] compared the effects of chronic treatment with clozapine, haloperidol, thioridazine and a number of other antipsychotics on the striatum levels of mRNA for protachykinin (from which substance P is derived) and found that all antipsychotics (including thioridazine and sulpiride) reduce these mRNA levels, with the only exception being clozapine. This clearly illustrates the danger in making conclusions about the group of the atypical antipsychotics solely on the basis of the effects of clozapine. When comparing repeated treatment with haloperidol, chlorpromazine, sulpiride and clozapine on mRNA for protachykinin, Shibata et al. [63] found that haloperidol and chlorpromazine reduced the levels in the neostriatum and increased them in the septum. Clozapine and sulpiride on the other hand increased the levels in the nucleus accumbens and the bed nucleus of the stria terminalis.

Haloperidol and clozapine have also been found to differentially affect other neuropeptides, such as neurotensin and enkephalin. Acute and chronic administration of haloperidol increase mRNA levels for neurotensin in both the dorsolateral part of the neostriatum as well as the shell region of the nucleus accumbens. Clozapine on the other hand only increased the levels of neurotensin mRNA in the shell. [64, 65]. On the other hand, acute administration of clozapine decreased mRNA levels of proenkephalin within the neostriatum, whereas haloperidol had no effect [66], although no differences between antipsychotics were found after chronic administration [67]. Clozapine and thioridazine, but not haloperidol and pimozide were also found to increase GABA turnover and efflux in the neostriatum, whereas all four antipsychotics increased turnover and efflux of GABA in the nucleus accumbens [68].

Differences in the biochemistry at the level of the nucleus accumbens and the neostriatum are likely to also result in differences at lower levels in the circuitry. In this respect it is interesting to see that clozapine and thioridazine, but not haloperidol, pimozide or chlorpromazine increase GABA turnover in the substantia nigra, whereas all drugs increased the efflux and turnover of GABA in the globus pallidus [68]. This increase in GABA efflux in the substantia nigra after clozapine treatment might also explain why these drugs decrease cell firing in this nucleus [37].

Regional selectivity in c-fos expression

When neuronal cells are activated, for instance by neurotransmitter agonists or antagonists, a number of intracellular processes are initiated. An important consequence of such activation is usually an increase in transcription of specific proteins. Several years ago it was found that a number of genes (already known as oncogenes) were rapidly and strongly activated by a number of neural signals [69]. These so-called immediate early genes include c-fos, Fra-1 (Fos related antigen-1), FosB, c-jun, junB and junD. From these immediate early genes, especially c-fos has been studied in relation to the regional selectivity of antipsychotic drugs.

Dragunow et al. [70] were probably the first to investigate the c-fos inducing effects of a number of antipsychotic drugs. When comparing the acute effects of haloperidol and clozapine, they found that both drugs activated c-fos in the nucleus accumbens, however, only haloperidol activated c-fos in the neostriatum. These findings were replicated and extended in a subsequent paper [71] showing that clozapine additionally activated c-fos in the medial prefrontal cortex and in the septum, whereas haloperidol had no effect on the medial prefrontal cortex, and only marginally activated the septum. This differential activation of the neostriatum by conventional antipsychotics such as haloperidol has been replicated by others [72, 73], and closer investigation of the patterns of activation indicated that within the nucleus accumbens, the more medial parts (i.e. the shell region) are more strongly activated by all antipsychotic drugs [74], which seems to be in agreement with previous studies on the dopaminergic system (see above). The selective activation of the prefrontal cortex by clozapine has also been replicated by others [75, 76], and has been taken to suggest that this might be the site of action of clozapine in therapy resistant patients (or on negative symptoms). Selective activation of c-fos in the nucleus accumbens has also been described for a number of other novel antipsychotics, including quetiapine, remoxipride and risperidone [77] and olanzapine [78]. Likewise, quetiapine, remoxipride and olanzapine, but not risperidone activated medial prefrontal c-fos [77, 78]. On the other hand, some studies found only marginal differences between haloperidol, clozapine and risperidone [79]. Sertindole seems to be relatively inactive in fos activation. A dose of 10 mg/kg only marginally activated fos in the nucleus accumbens and in the medial prefrontal cortex [79].

Summarising the biochemical data suggests that, as with the electrophysiological data, most evidence points in the direction of a differentiation between conventional and novel antipsychotics at the level of neostriatum and nucleus accumbens. Moreover, it appears that within the nucleus accumbens a subdivision can be made with respect to the shell region (which is activated by all antipsychotics) and the core region (which is activated by conventional antipsychotics only). In addition the fos data suggest that a number of novel antipsychotics selectively increase activity within the prefrontal cortex. It should however be kept in mind that the lack of c-fos in a particular neuronal structure does not necessarily imply that that structure is not influenced. First of all, the neuronal activity of that structure may be reduced, which does not lead to increased c-fos activity. Second, the activation of that specific structure may be accompanied by activation of other immediate early genes. In this respect it is important to recall that clozapine was found to induce JunB, Fra-1 and Krox24, but not c-fos within the neostriatum [80], suggesting that this drug is capable of activating neostriatal cells.

Behavioural studies

The number of studies investigating regional selectivity of antipsychotic drugs in behavioural paradigms is fairly limited, and usually restricted to only a few antipsychotic drugs. One of the few exceptions has been the original study by Costall and Naylor, who studied the effects of antipsychotics on locomotor activity induced by local application of dopamine into the neostriatum, nucleus accumbens or olfactory tubercle [81]. The results show that all antipsychotics were more potent in inhibiting the locomotor activity induced from the nucleus accumbens than from the neostriatum. However, whereas conventional antipsychotics like haloperidol and fluphenazine were equipotent in inhibiting the locomotor activity induced from the nucleus accumbens and the olfactory tubercle, antipsychotics such as clozapine and thioridazine were more effective against the locomotor activity induced from the nucleus accumbens.

A different result was obtained in a recent study comparing the effects of antipsychotics on locomotor activity induced from the nucleus accumbens or the olfactory tubercle [82]. These authors found that atypical antipsychotics were *more* effective in inhibiting locomotor activity induced from the olfactory tubercle. The two studies differ in two respects. First in the study of Cools et al. locomotor activity was induced by different agents in the nucleus accumbens (ergometrine) and the olfactory tubercle (dopamine), whereas in the study of Costall and Naylor the same drug (dopamine) was used in all brain regions. The second difference between the two studies is that in the study of Costall and Naylor antipsychotics were injected systemically, whereas in the Cools et al. study the antipsychotics were applied locally.

The preferential involvement of the olfactory tubercle and the nucleus accumbens in the action of novel antipsychotics is also supported by findings of the paw test. This test was specifically designed to differentiate between conventional and novel antipsychotics [8]. In a recent study, sulpiride was locally applied to the neostriatum, the nucleus accumbens or the olfactory tubercle [83]. The results show that local injection into the olfactory tubercle or the nucleus accumbens produced a behavioural profile similar to that seen after systemic injections of atypical antipsychotic drugs.

Mechanisms for regional selectivity

Summarising the data it seems that there are indeed regional differences between classical and atypical antipsychotic drugs. Although there are certainly some conflicting data the overall analysis suggests that all antipsychotics influence the nucleus accumbens (especially the shell region). Classical antipsychotics additionally strongly activate the neostriatum, whereas the atypical antipsychotics seem to more clearly influence the prefrontal cortex and the olfactory tubercle. An important question is, of course, which mechanisms are responsible for these differences in regional selectivity. A difference in regional binding to, for instance, dopamine receptors seems unlikely (as described in the first part of this chapter).

The c-fos technique has been used to investigate the neuropharmacological mechanisms involved in the activation of neuronal cells by antipsychotic drugs. It has been found that the c-fos activation within the neostriatum by haloperidol is due to its D_2 blocking properties [84, 85]. Dopamine D_3 and D_4 receptors, on the other hand, have been implicated in the clozapine-induced c-fos activation of the nucleus accumbens and the medial prefrontal cortex respectively [86], although the data are less convincing.

Of more interest is probably the role of serotonin and acetylcholine receptors, since both have been implicated in the differentiation of classical and atypical antipsychotics [12, 13]. Pre-treatment with scopolamine has been reported to reverse the haloperidol induced c-fos activation in the neostriatum [86], whereas pre-treatment with ritanserin did not [87]. These data are in agreement with electrophysiological studies showing that scopolamine can prevent the haloperidol induced depolarisation inactivation [88].

Relatively little is known about the pharmacological mechanisms underlying the specific clozapine induced increase in prefrontal cortex c-fos activity. Thus lesions of the noradrenergic system or the serotonergic system do not affect the clozapine induced c-fos activation [89]. Likewise application of SCH 23390, ritanserin, prazosin nor scopolamine induce increase in prefrontal c-fos [89]. Although these studies are generally taken to indicate that serotonergic and noradrenergic receptors do not play a role in the clozapine induced fos activation of the prefrontal cortex, this conclusion is not necessarily justified by the data. The prefrontal cortex activation by clozapine may be due to a combined action of, for instance dopamine, serotonin and noradrenaline blockade. If this is true, any single neurotransmitter antagonist may be incapable of activating c-fos by itself. In this respect results obtained with the paw test may be relevant. In this paradigm, it was shown that neither SCH 23390, nor ketanserin or phenoxybenzamine was capable of affecting the parameters measured in the paw test. Moreover, any combination of two of these three antagonists produced any significant effect. However, when all three were combined a profile similar to clozapine was observed [90]. Therefore, an alternative strategy may be to combine clozapine with selective agonists, to selectively reverse one component of the clozapine profile.

There is evidence suggesting that the serotonin receptors are involved in the selective blockade of olfactory tubercle induced locomotor activity by atypical antipsychotics. Thus, whereas the serotonin antagonist ritanserin is ineffective in reversing the ergometrine induced locomotor activity from the nucleus accumbens, it strongly reverses the effects of amphetamine within the olfactory tubercle [91]. This suggests that serotonin antagonists and dopamine antagonists work in a co-operative manner within the olfactory tubercle, whereas they work independently in the nucleus accumbens.

Conclusions

In conclusion, there is quite an extensive body of evidence that antipsychotics which produce many extrapyramidal side-effects influence other brain structures than antipsychotics that produce less side-effects. Although the data are far from unequivocal, the overall picture emerges that drugs which strongly activate the neostriatum produce more side-effects than drugs which do not activate the neostriatum. Likewise there is evidence that drugs which in addition to activating the nucleus accumbens (especially the shell region) also activate the medial prefrontal cortex may have additional beneficial action (possibly on negative symptoms or on therapy resistant patients). The mechanisms behind these regional differences remain, however, very much unclear so far, and much more research is needed to fully appreciate the differences between individual antipsychotic drugs. It is important that this future research takes two important points into account. First clozapine still appears to be a unique drug, and deducing generalisations on the basis of experiments done only with clozapine is dangerous. Secondly, a close inspection of the increasing clinical literature on possible therapeutic differences between antipsychotics drugs is essential for developing hypotheses on the possible involvement of brain structures in the clinical effects of these drugs.

References

1 National Institute of Mental Health (1964) Phenothiazine treatment in acute schizophrenics. *Arch Gen Psychiatr* 10: 246–261
2 Galbrecht C, Klett C (1968) Predicting response to phenothiazines: the right drug for the right patient. *J Nerv Ment Dis* 147: 173–183
3 Herman E, Pleasure H (1963) Clinical evaluation of thioridazine and chlorpromazine in chronic schizophrenics. *Dis Nerv Syst* 24; 54–59
4 Lasky J, Klett C, Caffey E, Bennett J, Rosenblum M, Hollister L (1962) A comparison evaluation of chlorpromazine, chlorprothixene, fluphenazine, reserpine, thioridazine and triflupromazine. *Dis Nerv Syst* 23: 1–8
5 Baldessarini R, Frankenburg F (1991) Clozapine: A novel antipsychotic agent. *N Eng J Med* 324: 646–754
6 Fitton A, Heel R (1990) Clozapine. A review of its pharmacological properties, and therapeutic use in schizophrenia. *Drugs* 40: 722–747
7 Sayers A, Amsler H (1977) Clozapine. In: M Goldberg (ed.): *Pharmacological and biochemical properties of drug substances vol. 1.* Amer Pharmaceut Ass 1–31
8 Ellenbroek BA (1993) Treatment of schizophrenia: A clinical and preclinical evaluation of neuroleptic drugs. *Pharmac Ther* 57: 1–78
9 Christensen A (1985) Classification of neuroleptics: Implications for tardive dyskinesia. *Pol J Pharm Pharmacol* 37: 295–309
10 Malmberg A, Jackson DM, Eriksson A, Mohell N (1993) Unique binding characteristics of antipsychotic agents interacting with human dopamine D_{2A}, D_{2B}, and D_3 receptors. *Mol Pharmacol* 43: 749–754
11 Köhler C, Hall H, Magnusson O, Lewander T, Gustafsson K (1990) Biochemical pharmacology of the atypical neuroleptic remoxipride. *Acta Psychiatr Scand* 82 (A suppl 358): 27–36
12 Snyder S, Greenberg D, Yamamura H (1974) Antischizophrenic drugs and brain cholinergic receptors. *Arch Gen Psychiatr* 31: 58–61
13 Meltzer HY, Matsubara S, Lee J (1989) Classification of typical ant atypical antipsychotic drugs on the basis of D_1, D_2 and serotonin pK_i values. *J Pharmacol Exp Ther* 251: 238–246
14 LeFur G, Burgevin M, Malgouris C, Uzan A (1979) Differential effects of typical and atypical neuroleptics on alpha-noradrenergic and dopaminergic receptors. *Neuropharmacol* 18: 591–594

15 Altar C, Wasley A, Neale R, Stone G (1986) Typical and atypical antipsychotic occupancy of D_2 and S_2 receptors: An autoradiographic analysis on rat brain. *Brain Res Bull* 16: 517–525
16 Meltzer H (1992) The importance of serotonin-dopamine interactions in the action of clozapine. *Br J Psychiat* 160 (Suppl 17): 22–29
17 Bischoff S, Christen P, Vassout A (1988) Blockade of hippocampal dopamine (DA) receptors: A tool for antipsychotics with low extrapyramidal side effect. *Prog Neuro-Psychopharmacol. Biol Psychiat* 12: 455–467
18 Wetzel H, Wiedemann K, Holsboer F, Benkert O (1991) Savoxepine: invalidation of an "atypical" neuroleptic response pattern predicted by animal models in an open clinical trial with schizophrenic patients. *Psychopharmacology* 103: 280–283
19 Chiodo L, Bunney B (1983) Typical and atypical neuroleptics: Differential effects of chronic administration on the activity of A_9 and A_{10} midbrain dopaminergic neurons. *J Neurosci* 3: 1607–1619
20 White F, Wang R (1983) Differential effects of classical and atypical antipsychotic drugs on A9 and A10 dopamine neurons. *Science* 211: 1054–1056
21 Skarsfeldt T (1988) Differential effects after repeated treatment with haloperidol, clozapine, thioridazine and tefludazine on SNC and VTA dopamine neurones in rats. *Life Sci* 42: 1037–1044
22 Goldstein J, Litwin L, Sutton E, Malick J (1989) Effects of ICI 169,369, a selective serotonin$_2$ antagonist, in electrophysiological tests predictive of antipsychotic activity. *J Pharmacol Exp Ther* 249: 673–680
23 Bunney BS (1984) Antipsychotic drug effects on the electric activity of dopaminergic neurons. *Trends Neurosci* 8: 212–215
24 Arnt J, Skarsfeldt T (1998) Do novel antipsychotics have similar pharmacological characteristics? A review of the literature. *Neuropsychopharmacol* 18: 63–101
25 Stockton ME, Rasmussen K (1996) Electrophysiological effects of olanzapine, a novel antipsychotic, on A9 and A10 dopamine neurons. *Neuropsychopharmacol* 14: 97–105
26 Gysling K, Wang R (1983) Morphine-induced activation of A10 dopamine neurons in the rat. *Brain Res* 277: 119–127
27 Ichikawa J, Meltzer H (1990) The effects of chronic clozapine and haloperidol on basal dopamine release and metabolism in rat striatum and nucleus accumbens studied by *in vivo* microdialysis. *Eur J Pharmacol* 176: 371–374
28 Kelland M, Freedman A, Chiodo L (1989) Chloral hydrate anaesthesia alters the responsiveness of identified midbrain dopamine neurons to dopamine agonist administration. *Synapse* 3: 30–37
29 Zhang W, Tilson H, Stackowiak M, Hong J (1989) Repeated haloperidol administration changes basal release of striatal dopamine and subsequent response to haloperidol challenge. *Brain Res* 484: 389–392
30 Mereu G, Lilliu V, Vargiu P, Muntoni AL, Diana M, Gessa GL (1995) Depolarization inactivation of dopamine neurons: an artifact? *J Neuroscience* 15: 1144–1149
31 Melis M, Mereu G, Lilliu V, Quartu M, Diana M, Gessa GL (1998) Haloperidol does not produce dopamine cell depolarization-block in paralyzed, unanesthetized rats. *Brain Res* 783: 127–132
32 Melis M, Gessa GL, Diana M (1998) Clozapine does activate nigrostriatal dopamine neurons in unanesthetized rats. *Eur J Pharmacol* 363: 135–138
33 Rebec GV, Alloway KD, Bashore TR (1991) Differential actions of classical and atypical antipsychotic drugs on spontaneous neuronal activity in the amygdala complex. *Pharmacol Biochem Behav* 14: 49–56
34 Wang Z, Rebec GV (1996) Amygdaloid neurons respond to clozapine rather than haloperidol in behaving rats pretreated with intra-amygdaloid amphetamine. *Brain Res* 711: 64–72
35 Morelli M, Porceddu ML, Imperato A, DiChiara G (1981) Role of substantia nigra pars reticulata neurons in expression of antipsychotic-induced catalepsy. *Brain Res* 217: 375–379
36 Ellenbroek BA, Schwarz M, Sontag KH, Cools AR (1985) The importance of the striato-nigro-collicular pathway in the expression of haloperidol-induced tonic electromyographic activity. *Neurosci Lett* 54: 189–194
37 Bruggeman R, Westerink BHC, Timmerman W (1997) Effects of risperidone, clozapine and haloperidol on extracellular recordings of substantia nigra pars reticulata neurons of the rat brain. *Europ J Pharmacol* 324: 49–56

38 Timmerman W, Heijmen M, Westerink BHC, Bruggeman R, den Boer JA (1999) Effects of acute and administration of olanzapine in comparison to clozapine and haloperidol on extracellular recordings of substantia nigra reticulata neurons in the rat brain. *Psychopharmacology* 144: 286–294
39 Van Rossum J (1966) The significance of dopamine-receptor blockade for the mechanism of action of neuroleptic drugs. *Arch Intern Pharmacodyn Ther* 160: 492–494
40 Westerink B, Korf J (1975) Influence of drugs on striatal and limbic homovanillic acid concentration in the rat brain. *Europ J Pharmacol* 33: 31–40
41 Bürki HR, Ruch W, Asper H (1975) Effects of clozapine, thioridazine, perlapine and haloperidol on the metabolism of the biogenic amines in the brain of the rat. *Psychopharmacology* 41: 27–33
42 Saller CF, Salama AI (1986) 3-Methoxytyramine accumulation: Effects of typical neuroleptics and various atypical compounds. *Naunyn Schmiedeb Arch Pharmacol* 334: 125–132
43 Lane RF, Blaha CD (1986) Electrochemistry *in vivo*: Application to CNS pharmacology. *Ann NY Acad Sci* 473: 50–69
44 Blaha CD, Lane RF (1987) Chronic treatment with classical and atypical antipsychotic drugs differentially decreases dopamine release in striatum and nucleus accumbens *in vivo*. *Neurosci Lett* 78: 199–204
45 Chen J, Parades W, Gardner EL (1991) Chronic treatment with clozapine selectively decreases basal dopamine release in nucleus accumbens but not in caudate-putamen as measured by *in vivo* brain microdialysis: further evidence for depolarization block. *Neurosci Lett* 122: 127–131
46 Maidment N, Marsden CA (1987) Acute administration of clozapine, thioridazine and metoclopramide increases extracellular DOPAC and decreases extracellular 5-HIAA, measured in the rat striatum of the rat using *in vivo* voltammetry. *Neuropharmacol* 26: 187–193
47 Maidment N, Marsden C (1987) Repeated atypical neuroleptic administration: effects on central dopamine metabolism monitored by *in vivo* voltammetry. *Europ J Pharmacol* 136: 141–149
48 Ichikawa J, Meltzer H (1990) The effects of chronic clozapine and haloperidol on basal dopamine release and metabolism in rat striatum and nucleus accumbens studied by *in vivo* microdialysis. *Eur J Pharmacol* 176: 371–374
49 Imperato A, Angelucci L (1989) The effects of clozapine and fluperlapine on the *in vivo* release and metabolism of dopamine in the striatum and in prefrontal cortex of freely moving rats. *Psychopharmacol Bull* 25: 383–389
50 Invernizzi R, Morally F, Pozzi L, Semanin R (1990) Effects of acute and chronic clozapine on dopamine release and metabolism in the striatum of conscious rats. *Br J Pharmacol* 100: 774–778
51 Chang W, Chen T, Yeh E (1987) Time-response curves of homovanillic acid in caudate and pre-frontal cortex following acute neuroleptic administration. *Psychopharmacology* 93: 403–404
52 Li XM, Perry KW, Wong DT, Bymaster FP (1998) Olanzapine increases *in vivo* dopamine and norepinephrine release in rat prefrontal cortex, nucleus accumbens and striatum. *Psychopharmacology* 136: 153–161
53 Graybiel AM (1990) Neurotransmitters and neuromodulation in the basal ganglia. *Trends Neurosci* 13: 244–254
54 Groenewegen HJ, Meredith GE, Berendse HW, Voorn P, Wolters JG (1987) The compartmental organization of the ventral striatum. In: AR Crossman, MA Sambrook (eds): *Neural mechanisms in disorders of movement*, London, John Libbey, 45–54
55 Groenewegen HJ, Berendse HW, Meredith GE, Haber SH, Voorn P, Wolters JG, Lohman AHM (1991) Functional anatomy of the ventral, limbic system-innervated striatum. In: P Willner, J Scheel-Krüger (eds): *The mesolimbic dopamine system: From motivation to action*. John Wiley and Sons, Chichester 19–59
56 Deutch AY, Cameron DS (1992) Pharmacological characterization of dopamine system in the nucleus accumbens core and shell. *Neuroscience* 46: 49–56
57 Marcus MM, Nomikos GG, Svensson TH (1996) Differential actions of typical and atypical antipsychotic drugs on dopamine release in the core and shell of the nucleus accumbens. *Eur Neuropsychopharmacol* 6: 29–38

58 Westerink BH, deBoer P, deVries JB, Kruse CG, Long SK (1998) Antipsychotic drugs induce similar effects on the release of dopamine and noradrenaline in the medial prefrontal cortex. *Eur J Pharmacol* 361: 27–33
59 Moghaddam B, Bunney BS (1990) Acute effects of typical and atypical antipsychotic drugs on the release of dopamine from prefrontal cortex, nucleus accumbens, and striatum of the rat: an *in vivo* microdialysis study. *J Neurochem* 54: 1755–1760
60 Pehek EA, Yamamoto BK (1994) Differential effects of locally administered clozapine and haloperidol on dopamine efflux in the rat prefrontal cortex and caudate-putamen. *J Neurochem* 63: 2118–2124
61 Nylander I, Terenius L (1986) Chronic haloperidol and clozapine differentially affect dynorphin peptides and substance P in basal ganglia of the rat. *Brain Res* 380: 34–41
62 Angulo JA, Cadet JL, McEwen BS (1990) Effects of typical and atypical neuroleptic treatment on protachykinin mRNA levels in the striatum of the rat. *Neurosci Lett* 113: 217–221
63 Shibata K, Haverstick DM, Bannon MJ (1990) Tachykinin gene expression in rat limbic nuclei: Modulation by dopamine antagonists. *J Pharmacol Exp Ther* 255: 388–392
64 Merchant KM, Dobner PR, Dorsa DM (1992) Differential effects of haloperidol and clozapine on neurotensin gene transcription in rat neostriatum. *J Neuroscience* 12: 652–663
65 Merchant KM, Dobie DJ, Filloux FM, Totzke M, Aravagiri M, Dorsa DM (1994) Effects of chronic haloperidol and clozapine treatment on neurotensin and c-fos mRNA in rat nesotriatal subregions. *J Pharmacol Exp Ther* 271: 460–471
66 Mercugliano M, Chesselet MF (1992) Clozapine decreases enkephalin mRNA in rat striatum. *Neurosci Lett* 136: 10–14
67 Angulo JA, Cadet JL, Woolley CS, Suber F, McEwen BS (1990) Effects of chronic typical and atypical neuroleptic treatment on proenkephalin mRNA levels in the striatum and nucleus accumbens of the rat. *J Neurochem* 54: 1889–1894
68 Marco E, Mao CC, Revuelta A, Pealta E, Costa E (1978) Turnover rates of gamma-aminobutyric acid in substantia nigra, n. caudatus, globus pallidus and n. accumbens of rats injected with cataleptogenic antipsychotics. *Neuropharmacol* 17: 589–596
69 Morgan JI, Curran T (1989) Stimulus-transcription coupling in neurons: role of cellular immediate-early genes. *Trends Neurosci* 12: 459–462
70 Dragunow M, Robertson GS, Faull RLM, Robertson HA, Jansen K (1990) D_2 dopamine receptor antagonists induce fos and related proteins in striatal neurons. *Neuroscience* 37: 287–294
71 Robertson GS, Fibiger HC (1992) Neuroleptics increase c-fos expression in the forebrain: Contrasting effects of haloperidol and clozapine. *Neuroscience* 46: 315–328
72 Nguyen TV, Kasofsky B, Birnbaum R, Cohen BM, Hyman SE (1992) Differential expression of c-fos and Zif 268 in rat striatum following haloperidol, clozapine and amphetamine. *Proc Natl Acad Sci* 89: 4270–4274
73 Dilts RP Jr, Helton TE, McGinty JF (1993) Selective induction of fos and FRA immunoreactivity with the mesolimbic and mesostriatal dopaminergic terminal fields. *Synapse* 13: 251–263
74 Deutch AY, Lee MC, Iadarola MJ (1992) Regionally specific effects of atypical antipsychotic drugs on striatal fos expression: the nucleus accumbens shell as a locus of antipsychotic action. *Mol Cell Neurosci* 3: 332–341
75 Deutch AY, Duman RS (1996) The effects of antipsychotics on prefrontal cortical fos expression: cellular localization and pharmacological characterization. *Neuroscience* 70: 377–389
76 Merchant KM, Figur LM, Evans DL (1996) Induction of c-fos mRNA in rat medial prefrontal cortex by antipsychotic drugs: role of dopamine D_2 and D_3 receptors. *Cereb Cortex* 6: 561–570
77 Robertson GS, Matsumura H, Fibiger HC (1994) Induction patterns of fos-like immunoreactivity in the forebrain as predictors of atypical antipsychotic activity. *J Pharmacol Exp Ther* 271: 1058–1066
78 Robertson GS, Fibiger HC (1996) Effects of olanzapine on regional c-fos expression in rat forebrain. *Neuropsychopharmacol* 14: 105–110
79 Fink-Jensen A, Kristensen P (1994) Effects of typical and atypical neuroleptics on Fos protein expression in the rat forebrain. *Neurosci Lett* 182: 115–118
80 MacGibbon GA, Lawlor PA, Bravo R, Dragunow M (1994) Clozapine and haloperidol produce a differential pattern of immediate early gene expression in rat caudate-putamen, nucleus accumbens, lateral septum and islands of Calleja. *Mol Brain Res* 23: 21–32

81 Costall B, Naylor RJ (1976) A comparison of the abilities of typical neuroleptic agents and of thioridazine, clozapine, sulpiride and metoclopramide to antagonise the hyperactivity induced by dopamine applied intracerebrally to areas of the extrapyramidal and mesolimbic system. *Europ J Pharmacol* 40: 9–19
82 Cools AR, Prinssen EPM, Ellenbroek BA (1995) The olfactory tubercle as a site of action of neuroleptics with an atypical profile in the paw test: effect of risperidone, prothipendyl, ORG 5222, sertindole and olanzapine. *Psychopharmacology* 119: 428–439
83 Prinssen EPM, Ellenbroek BA, Stamatovic B, Cools AR (1995) Role of striatal dopamine D_2 receptors in the paw test, an animal model for the therapeutic efficacy and extrapyramidal side-effects of neuroleptic drugs. *Brain Res* 673: 283–289
84 Miller JC (1990) Induction of c-fos mRNA expression in rat striatum by neuroleptic drugs. *J Neurochem* 54: 1453–1455
85 Rogue P, Vincendon G (1992) Dopamine D2 receptor antagonists induce immediate early genes in the rat striatum. *Brain Res Bull* 29: 469–472
86 Guo N, Robertson GS, Fibiger HC (1992) Scopolamine attenuated haloperidol induced c-fos expression in the striatum. *Brain Res* 588: 164–167
87 Guo N, Klitenick MA, Tham CS, Fibiger HC (1995) Receptor mechanisms mediating clozapine-induced c-fos expression in the forebrain. *Neuroscience* 65: 747–756
88 Chiodo LA, Bunney BS (1985) Possible mechanisms by which repeated clozapine administration differentially affects the activity of two subpopulations of midbrain dopamine neurons. *J Neuroscience* 5: 2539–2544
89 Deutch AY, Duman RS (1996) The effects of antipsychotic drugs on fos protein expression in the prefrontal cortex: Cellular localization and pharmacological characterization. *Neuroscience* 70: 377–389
90 Prinssen EPM, Ellenbroek BA, Cools AR (1994) Combined antagonism of adrenoceptors and dopamine and 5-HT receptors underlies the atypical profile of clozapine. *Europ J Pharmacol* 262: 167–170
91 Cools AR, Prinssen EPM, Ellenbroek BA, Heeren DJ (1994) Role of olfactory tubercle and nucleus accumbens in the effects of classical and atypical neuroleptics: search for regional specificity. In: T Palamo, T Archer, R Beninger (eds): *Strategies for studying brain disorders. vol 2,* Madrid, Farrand Press 33–53

Atypical Antipsychotics
ed. by B.A. Ellenbroek and A.R. Cools

Screening models for antipsychotic drugs

Jørn Arnt

Department of Psychopharmacology, Psychopharmacological Research, H. Lundbeck A/S, Ottiliavej 9, DK 2500 Copenhagen-Valby, Denmark

Introduction

Development of effective screening strategies for improved antipsychotic drugs (APDs) rely primarily on the actual hypotheses for mechanism of action of these compounds. In the early times of the dopamine (DA) hypothesis of schizophrenia animal models were designed to detect compounds which blocked the behavioural effects of high doses of dopaminergic drugs (e.g. amphetamine-, apomorphine- and methylphenidate-induced stereotyped behaviour). When *in vitro* receptor binding methods became available it was routinely demonstrated that the behavioural models identified compounds with potent DA receptor blocking activity (e.g. phenothiazines, like chlorpromazine and fluphenazine; thioxanthenes such as cis(Z)-flupentixol; butyrophenones such as haloperidol). Furthermore, the same compounds all blocked conditioned avoidance responses (e.g. shuttle-box active avoidance), another conventional model for measuring antipsychotic activity. However, these compounds also induced catalepsy in rodents, a model with close symptom analogy of Parkinsonism in humans. This example illustrates the inherent problem using these models in drug discovery, since they pick up compounds which have putative antipsychotic activity *and* extrapyramidal side-effects (EPS) at the same time. In addition, these methods will detect drugs with similar activity profiles as those already known. The potencies of APDs correlate with DA receptor affinities (D_2 subtype) and with clinical dose range [1].

A breakthrough came with the discovery of clozapine, which has antipsychotic activity, but fails to show efficacy in the stereotypy and catalepsy tests, though it inhibits conditioned avoidance response. Clozapine has subsequently been used as tool to improve the understanding of the mechanism of action of APDs (for review see [2]). Two different and complementary drug screening strategies were successfully developed based on the pharmacological differences between conventional APDs and clozapine:

1) Limbic selectivity: Clozapine was found to influence the DA system selectively in limbic brain regions (see next section and Ellenbroek and

Cools, Regional selectivity of antipsychotic drugs, this volume for further discussion). Therefore development of models optimising inhibitory effect on limbic DA function (believed to be responsible for antipsychotic activity) and minimising inhibitory effect on nigrostriatal DA function (responsible for EPS) is important for discovery of new drugs. The profile of a compound in such models does not necessarily depend on a specific receptor mechanism (i.e. DA receptor blockade), and the model can accordingly be used for broad *in vivo* screening.

2) Receptor Profiles: Clozapine has a mixed receptor activity profile, and numerous hypotheses have been formulated that suggest a major role of inhibiting either DA D_1, D_2 and/or D_4, muscarinic, 5-$HT_{2A/2C}$ receptor and/or α_1-adrenoreceptor antagonism to account for its selective antipsychotic effect [2]. Models determining the relative potencies of compounds on these receptors in CNS *in vitro* and *in vivo* have been used extensively in the search for novel APDs. Moreover, specific antagonists at these receptors have been identified using receptor screening methodology and have become important research tools in the attempts of understanding the mechanisms involved in antipsychotic activity and mediating the effects in the symptom based models mentioned in the previous section.

In addition to the theoretical rationale for a model (see Ellenbroek and Cools, Animal models, this volume), another important aspect to consider is the predictive validity of each model. This can be described by some key characteristics: (1) The model should give limited number of false positive and negative results; (2) An effect of a putative APD in a model of antipsychotic activity should be insensitive to co-treatment with an antimuscarinic drug, while effects in EPS-related models should be reversed by antimuscarinic drugs (used clinically to treat APD-induced EPS); (3) A model for antipsychotic effect should ideally mimic the slow onset of antipsychotic activity. The latter criterion, however, is seldom fulfilled.

The chapter will discuss some of the important animal models which have been instrumental in the discovery of the second generation of APDs, the group to which clozapine, risperidone, olanzapine, sertindole, quetiapine and ziprasidone among others belong to. In addition, the effect on cognitive function will briefly be addressed, since this symptom dimension recently has attracted increasing focus. The complimentary chapter on simulation models for APDs further discuss potential screening methods with improved face and/or construct validity, including evaluation of potential effects on negative symptoms. Finally, the chapter on regional effects of APDs will discuss possibilities of relating e.g., for example, effects of APDs to prefrontal cortex mechanisms.

Test capacity of a screening model has not been mentioned, but is of course of importance. However, this parameter is always a compromise compared with the predictive value of the model in question.

Screening strategies for antipsychotic drugs

The concept of limbic vs striatal selectivity

The most widely accepted hypothesis is that antipsychotic activity is related to reduction of DA function in limbic brain regions (though not necessarily by blocking the receptors), while EPS are mediated by inhibition of nigrostriatal DA function; for a review, see [3, 4]. However, it should be emphasised that the hypothesis includes limbic as well as cortical DA systems. There are many examples of abnormalities of prefrontal-temporolimbic cortices in schizophrenia [5–8], which are hypothesised to be involved in the pathophysiology of psychosis, including negative symptomatology and cognitive deficits.

Selective inhibition of limbic *versus* striatal DA activity can be achieved in different ways: It is possible, but unlikely, that an APD accumulates selectively in the relevant brain area(s).

Another possible strategy is to develop compounds with preferential or selective affinity for the subtypes of the D_2 receptor family mainly expressed in the limbic system [9]. This strategy is under active investigation, for example, by development of specific D_3 [10] and D_4 ligands [11–13] though clinical data so far are scarce. However, there is no evidence for selective binding to D_2 receptor subtypes of the present generation of novel APDs in clinical use.

The most widely accepted hypothesis for obtaining functional limbic and/or cortical selectivity is that a delicately balanced effect on several neurotransmitter receptors, particularly DA D_2 and 5-HT_2 receptors as well as α_1-adrenoceptors and muscarinic receptors, leads to a selective inhibition of limbic/cortical DA function [3, 14, 15]. This hypothesis is attractive, though probably a simplification, since it is difficult to incorporate the hypothesis into profiles of all available compounds and sometimes difficult to reproduce limbic selectivity by combination of conventional APDs with other selective antagonists [16].

Mechanistic receptor models

Relative in vivo effects on neurotransmitter receptors

As previously mentioned putative APDs can be identified on the basis of a specified affinity profile for a large number of receptor targets *in vitro* and *ex vivo* [17], see also Leysen, this volume). A similar strategy can be chosen to demonstrate the relative *in vivo* potencies and efficacies on the target receptors, in order to confirm the *in vitro* effects in the living animal. This is done by selecting *in vivo* effects (preferentially CNS-mediated) which are as specific as possible for the receptor in question, most often by using a selective agonist as a tool. For example, DA D_2 antagonism can be measured by inhibition of pergolide-induced circling behaviour in 6-hydroxy-DA-lesioned rats [18] and 5-HT_2 antagonism can be measured by inhibition of head twitches induced by a 5-HT_2 agonist or the 5-HT precursor, l-5-HTP [19, 20]. A simple but illustrative way to compare activity profiles of different APDs is to express *relative* affinities/potencies as pie charts, disregarding absolute potencies [4].

When this method is applied to haloperidol and second generation APDs it appears that for some compounds there are large discrepancies between the *in vitro* and *in vivo* effects: For example, while haloperidol and risperidone has preferential D_2 activity in both conditions, sertindole shows unexpectedly weak D_2 antagonism *in vivo*. Although the mechanism behind the apparent lack of D_2 blockade of sertindole is not understood, such results are of potential importance for understanding the activity profile in symptom models of antipsychotic activity and EPS as well as clinical effects. It also indicates the importance of doing parallel *in vitro* and *in vivo* studies of new lead compounds.

Drug discrimination

Discrimination between a given drug and its vehicle is a powerful *in vivo* assay, since the technique usually combines high pharmacological specificity with objectivity (the animal decides the result of the experiment, not the researcher). The limitation of the technique is the low capacity, due to long initial acquisition period and the need for maintenance of stable discrimination accuracy by regular training of animals. Drug discrimination has been extensively used in rats, monkeys and even humans [21]. Two main principles have been used, 1) to use a stimulus drug with selectivity for a given neurotransmitter function (an agonist, neurotransmitter-releasing compound or, less often, an antagonist) or 2) to use a stimulus drug with mixed effects on a variety of receptors (e.g. clozapine), in order to reveal similarities to or differences from this drug by the test compounds. An important variable in drug discriminations assays is choice of training dose of the stimulus drug. Particularly when using stimulus drugs with mixed effects on several receptors the relative balance of these effects differ markedly, depending on dose. Furthermore, training dose is important for the outcome of studies of partial agonists which may be recorded as agonists and antagonists against a low and high dose of the stimulus drug, respectively [22, 23].

The discriminative stimulus properties of d-amphetamine (AMPH) in rats have previously been suggested to be a relevant animal model for evaluation of antipsychotic effect, since the model detects the effects of conventional APDs as well as clozapine [24]. The AMPH stimulus is blocked by selective DA D_1 and D_2 receptor antagonists, while α_1-adrenoceptor and 5-HT_2 antagonists are ineffective [25]. Furthermore, the AMPH response is mediated by the limbic DA system: It can be elicited by local injection of AMPH into nucleus accumbens, but not striatum [26], and the response to systemic administration of AMPH is abolished by previous 6-OHDA lesion of the same nucleus [27]. The predictability of AMPH discrimination as a model of antipsychotic activity has, however, recently been questioned by the finding that sertindole is unable to inhibit the AMPH response, while clozapine has the expected inhibitory effect [28]. Subsequently, it was observed that novel APDs differ in their ability to inhibit the AMPH stimulus effect as summarised in Table 1: Sertindole and quetiapine have no significant effects, remoxipride and risperidone have weak efficacies, while olanzapine and clozapine produce more complete inhibition [25]. It should, however, be mentioned that risperidone in another study of AMPH discrimination shows higher inhibitory activity, but no other novel APDs were included for comparison [29]. Since definite antipsychotic activity has been demonstrated with both sertindole (e.g. [30]) and quetiapine (e.g. [31]), this indicates that AMPH discrimination is not an animal model of schizophrenia. Instead it has been suggested that it is a measure of inhibitory effects on the DA reward system and accordingly that the model may be relevant for evaluation of the potential to induce the neuroleptic-induced deficit syndrome [21, 25].

In parallel studies of DOI (a 5-HT_2 agonist) and St 587 (an α_1-adrenoceptor agonist) discrimination, sertindole shows marked and moderate antagonistic activity, respectively, corresponding to its inhibitory effects on these receptors. Other APDs generally inhibit DOI and St 587 discrimination according to their effects on 5-HT_2 and α_1-adrenoceptors [25, 28]. Thus, the relative effects in these models can be used as an indicator for the mixed effects on these receptors *in vivo* under identical experimental conditions.

The non-competitive NMDA antagonists phencyclidine (PCP) and dizocilpine (MK-801) induce psychotomimetic effects in animals and humans. Thus, it would be interesting to study inhibition of PCP or dizocilpine discrimination as an alternative model for detection of antipsychotic activity, but only a few results are available. Though it has been suggested that clozapine, but not haloperidol, can reverse dizocilpine discrimination, the relevant study lacked information on response rates necessary for evaluation of specificity [32].

As mentioned above drug discrimination can be used for comparison of similarities *between* APDs. Clozapine, in contrast to conventional APDs, can function as an effective discriminative stimulus: It has been shown that olanzapine can generalise to the clozapine stimulus within a narrow dose range, while haloperidol is ineffective [33]. In another study [34], risperidone fails to generalise to clozapine. A larger study of clozapine discrimination in rats shows that second generation APDs differ markedly in their ability to generalise to clozapine: Quetiapine produces nearly full substitution, while sertindole, risperidone, olanzapine and amisulpiride are ranked by decreasing efficacy to no substitution at all [35].

In squirrel monkeys it was also demonstrated that quetiapine can substitute for clozapine, olanzapine partially substituted, while risperidone, sertindole and remoxipride fail to show generalisation [36]. These results indicate pharmacological differences between novel APDs, even between the close analogues clozapine and olanzapine.

The clozapine discrimination is complex, involving muscarinic and 5-HT_2 antagonism as well as possibly α_1-adrenoceptor blockade [34, 37].

It has recently been shown that olanzapine in rats can function as a discriminative stimulus, to which clozapine generalises, thus suggesting similar profiles. However, other APDs need to be studied [38].

Symptom models of antipsychotic activity and EPS

Conditioned avoidance response (CAR)

Selective inhibition of CAR *versus* unconditioned escape responses has been used for characterisation of APDs for more than 25 years, but has declined in popularity as a screening procedure, probably because of its low capacity. Inhibition by APDs of the *acquisition* of CAR has also been used [39]. CARs are inhibited by all classes of APDs, including clozapine, and are from a mechanistic viewpoint sensitive to DA and α_1-adrenoceptor antagonists, but also to benzodiazepines, GABA agonists and morphine, compounds which in rats inhibit motor activity ([40]; see also review by Ellenbroek [41]). A procedure which eliminates diazepam as false positive has been described [42]. CAR inhibition induced by a selective D_2 antagonist is moderately reversed by co-treatment with antimuscarinic, but not by 5-HT_2 and α_1-adrenergic antagonists, suggesting that it is neither a pure psychosis nor EPS model [43, 44]. However, co-treatment with a D_2 antagonist and a 5-HT_{1A} agonist *increases* the inhibitory effect on CAR [44, 45]. These interactions are further discussed in the later section on drug-induced hypermotility.

Only few studies of novel APDs are available: olanzapine, quetiapine, risperidone, remoxipride, and ziprasidone inhibit the response [46–48]. Sertindole shows inhibitory effects at high doses [49]. Inhibition of CAR by APDs is seen at doses below those inducing catalepsy, but similar to those inhibiting hypermotility induced by DA stimulants and to doses which depress spontaneous locomotor activity. Since α_1-adrenoceptor antagonists are inhibitors of the CAR, antagonism of this receptor likely contributes to the activity of second generation APDs, while 5-HT_2 receptor blockade is without importance.

Inhibition of drug-induced hypermotility and stereotypy; cataleptogenic activity

These models are often used as the first *in vivo* screening of putative APDs and are therefore discussed in parallel. The rationale is the evidence from lesion and intracerebral drug injection studies that drug-induced hypermotility is mediated by the limbic DA system (particularly nucleus accumbens and tuberculum olfactorium, but cortical regions are also involved) [50–52], while stereotyped behaviour and catalepsy are associated with increased and decreased striatal DA function, respectively. Obviously the goal of a basic screening program is to optimise inhibitory effect on dopaminergic hypermotility, while minimising antistereotypic as well as cataleptogenic activity.

However, there are also several problems arising by using hypermotility models: First it is important to ensure that a test compound is effective at a dose which does not block spontaneous locomotor activity – in order to exclude non-specific effects (e.g. [53]). Second, inhibition of hypermotility is not a sufficient criterion for an APD, since false positives are known, e.g. GABA agonists [54]. Third, the effects can be demonstrated acutely within minutes to hours, in contrast to the slow onset of antipsychotic activity.

Despite the limitations useful information on the activity profiles of APDs has been gained from these models: Conventional APDs inhibit hypermotility and stereotypies induced by dopaminergic drugs (e.g. AMPH) and induce catalepsy at similar dose levels in rats [19, 53, 55]. Results from our own laboratory are summarised in Table 1. Stereotypy and catalepsy results correlate closely, in agreement with their presumed similar neuronal substrates, striatal DA blockade [56]. In contrast second generation APDs have very different activity profiles: Sertindole, clozapine and ziprasidone selectively inhibit hypermotility induced by AMPH without effects on stereotyped behaviour and catalepsy.

Inhibition of AMPH-induced hypermotility has been studied in parallel using two doses of AMPH (0.5 and 2.0 mg/kg), further adding to the complexity (see Table 1). While the conventional APDs inhibit hypermotility induced by both doses of AMPH with similar potencies, the effects of most novel APDs are much more potent against the low AMPH dose. Quetiapine and the 5-HT_{2A} antagonist MDL 100.151 (the racemic form of MDL 100.907 (now termed M100907) [57] which is in phase II/III clinical development) lack effects on catalepsy, stereotypy and on hypermotility induced by AMPH 2 mg/kg, but inhibit selectively the hypermotility induced by the low AMPH dose, thus differentiating these compounds from sertindole, clozapine and ziprasidone [4, 53].

Some second generation of APDs can be placed in an intermediate group between the above-mentioned and conventional APDs: Remoxipride fails to produce catalepsy in our experimental conditions, but inhibits only with marginal selectivity the AMPH-induced hypermotility *versus* stereotypy.

Table 1. Summary of potencies of haloperidol, second generation APD_s and the $5\text{-}HT_{2A}$ antagonist MDL 100.151 in models of antipsychotic activity and EPS. All data, except when noted, are from H. Lundbeck A/S. All values are in µmol/kg and indicate ED_{50} values in rats, except dystonia, which is expressed as minimal effective dose. For methods, see appropriate references

Compound	Inhibited spontaneous locomotor activity[a,b]	D-amphetamine (AMPH dose in parentheses)				Catalepsy[b]	Dystonia monkeys[b,d]	VTA** inhibition[e,f,g]	SNC** inhibition[e,f,g]
		Hypermotility (0.5 mg/kg[a])	Hypermotility (2.0 mg/kg[a])	Discrimination (1.0 mg/kg[c])	Stereotypy (13 mg/kg[b])				
Haloperidol	0.41	2.4	0.24	0.30	0.15	0.34	0.067	0.043	0.033
Sertindole	12	0.25	4.6	>23 ns	>45	>91	1.1–2.3	0.015	1.6
Clozapine	7.8	1.2	12	7.2	>120	>120	>76	56	>120
Risperidone	2.6	0.35	3.5	>6.1	11	17	0.061	0.2	0.3
Olanzapine	8.7	1.4	9.1	5.9	36	37	0.51	35	>32
Quetiapine	72	4.6	>40	>20 ns	>80	>80	14	38	29
Ziprasidone	12	0.47	5.7	nt	>190	>48	0.38	0.2	0.2
Remoxipride	>47	2.9	4.8	>47	15	>47	12	1.9	>12
MDL 100.151*	>54	0.64	>13	>13	>54	>54	nt	>0.83 (41% at 0.083)	0.8 (70% at 0.83)

ns: Indicates no significant inhibition.
nt: Not tested.
* Racemic form of MDL 100.907 (now M100907).
** Several of these ED_{50} values are calculated on ascending part of dose-response curves which often show biphasic shape; please refer to original articles.

Data taken from: [a] [53] [b] [4] [c] [25] [d] [95] [e] [91] [f] [93] [g] [107].

Others have similar results, including additional observation of catalepsy after high doses of remoxipride [55]. Finally, risperidone and olanzapine are effective in all models, but in contrast to conventional APDs they show some preference in blocking the hypermotility *versus* stereotypy response to AMPH, particularly when the low AMPH dose is used. Similar results indicating slight selectivity of olanzapine [33, 58] and risperidone [58–60] in these models have been published by others.

Comparisons between inhibitory potencies on spontaneous locomotor activity and on AMPH-induced hypermotility indicate that the effects on the AMPH 2 mg/kg dose are of questionable specificity. Only remoxipride and to some extent sertindole and ziprasidone have preferential effects on AMPH *versus* spontaneous locomotor activity. Much larger separation to the inhibition of spontaneous motility is obtained using the low AMPH dose, except for the conventional compounds.

It is difficult to explain all differences in drug profiles, as numerous mechanisms are involved. The non-selective inhibitory effects of conventional APDs across models can be explained by predominant DA D_2 receptor antagonism. This is the only receptor blockade that both leads to catalepsy and inhibition of AMPH stereotyped behaviour. In contrast, inhibition of AMPH-induced hypermotility can be achieved by different mechanisms: The effect of both doses of AMPH is inhibited by a selective α_1-adrenoceptor antagonist, e.g. prazosin, with marginal selectivity for inhibition of the lower AMPH dose [53]. Selective 5-HT_2 antagonists, e.g. ritanserin (5-$HT_{2A/2C}$) and MDL 100.151 (5-HT_{2A}) inhibit the effect of the low AMPH dose only [53]. In addition to the direct effects of selective receptor blockers, receptor interactions influence the actual potencies of individual compounds in these models. Unpublished observations in the author's laboratory suggest that combined α_1-adrenoceptor and 5-HT_{2A} receptor blockade enhances the inhibitory effect in the AMPH hypermotility models. Thus weak inhibitory effects on DA receptors, combined with marked α_1-adrenoceptor and/or 5-HT_2 antagonism will enhance limbic preference in hypermotility models.

Furthermore, additional antimuscarinic effect will reverse or weaken the functional consequences, particularly, of nigrostriatal DA receptor blockade (catalepsy, inhibition of stereotyped behaviour), while having less influence on behaviours mediated by DA receptors in the limbic system, e.g. drug-induced hypermotility [41, 43, 61]. The net effect of DA antagonism plus muscarinic antagonism is thus a separation of the potencies to block responses mediated by the limbic and nigrostriatal DA system. A similar result is obtained by combining a DA antagonist with a 5-HT_{1A} *agonist*, as demonstrated by interaction studies with 8-OH-DPAT, showing reversal of catalepsy induced by the conventional APD, haloperidol, and raclopride, while *enhancing* other effects of APDs [45, 62, 63].

The activity profiles of sertindole, clozapine and ziprasidone may thus be explained by their weak DA D_2 antagonism combined with potent α_1-

adrenoceptor and 5-$HT_{2A/2C}$ receptor blockade (all three compounds), with additional contribution of antimuscarinic activity (clozapine) and/or possibly 5-HT_{1A} agonism (ziprasidone, clozapine). Ziprasidone and clozapine have shown significant 5-HT_{1A} agonist activity *in vitro* [48, 64]. The 5-HT_{1A} agonism *in vivo* is controversial – it has been demonstrated by microdialysis experiments in frontal cortex [65], but not in hippocampus [66], and has been challenged in behavioural studies, including catalepsy experiments [62, 66, 67]. It should be noted that clozapine has agonist activity at the m4 subtype of muscarinic receptors which are abundant in basal ganglia [68]. The importance for its activity profile is unknown.

For the 5-HT_{2A} antagonist MDL 100.907 specific inhibition of drug-induced hypermotility *versus* stereotyped behaviour is also one of the main findings [57, 69]. Surprisingly, quetiapine has also a profile similar to a selective 5-HT_2 antagonist which does not correspond to its broad antagonist activity *in vivo* including potent α_1-adrenoceptor activity [4, 70].

The lower selectivity (hypermotility *versus* stereotypy blockade) of risperidone and olanzapine compared with clozapine is most likely caused by their more predominating DA antagonism compared with clozapine and sertindole. The partial selectivity is likely obtained by additional α_1-adrenoceptor and 5-HT_2 receptor blockade. It could be expected that the high *in vitro* and *ex vivo* muscarinic affinity of olanzapine would further enhance selectivity [71, 72], but the *in vivo* antimuscarinic activity is rather weak in our hands [4].

Finally, the profile of remoxipride is different from all other APDs. The failure to differentiate between the inhibitory potencies against the two doses of AMPH can be explained by its lack of effects on α_1-adrenergic and 5-HT_2 receptors, but the preferential inhibition of AMPH hypermotility compared with stereotypy and catalepsy is unexplained due to D_2 selective effects. However, there is some evidence for limbic selectivity demonstrated by *in vivo* binding studies at D_2 receptors to different brain regions [73].

Differential effects of novel APDs and the 5-HT_2 antagonist ritanserin have also been demonstrated after DA-stimulant-induced hyperactivity elicited by intracerebral injections into nucleus accumbens and tuberculum olfactorium, two regions belonging to the limbic system. The olfactory tubercle is particularly sensitive to 5-HT_2 antagonism (including the novel APDs sertindole, risperidone and olanzapine), while haloperidol is more potent in nucleus accumbens [52, 74]. While it is not clear how these results are related to the clinical profiles of the compounds, they do indicate that the hyperactivity models are more complex than generally assumed. These results, together with the previously discussed results with different AMPH doses, point to a heterogeneous regulation of dopaminergic hypermotility, shown both pharmacologically and anatomically. Even α_1-adrenoceptors in frontal cortex influence AMPH-induced hypermotility [51].

Non-competitive NMDA antagonists (phencyclidine (PCP) or dizocilpine (MK-801)) also induce hypermotility and stereotyped behaviour in rodents (though of different phenotype than that of AMPH), and this model is used for evaluation of APDs. The rationale is that PCP induces both positive and negative symptoms in humans, and inhibition of PCP-induced hypermotility might accordingly be a broader model of psychotic symptoms. However, this is probably an oversimplification, since other PCP-induced behavioural parameters (e.g. social withdrawal) have better face validity to negative symptoms than hypermotility [75]; see Ellenbroek et al., this volume).

The dose of PCP and dizocilpine used in hypermotility experiments should be carefully selected, since high doses lack behavioural specificity [76] and induce neurotoxicity [77]. At high doses no co-ordinated motor activity remains, which makes questionable the validity of antagonist experiments (e.g. [78]). No marked differences between the potencies for inhibition of AMPH- or PCP-induced hypermotility in rats are found with remoxipride, sertindole, risperidone, clozapine and haloperidol. Remoxipride and sertindole are the only APDs showing PCP inhibition in the absence of suppression of spontaneous motor behaviour, while sertindole as the only APD that has a marginally selective antagonistic effect against PCP compared with AMPH [79]. In a study in mice haloperidol and risperidone show similar potencies for inhibition of apomorphine-induced climbing behaviour and of dizocilpine-induced locomotion, while clozapine and olanzapine have 10-fold preference against inhibition of dizocilpine [80]. The 5-$HT_{2A/2C}$ antagonist ritanserin and the α_1-adrenoceptor antagonist prazosin are weak or ineffective in both studies.

The lack of effect of ritanserin is in contrast to results of two other studies in mice in which 5-HT_2 antagonists (ritanserin, ketanserin and MDL 100.907) preferentially the effect of PCP [81]. In this study also olanzapine and clozapine have PCP-antagonistic effects at doses below those affecting spontaneous locomotor activity. These results are consistent with those of Carlsson [82] who showed that MDL 100.907 and ritanserin inhibit hypermotility induced by a high dose of dizocilpine in mice. A more recent study suggests that the 5-HT_{2A} rather than the 5-HT_{2C} receptor is important, since the inhibition of dizocilpine-induced hypermotility is *reversed* by cotreatment with ritanserin [83]. This result may indicate that 5-HT_{2C} antagonism has a negative impact for antipsychotic activity, but the study needs confirmation by others.

The role of α_1-adrenoceptors in PCP- and dizocilpine-induced hypermotility is also controversial. In contrast to the above-mentioned negative results with prazosin there is also opposite results, where prazosin prevents both dizocilpine-induced hypermotility and DA release in nucleus accumbens, while being ineffective in the absence of dizocilpine [84].

In summary the hypermotility models (both those based on DA and glutamatergic mechanisms) are complex and suggest that the effects of conventional and novel APDs as well as α_1-adrenoceptor and 5-HT_2 antagonists depend critically on the experimental conditions (challenge dose of behavioural stimulant, animal species and possibly even strain). A critical evaluation of the effect of an APD on normal motor activity when given alone and of the behavioural specificity of the drug-induced hypermotility is warranted when interpreting experiments on drug-induced hypermotility. The results also illustrate the complex interaction between DA, α_1-adrenergic, glutamate and 5-HT receptors for regulation of motor activity. However, direct comparisons of APDs require that they are evaluated using identical experimental conditions.

As a general conclusion, the results confirm the hypotheses that 5-HT_2 receptor and α_1-adrenoceptor antagonism addition to the DA D_2 antagonism of second generation APDs are important for their limbic-selective profile.

Paw test

Still another approach to differentiate between conventional and novel APDs is the paw test described by Cools, Ellenbroek and colleagues [85]. Cataleptic responses are measured in rats separately as inhibition of retraction times of fore- and hindpaws after placing the rat in a four-hole box, and it is suggested that the responses are an indication of EPS potential and antipsychotic activity, respectively. A study of the limbic vs. striatal mediation of the two responses indicated limited regional selectivity between effects elicited by injection of sulpiride in dorsal striatum and nucleus accumbens, respectively [86].

Consistent with the discussion in the previous section haloperidol is equally effective in both paradigms, while the second generation APDs (sertindole, risperidone, olanzapine, quetiapine) have a four- to 20-fold selectivity on hindlimb retraction times [52, 87]. There is evidence for complex interactions between DA, 5-HT_{1A}, 5-HT_2 and α_1-adrenergic receptors in the regulation of these effects [88–90]. Thus, the paw model appears to give qualitatively similar differentiation between APDs as did the previously discussed hypermotility/stereotypy models, though only results from a few laboratories are available.

Electrophysiological effects on DA neurones in VTA and SNC

The screening models so far mentioned utilise acute drug treatment and as such fail to parallel the slow onset of antipsychotic activity (2–4 weeks) routinely demonstrated in clinical trials. However, the demonstration of a non-selective decrease in the number of spontaneously active DA neurones in ventral tegmental area (VTA) and substantia nigra, pars compacta (SNC) after repeated treatment with haloperidol for at least 3 weeks, and the selective inhibition of limbic DA neurones in VTA after clozapine treatment has prompted the use of the VTA/SNC model for characterisation of lead compounds in several laboratories. The mechanism is induction of a depolarisation blockade of the DA neurones and is most often, but not exclusively, induced by prolonged DA receptor blockade [15, 91].

The advantage of the model, in addition to its modelling of the time-course of APD treatment, is that limbic *versus* striatal selectivity ratio of the drug effect can be evaluated in the same group of animals. Furthermore, it fulfils the criteria that co-treatment with an antimuscarinic drug selectively reverses the effect in SNC, a parallel to the clinical use of antimuscarinic drugs for treatment of EPS [14]. A disadvantage is obviously the limited capacity.

Conventional APDs inhibit DA neurone activity similarly in both structures, while the second generation APDs have heterogeneous profiles as summarised in Table 1: Selective activity in VTA is provided by clozapine, olanzapine and sertindole. Quetiapine and MDL 100.151 (MDL 100.907) are non-selective in our laboratory, but show VTA selectivity at one dose level in another study [57, 92]. Risperidone and ziprasidone fail to show selectivity, and have not been studied elsewhere [93]. The reason for these differences cannot be explained based on the receptor profiles of the compounds, but most authors assume that selectivity depends on a delicate balance between the effects on DA, 5-HT, α_1-adrenergic and muscarinic receptors.

Dystonia in non-human primates

The ability of APDs to induce acute dystonia and other EPS symptoms in non human primates is considered to be the most predictive model of EPS in humans. Expression of symptoms is varied and they are analogous to those seen in humans. Furthermore, the model has high sensitivity when using monkeys primed to the dystonia effect of conventional APDs by long-term treatment. Casey [94, 95] used the potency of haloperidol to develop a criterion for predicting the dose level producing EPS in schizophrenic patients by correlating results in monkeys with the accepted dose-range of haloperidol for EPS in the clinic. Multiplication of the minimal effective dystonia dose in the monkeys by the factor 200 and 800 to obtain a dose interval gave valid predictions of EPS dose ranges for a number of marketed APDs. When this is done for novel APDs it appears that the antipsychotic dose-response curve could be dissociated from the EPS dose-response curve for some of the second generation APDs.

Clozapine is the only known APD that does not induce dystonia, while other second generation APDs all have potential to induce EPS at a certain dose level. However, large potency differences are apparent as summarised in Table 1: Sertindole has a large separation between predicted EPS dose and clinically effective dose [95]. Olanzapine, quetiapine and remoxipride are less selective, but still have reasonable margins with respect to clinically recommended dose range [96], while it is predicted that risperidone and ziprasidone have little or no separation. It should be mentioned that the dystonia thresholds with olanzapine, quetiapine and ziprasidone have been determined using a monkey colony at the laboratories of J. Gerlach in Denmark. Though of the same species, these monkeys have a marginally higher sensitivity than those at D. Casey's site (J. Gerlach, personal communication; [96]), and may thus lead to a slight underestimation of EPS safety indexes for these compounds.

There are only few comparative reports on novel APDs in the literature. One study [70] showed very weak effects of quetiapine. Unfortunately it is difficult to compare the studies, since oral administration was used in the latter study *versus* subcutaneous or intramuscular injection in other studies. Quetiapine has also been administered weekly to drug-naïve monkeys and induces less dystonia compared with that seen in a haloperidol-treated group [70].

The mechanism underlying the differences in dystonia-inducing potencies between novel APDs is not known, but it appears that all APDs with DA D_2 antagonistic effect *in vivo* induce dystonia. Dystonia is effectively reversed by additional treatment with a muscarinic antagonist. The muscarinic antagonism may thus contribute to the activity profile of clozapine and olanzapine. In contrast 5-HT_2 antagonist only weakly or does not influence the response, as demonstrated by combination experiments with haloperidol and ritanserin [97]. Agonism at 5-HT_{1A} receptors can also diminish haloperidol- induced dystonia (loc. cit.). No published evidence has evaluated the role of α_1-adrenoceptor antagonism in the dystonia response, but our own unpublished studies of the combination of haloperidol and the α_1-adrenoceptor antagonist aceperone do not suggest any reversal of haloperidol- induced dystonia.

Cognitive function

While the main focus in the search for novel APDs so far has been to diminish EPS liability, the influence on cognitive function has been relatively neglected. Schizophrenic patients show impairment of cognitive function, i.e. compromised attention, information processing and memory. Some symptoms can be exacerbated by treatment with classical APDs, while others are improved slightly [98]. Thus it becomes important to develop new APDs that do not induce cognitive impairment or even drugs that improve already existing deficits in the patients.

Very few comparative studies of cognitive effects of APDs have been published. The effect on spatial learning and memory in the Morris' water maze [99] has been studied. Haloperidol, risperidone and ziprasidone potently inhibit spatial performance, while sertindole, clozapine and quetiapine are ineffective. Olanzapine inhibits spatial performance after administration of high doses [100].

The delayed non-match to position (DNMTP) task can be used for evaluation of working and reference memory, which involves frontal cortical structures and hippocampus [101–103]. The same series of APDs have been tested in a visual-spatial version of the DNMTP paradigm ([104] and unpublished observations). Animals are trained to perform the test with a performance accuracy decreasing from 90–100% to approximately 60–70% with increasing delay time between 0 and 12 s. Most APDs induce marked inhibitory effects: Risperidone and haloperidol potently decrease performance, whereas olanzapine, ziprasidone and clozapine have lower potency. Sertindole and quetiapine are inactive. Haloperidol, clozapine and sertindole have also been studied after daily treatment for 3 weeks: Haloperidol retains its marked inhibitory effect, while tolerance develops to the effect of clozapine. Sertindole induces no deficits, similar to the results obtained after acute administration [105]. This indicates that different mechanisms are involved in the deficits induced by haloperidol and clozapine, since tolerance only develops to the latter.

The rank order of potencies of the APDs in the two models is identical, although different cognitive processes are required to perform the tasks. It is suggested that a marked DA D_2 receptor antagonism *in vivo* is mainly responsible for the APD-induced deficits. Selective inhibition of 5-HT_2 and α_1-adrenergic receptors do not induce deficits [104]. The differences between APDs might be of clinical significance as several of the novel APDs are weak or relatively weak DA D_2 receptor antagonists and hence, do not exacerbate cognitive deficits in schizophrenic patients.

Improvement of the cognitive disturbances in schizophrenic patients will be an important target for future development of better APDs. However, the above-mentioned studies have little chance to predict such effects, since cognitive performance is near-optimal in normal rodents. Availability of animals with baseline cognitive deficits relevant for schizophrenia will be of crucial importance for development of new screening procedures. One such possibility is the model of neonatal hippocampal lesions [6], where cognitive deficits have been described in the adult rats [106].

Conclusions

The results show that the second generation APDs clearly differ from the conventional drugs in pharmacological profile. Although they have similar profiles in many models, they also possess many differences, as is indicated throughout the text and in Table 1. Therefore, I will emphasise a need to choose a broad battery of *in vivo* screening models to get a valid characterisation of lead compounds. Furthermore, due to the many discrepant findings in the literature – of which a few have been mentioned and likely depend on experimental details – it is necessary to validate the models thoroughly with reference APDs. Selection of APDs based solely on *in vitro* receptor screening can be successful, but I would not recommend it, due to the unexplained differences between activity profile *in vitro* and *in vivo* seen with some drugs.

The proof of concept for the models described in this review is how well the models are able to predict the clinical efficacy and adverse effect profile of an APD. The second generation APDs have been on the market for a relatively short time (even some have not reached the market yet), so it is difficult to judge whether the individual differences between these compounds in animals will be confirmed by clinical experience. However, the differentiation between effects in models of antipsychotic activity and EPS that are obtained in animal models has been confirmed by phase III trials of clozapine, sertindole, quetiapine and olanzapine which generally show antipsychotic activity in the absence of EPS when using recommended dosages. Furthermore, the limited limbic selectivity of risperidone is also confirmed by clinical experience (see chapter for further discussion). No complete studies of ziprasidone and M100907 have been published so far.

For prediction of effects on negative symptoms the reader is referred to other chapters. Finally, the clinical predictability of the results obtained in cognitive test models in animals remains to be determined, and in addition the animal models need to be improved in order to be useful for evaluation of reversal of cognitive deficits.

Another important question is whether the animal models can be used to screen for the next generation of APDs with completely different mechanisms of action. This remains to be seen, but may be possible as long as new drug targets mediate their effects through some kind of interaction with the DA system.

References

1 Creese I, Burt DR, Snyder SH (1976) Dopamine receptor binding predicts clinical and pharmacological potencies of antischizophrenic drugs. *Science* 192: 481–483
2 Ashby CR, Wang RY (1996) Pharmacological actions of the atypical antipsychotic drug clozapine – a review [review]. *Synapse* 24: 349–394
3 Kinon BJ, Lieberman JA (1996) Mechanisms of action of atypical antipsychotic drugs – a critical analysis. *Psychopharmacol* 124: 2–34
4 Arnt J, Skarsfeldt T (1998) Do novel antipsychotics have similar pharmacological characteristics? A review of the evidence. *Neuropsychopharmacol* 18: 63–101
5 Pearlson GD, Petty RG, Ross CA, Tien AY (1996) Schizophrenia: A disease of heteromodal association cortex? *Neuropsychopharmacol* 14: 1–17
6 Weinberger DR, Lipska BK (1995) Cortical maldevelopment, anti-psychotic drugs, and schizophrenia – a search for common ground. *Schizophr Res* 16: 87–110
7 Shapiro RM (1993) Regional neuropathology in schizophrenia: Where are we? Where are we going? *Schizophr Res* 10: 187–239
8 Gray JA, Feldon J, Rawlins JNP, Hemsley DR, Smith AD (1991) The neuropsychology of schizophrenia. *Behav Brain Sci* 14: 1–84

9 Lahti RA, Roberts RC, Tamminga CA (1995) D_2-family receptors distribution in human *post mortem* issue – an autoradiographic study. *Neuroreport* 6: 2505–2512

10 Millan MJ, Peglion JL, Vian J, Rivet JM, Brocco M, Gobert A, Newmantancredi A, Dacquet C, Bervoets K, Girardon S et al. (1995) Functional correlates of dopamine D-3 receptor activation in the rat *in vivo* and their modulation by the selective antagonist, (+)-S 14297. 1. Activation of postsynaptic D-3, receptors mediates hypothermia, whereas blockade of D-2 receptors elicits prolactin secretion and catalepsy. *J Pharmacol Exp Ther* 275: 885–898

11 Merchant KM, Gill GS, Harris DW, Huff RM, Eaton MJ, Lookingland K, Lutzke BS, Mccall RB, Piercey MF, Schreur PJKD et al. (1996) Pharmacological characterization of U-101387, a dopamine D_4 receptor selective antagonist. *J Pharmacol Exp Ther* 279: 1392–1403

12 Patel S, Freedman S, Chapman KL, Emms F, Fletcher AE, Knowles M, Markwood R, Mcallister G, Myers J, Curtis N et al. (1997) Biological profile of L-745,870, a selective antagonist with high affinity for the dopamine D_4 receptor. *J Pharmacol Exp Ther* 283: 636–647

13 Tallman JF, Primus RJ, Brodbeck R, Cornfield L, Meade R, Woodruff K, Ross P, Thurkauf A, Gallager DW (1997) Ngd 94-1 – identification of a novel, high-affinity antagonist at the human dopamine D-4 receptor 1. *J Pharmacol Exp Ther* 282: 1011–1019

14 Chiodo LA, Bunney BS (1985) Possible mechanisms by which repeated clozapine administration differentially affects the activity of two subpopulations of midbrain dopamine Neurons. *J Neurosci* 5: 2539–2544

15 Grace AA, Bunney BS, Moore H, Todd CL (1997) Dopamine-cell depolarization block as a model for the therapeutic actions of antipsychotic drugs. *Trends Neurosci.* 20: 31–37

16 Gardner EL, Walker LS, Paredes W (1993) Clozapine's functional mesolimbic selectivity is not duplicated by the addition of anticholinergic action to haloperidol: A brain stimulation study in the rat. *Psychopharmacology* 110: 119–124

17 Schotte A, Janssen PFM, Gommeren W, Luyten WHML, Vangompel P, Lesage AS, Deloore K, Leysen JE (1996) Risperidone compared with new and reference antipsychotic drugs – *in vitro* and *in vivo* receptor binding. *Psychopharmacology* 124: 57–73

18 Arnt J, Hyttel J (1986) Inhibition of SK and F 38393 – and pergolide-induced circling in rats with unilateral 6-OHDA lesion is correlated to dopamine D-1 and D-2 receptor affinities *in vitro*. *J Neural Transmission* 67: 225–240

19 Sánchez C, Arnt J, Dragsted N, Hyttel J, Lembøl HL, Meier E, Skarsfeldt T (1991) Neurochemical and *in vivo* pharmacological profile of sertindole, a limbic-selective neuro leptic compound. *Drug Dev Res* 22: 239–250

20 Arnt J, Hyttel J, Larsen J-J (1984) The citalopram/5-HTP-induced head-shake syndrome is correlated to $5\text{-}HT_2$ receptor affinity and also influenced by other transmitters. *Acta pharmacol et toxicol* 55: 363–372

21 Brauer LH, Goudie AJ, de Wit H (1997) Dopamine ligands and the stimulus effects of amphetamine: Animal models vs. human laboratory data. *Psychopharmacology* 130: 2–13

22 Arnt J, Hyttel J (1990) Dopamine D-2 agonists with high and low efficacies: differentiation by behavioral techniques. *J Neural Trans* 80: 33–50

23 Shannon HE, Holtzman SG (1979) Morphine training dose: a determinant of stimulus generalization to narcotic antagonists in the rat. *Psychopharmacology* 61: 239–244

24 Nielsen EB, Jepsen SA (1985) Antagonism of the amphetamine cue by both classical and atypical antipsychotic drugs. *Eur J Pharmacol* 111: 167–176

25 Arnt J (1996) Inhibitory effects on the discriminative stimulus properties of D-amphetamine by classical and newer antipsychotics do not correlate with antipsychotic activity. Relation to effects on the reward system? *Psychopharmacology* 124: 117–125

26 Nielsen EB, Scheel-Krüger J (1986) Cueing effects of amphetamine and LSD: elicitation by direct microinjections of the drugs into the nucleus accumbens. *Eur J Pharmacol* 125: 85–92

27 Dworkin S, Bimle C (1989) 6-hydroxydopamine lesions of the nucleus accumbens attenuate the discriminative stimulus effects of amphetamine. *Drug Dev Res* 16: 435–441

28 Arnt J (1992) Sertindole and several antipsychotic drugs differentially inhibit the discriminative stimuluseffects of amphetamine, LSD and St 587 in rats. *Behav Pharmacol* 3: 11–18

29 Meert TF, De Haes PLAJ, Vermote PCM, Janssen PAJ (1990) Pharmacological validation of ritanserin and risperidone in the drug discrimination test procedure in the rat. *Drug Dev Res* 19: 353–373
30 Zimbroff DL, Kane JM, Tamminga CA, Daniel DG, Mack RJ, Wozniak PJ, Sebree TB, Wallin BA, Kashkin KB, Adan F et al. (1997) Controlled, dose-response study of sertindole and haloperidol in the treatment of schizophrenia. *Am J Psychiatry* 154: 782–791
31 Arvanitis LA, Miller BG, Borison RL, Pitts WM, Sharif ZA, Hamner MB, Herz MI, True JE, Velligan D, Knesevich MA et al. (1997) Multiple fixed doses of seroquel (quetiapine) in patients with acute exacerbation of schizophrenia – a comparison with haloperidol and placebo. *Biol Psychiatry* 42: 233–246
32 Corbett R (1995) Clozapine but not haloperidol antagonizes an MK-801 discriminative stimulus cue. *Pharmacol Biochem Behav* 51: 561–564
33 Moore NA, Calligaro DO, Wong DT, Bymaster F, Tye NC (1993) The pharmacology of olanzapine and other new antipsychotic agents. *Curr Opin Invest Drugs* 2: 281–293
34 Hoenicke EM, Vanecek SA, Woods JH (1992) The discriminative stimulus effects of clozapine in pigeons: Involvement of 5-hydroxytryptamine$_{1C}$ and 5-hydroxytryptamine$_2$ receptors. *J Pharm Exp Ther* 263: 176–284
35 Goudie A, Taylor A (1998) Comparative characterisation of the discriminative stimulus properties of clozapine and other antipsychotics in rats. *Psychopharmacology* 135: 392–400
36 Carey GJ, Bergman J (1997) Discriminative-stimulus effects of clozapine in squirrel monkeys – comparison with conventional and novel antipsychotic drugs. *Psychopharmacology* 132: 261–269
37 Nielsen EB (1988) Cholinergic mediation of the discriminative stimulus properties of clozapine. *Psychopharmacology* 94: 115–118
38 Porter JH, Strong SE (1996) Discriminative stimulus control with olanzapine – generalization to the atypical antipsychotic clozapine. *Psychopharmacology* 128: 216–219
39 Davidson AB, Weidley E (1976) Differential effects of neuroleptic and other psychotropic agents on acquisition of avoidance in rats. *Life Sci* 18: 1279–1284
40 Arnt J (1982) Pharmacological specificity of conditioned avoidance response inhibition in rats: Inhibition by neuroleptics and correlation to dopamine receptor blockade. *Acta pharmacol et toxicol* 51: 321–329
41 Ellenbroek BA (1993) Treatment of schizophrenia: a clinical and preclinical evaluation of neuroleptic drugs. *Pharmacol Ther* 57: 1–78
42 van der Heyden JAM, Bradford LD (1988) A rapidly acquired one-way conditioned avoidance procedure in rats as a primary screening test for antipsychotics: influence of shock intensity on avoidance performance. *Behav Brain Res* 31: 61–67
43 Arnt J, Christensen AV (1981) Differential reversal by scopolamine and THIP of the antistereotypic and cataleptic effects of neuroleptics. *Eur J Pharmacol* 69: 107–111
44 Prinssen EPM, Kleven MS, Koek W (1996) Effects of dopamine antagonists in a two way active avoidance procedure in rats – interactions with 8-OH-DPAT, ritanserin, and prazosin. *Psychopharmacology* 128: 191–197
45 Wadenberg M-L, Ahlenius S (1995) Antipsychotic-like profile of combined treatment with raclopride and 8-OH-DPAT in the rat: enhancement of antipsychotic-like effects without catalepsy. *Eur J Pharmacol* 294: 247–251
46 Moore NA, Tye NC, Axton MS, Risius FC (1992) The behavioral pharmacology of olanzapine, a novel "atypical" antispychotic agent. *J Pharm Exp Ther* 262: 545–551
47 Ögren SO, Archer T (1994) Effects of typical and atypical antipsychotic drugs on two-way active avoidance. Relationship to DA receptor blocking profile. *Psychopharmacology* 114: 383–391
48 Seeger TF, Seymour PA, Schmidt AW, Zorn SH, Schulz DW, Lebel LA, Mclean S, Guanowsky V, Howard HR, Lowe JA et al. (1995) Ziprasidone (CP-88,059): a new antipsychotic with combined dopamine and serotonin receptor antagonist activity. *J Pharm Exp Ther* 275: 101–113
49 Fagerquist MV, Wadenberg M-L, Svensson TH (1998) Effects of sertindole on conditioned avoidance response behaviour in rats. *Nord J Psychiatry* 52: 98
50 Kelly PH, Seviour PW, Iversen SD (1975) Amphetamine and apomorphine responses in the rat following 6-OHDA lesions of the nucleus accumbens septi and corpus striatum. *Brain Res* 94: 507–522

51 Blanc G, Trovero F, Vezina P, Hervé D, Godeheu A-M, Glowinski J, Tassin J-P (1994) Blockade of prefronto-cortical α_1-adrenergic receptors prevents locomotor hyperactivity induced by subcortical d-amphetamine Injection. *Eur J Neurosci* 6: 293–298
52 Cools AR, Prinssen EPM, Ellenbroek BA (1995) The olfactory tubercle as a site of action of neuroleptics with an atypical profile in the paw test – effect of risperidone, prothipendyl, ORG 52222, sertindole and olanzapine. *Psychopharmacology* 119: 428–439
53 Arnt J (1995) Differential effects of classical and newer antipsychotics on the hypermotility induced by two dose levels of d-amphetamine. *Eur J Pharmacol* 283: 55–62
54 Scheel-Krüger J, Christensen AV, Arnt J (1978) Muscimol differentially facilitates stereotypy but antagonizes motility induced by dopaminergic drug: A complex GABA dopamine interaction. *Life Sci* 22: 75–84
55 Ögren SO, Hall H, Köhler C, Magnusson O, Lindblom L-O, Ängeby K, Florvall L (1984) Remoxipride, a new potential antipsychotic compound with selective antidopaminergic actions in the rat brain. *Eur J Pharmacol* 102: 459–474
56 Arnt J, Creese I, Fraser CM (eds) (1987) *Structure and function of dopamine receptors.* New York: Liss, Alan R. Behavioural studies of dopamine receptors: evidence for regional selectivity and receptor multiplicity. 199–231
57 Sorensen SM, Kehne JH, Fadayel GM, Humphreys TM, Ketteler HJ, Sullivan CK, Taylor VL, Schmidt CJ (1993) Characterization of the 5-HT_2 receptor antagonist MDL 100907 as a putative atypical antipsychotic: behavioral, electrophysiological and neurochemical studies. *J Pharm Exp Ther* 266: 684–691
58 Hoffman DC, Donovan H (1995) Catalepsy as a rodent model for detecting antipsychotic drugs with extrapyramidal side effect liability. *Psychopharmacology* 120: 128–133
59 Janssen PAJ, Niemegeers CJE, Awouters F, Schellekens KHL, Megens AAHP, Meert TF (1988) Pharmacology of risperidone (R 64766), a new antipsychotic with serotonin-S2 and dopamine-D_2 antagonistic properties. *J Pharm Exp Ther* 244: 685–693
60 Megens AAHP, Awouters FHL, Schotte A, Meert TF, Dugovic C, Niemegeers CJE, Leysen JE (1994) Survey of the pharmacodynamics of the new antipsychotic risperidone. *Psychopharmacology* 114: 9–23
61 Arnt J, Christensen AV, Hyttel J (1981) Differential reversal by scopolamine of effects of neuroleptics in rats. Relevance for evaluation of therapeutic and extrapyramidal side-effect potential. *Neuropharmacology* 20: 1331–1334
62 Bartoszyk GD, Roos C, Ziegler H (1996) 5-HT_{1A} receptors are not involved in clozapines lack of cataleptogenic potential. *Neuropharmacology* 35: 1645–1646
63 Lucas G, Bonhomme N, Dedeurwaerdere P, Lemoal M, Spampinato U (1997) 8-OH-DPAT, a 5-HT_{1A} agonist and ritanserin, a 5-$HT_{2A/C}$ antagonist, reverse haloperidol induced catalepsy in rats independently of striatal dopamine release. *Psychopharmacology* 131: 57–63
64 Newman-Tancredi A, Chaput C, Verriele L, Millan MJ (1996) Clozapine increases dopamine release in profrontal cortex by 5-HT_{1A} receptors. *Neuropharmacology* 35: 119–121
65 Rollema H, Lu Y, Schmidt AW, Zorn SH (1997) Clozapine increases dopamine release in prefrontal cortex by 5-HT_{1A} receptor activation. *Eur J Pharmacol* 338: R3–R5
66 Assie MB, Cosi C, Koek W (1997) 5-HT_{1A} receptor agonist properties of the antipsychotic, nemonapride – comparison with bromerguride and clozapine. *Eur J Pharmacol* 334: 141–147
67 Kleven M, Prinssen EPM, Koek W (1996) Role of 5-HT_{1A} receptors in the ability of mixed 5-HT_{1A} receptor agonist/dopamine D-2 receptor antagonists to inhibit methylphenidate-induced behaviors in rats. *Eur J Pharmacol* 313: 25–34
68 Zeng XP, Le F, Richelson E (1997) Muscarinic m4 receptor activation by some atypical antipsychotic drugs. *Eur J Pharmacol* 321: 349–354
69 Kehne JH, Baron BM, Carr AA, Chaney SF, Elands J, Feldman DJ, Frank RA, Vangiersbergen PLM, Mccloskey TC, Johnson MP et al. (1996) Preclinical characterization of the potential of the putative atypical antipsychotic MDL 100,907 as a potent 5-HT_{2A} antagonists with a favorable CNS safety profile. *J Pharm Exp Ther* 277: 968–981
70 Migler BM, Warawa EJ, Malick JB (1993) Seroquel: Behavioral effects in conventional and novel tests for atypical antipsychotic drug. *Psychopharmacology* 112: 299–307
71 Bymaster FP, Calligaro DO, Falcone JF, Marsh RD, Moore NA, Tye NC, Seeman P, Wong DT (1996) Radioreceptor binding profile of the atypical antipsychotic olanzapine. *Neuropsychopharmacology* 14: 87–96

72 Bymaster FP, Hemrickluecke SK, Perry KW, Fuller RW (1996) Neurochemical evidence for antagonism by olanzapine of dopamine, serotonin, α_1-adrenergic and muscarinic receptors *in vivo* in rats. *Psychopharmacology* 124: 87–94
73 Köhler C, Radesater AC, Karlsson-Boethius G, Bryske B, Widman M (1992) Regional distribution and invivo binding of the atypical antipsychotic drug remoxipride – a biochemical and autoradiographic analysis in the rat brain. *J Neural Transm* 87: 49–62
74 Cools AR, Prinssen EPM, Ellenbroek BA, Heeren DJ. Palomo T, Archer T, Beninger R, editors (1994) *Strategies for studying brain disorders.* Madrid: editorial complutense; 2, Role of olfactory tubercle and nucleus accumbens in the effects of classical and atypical neuroleptics: Search for regional specificity 33–53
75 Sams-Dodd F (1997) Effect of novel antipsychotic drugs on phencyclidine-induced stereotyped behaviour and social isolation in the rat social interaction test. *Behav Pharmacol* 8: 196–215
76 Sams-Dodd F (1996) Phencyclidine-induced stereotyped behaviour and social isolation in rats: a possible animal model of schizophrenia. *Behav Pharmacol* 7: 3–23
77 Farber NB, Foster J, Duhan NL, Olney JW (1996) Olanzapine and fluperlapine mimic clozapine in preventing MK-801 neurotoxicity. *Schizophr Res* 21: 33–37
78 Maurel-Remy S, Bervoets K, Millan MJ (1995) Blockade of phencyclidine-induced hyperlocomotion by clozapine and MDL 100,907 in rats reflects antagonism of 5-HT_{2A} receptors. *Eur J Pharmacol* 280: R9–R11
79 Jackson DM, Johansson C, Lindgren L-M, Bengtsson A (1994) Dopamine receptor antagonists block amphetamine and phencyclidine-induced motor stimulation in rats. *Pharm Biochem and Behav* 48, 2: 465–471
80 Corbett R, Camacho F, Woods AT, Kerman LL, Fishkin RJ, Brooks K, Dunn RW (1995) Antipsychotic agents antagonize non-competitive N-methyl-D-aspartate antagonist induced behaviors. *Psychopharmacology* 120: 67–74
81 Gleason SD, Shannon HE (1997) Blockade of phencyclidine-induced hyperlocomotion by olanzapine, clozapine and serotonin receptor subtype selective antagonists in mice. *Psychopharmacology* 129: 79–84
82 Carlsson ML (1995) The selective 5-HT_{2A} receptor antagonist MDL 100,907 counteracts the psychomotor stimulation ensuing manipulations with monoaminergic, glutamatergic or muscarinic neurotransmission in the mouse – implications for psychosis. *J Neural Trans Gen Sect* 100: 225–237
83 Martin P, Waters N, Carlsson A, Carlsson ML (1997) The apparent antipsychotic action of the 5-HT_{2A} receptor antagonist MDL 100,907 in a mouse model of schizophrenia is counteracted by ritanserin – rapid communication. *J Neural Transm* 104: 561–564
84 Mathé JM, Nomikos GG, Hildebrand BE, Hertel P, Svensson TH (1996) Prazosin inhibits MK-801-induced hyperlocomotion and dopamine release in the nucleus accumbens. *Eur J Pharmacol* 309: 1–11
85 Ellenbroek BA, Peeters BW, Honig WM, Cools AR (1987) The paw test: a behavioural paradigm for differentiating between classical and atypical neuroleptic drugs. *Psychopharmacology* 93: 343–348
86 Prinssen EPM, Ellenbroek BA, Stamatovic B, Cools AR (1995) Role of striatal dopamine D_2 receptors in the paw test, an animal model for the therapeutic efficacy and extrapyramidal side-effects of neuroleptic drugs. *Brain Res* 673: 283–289
87 Ellenbroek BA, Lubbers LJ, Cools AR (1996) Activity of seroquel (ICI 204,636) in animal models for atypical properties of antipsychotics – a comparison with clozapine. *Neuropsychopharmacol* 15: 406–416
88 Ellenbroek BA, Prinssen EPM, Cools AR (1994) The Role of serotonin receptor subtypes in the behavioural effects of neuroleptic drugs. A paw test study in rats. *Eur J Neurosci* 6: 1–8
89 Prinssen EPM, Ellenbroek BA, Cools AR (1994) Combined antagonism of adrenoceptors and dopamine and 5-HT receptors underlies the atypical profile of clozapine. *Eur J Pharmacol* 262: 167–170
90 Prinssen EPM, Ellenbroek BA, Cools AR (1994) Peripheral and central adrenoceptor modulation of the behavioural effects of clozapine in the paw test. *Br J Pharmacol* 112: 769–774
91 Skarsfeldt T (1992) Electrophysiological profile of a new atypical neuroleptic, sertindole, on midbrain dopamine neurones in rats: Acute and repeated treatment. *Synapse* 10: 25–33

92 Goldstein JM, Litwin LC, Sutton EB, Malich JB (1993) Seroquel: electrophysiological profile of a potential atypical antipsychotic. *Psychopharmacology* 112: 293–298
93 Skarsfeldt T (1995) Differential effects of repeated administration of novel antipsychotic drugs on the activity of midbrain dopamine neurons in the rat. *Eur J Pharmacol* 281: 289–294
94 Casey DE (1993) Serotonergic and dopaminergic aspects of neuroleptic-induced extrapyramidal syndromes in nonhuman primates. *Psychopharmacology* 112: 55–59
95 Casey DE (1996) Behavioral effects of sertindole, risperidone, clozapine and haloperidol in cebus monkeys. *Psychopharmacology* 124: 134–140
96 Gerlach J, Peacock L (1995) New antipsychotics – the present status. *Int Clin Psychopharmacol* 10: 39–48
97 Casey DE, Fog R, Gerlach J, Hemmingsen R (eds) (1995) *Schizophrenia:* Alfred Benzon Symposium 38. Copenhagen: Munksgaard; The nonhuman primate model: Focus on dopamine D_2 and serotonin mechanisms. 287–297
98 Green MF (1996) What are the functional consequences of neurocognitive deficits in schizophrenia? *Am J Psychiatry* 153: 321–330
99 Morris RGM (1984) Development of a water maze procedure for studying spatial learning in the rat. *J Neurosci Methods* 11: 47–60
100 Skarsfeldt T (1996) Differential effect of antipsychotics on place navigation of rats in the Morris water maze – a comparative study between novel and reference antipsychotics. *Psychopharmacology* 124: 126–133
101 Dunnett SB, Evenden JL, Iversen SD (1988) Delay-dependent short-term memory deficits in aged rats. *Psychopharmacology* 96: 174–180
102 Dunnett SB, Wareham AT, Torres EM (1990) Cholinergic blockade in prefrontal cortex and hippocampus disrupts short-term memory in rats. *Neuroreport* 1: 61–64
103 Sawaguchi T (1996) Functional modular organization of the primate prefrontal cortex for representing working memory process. *Cogn Brain Res* 5: 157–163
104 Didriksen M (1995) Effects of antipsychotics on cognitive behavior in rats using the delayed non-match to position paradigm. *Eur J Pharmacol* 281: 241–250
105 Didriksen M, Sams-Dodd F (1997) Effects of haloperidol, clozapine, and sertindole on cognitive function in rats after chronic treatment. *Society for Neuroscience Abstracts.* Vol 23, Abstr 747, 24
106 Chambers RA, Moore J, Mcevoy JP, Levin ED (1996) Cognitive effects of neonatal hippocampal lesions in a rat model of schizophrenia. *Neuropsychopharmacol* 15: 587–594
107 Skarsfeldt T (1993) Comparison of the effect of substituted benzamides on midbrain dopamine neurones after treatment of rats for 21 days. *Eur J Pharmacol* 240: 269–275

Atypical Antipsychotics
ed. by B. A. Ellenbroek and A. R. Cools

Simulation models for schizophrenia

Bart A. Ellenbroek [1], Frank Sams-Dodd [2] and Alexander R. Cools [1]

[1] *Department of Psychoneuropharmacology, University of Nijmegen, P.O. Box 9101, 6500 HB Nijmegen, The Netherlands*
[2] *Department of Psychopharmacology, Pharmacological Research, H. Lundbeck A/S, Ottiliavej 9, DK 2500 Copenhagen-Valby, Denmark*

Introduction

As discussed in Ellenbroek and Cools, Animal models, this volume, the development of simulation models for schizophrenia has gained momentum in the last decade through the recognition that not only symptoms, but also psychophysiological and psychological disturbances of the disease can be used. This has led to the development of models like prepulse inhibition (PPI), P_{50} gating and latent inhibition. However, the development of models simulating schizophrenic symptomatology has also improved considerably. Apart from the classical models, such as apomorphine induced stereotypy, models studying social withdrawal and models analysing aspects of anhedonia have been developed. Unfortunately, only few of these models have so far been used to evaluate the effects of (atypical) antipsychotic drugs. This chapter will therefore predominantly focus on the various models that have been developed and only describe the effects of (atypical) antipsychotics when rigorous screening has been performed.

An important issue with regard to the development of simulation models is the induction of a "*schizophrenia-like*" condition, since the aetiology and the pathophysiology of schizophrenia are still largely unknown. Simulation models have therefore, in the past generally resorted to the use of psychotomimetic drugs to induce a "*schizophrenia-like*" condition in animals. The most often used drugs are amphetamine and phencyclidine and their analogues.

Amphetamine ("*speed*") is known to induce a psychotic state [1, 2] in many individuals. Although it is generally thought that this psychosis only occurs after long-term treatment, Angrist clearly showed that dosage is a much more important factor [3]. Thus a single large dose may already induce an amphetamine psychosis [1, 2]. Moreover, Kalant pointed out that the psychosis seen after acute amphetamine intoxication was indistinguishable from that seen in chronic amphetamine abusers [2]. Studies performed predominantly in Japan showed that the amphetamine analogue methamphetamine produces very similar psychoses [4, 5]. When given to schizophrenic patients, amphetamine and analogues generally exacerbate the existing symptomatology. In an extensive review of the literature encompassing almost 1000 patients, Lieberman and colleagues found that 40% of the patients worsened after the application of psychotomimetics. In the nonschizophrenic patients only 19% showed a worsening [6], suggesting that schizophrenic patients are much more sensitive to drugs such as amphetamine. Recent studies have further substantiated this enhanced sensitivity of schizophrenic patients to dopaminergic agonists [7, 8]. Although there is little debate about the induction of paranoid hallucinatory behaviour by amphetamine, the induction of negative symptoms such as social withdrawal or anhedonia is less evident. Nevertheless some authors have reported signs of apathy and social withdrawal after (meth)amphetamine abuse [3, 4]. Griffith and colleagues reported that volunteers became depressed, spent most time in bed and lost interest in their surrounding and in their usual activities, and subjects became reserved and negativistic [9], a finding also reported by others [10].

Phencyclidine (PCP, "*angel dust*") was originally developed as a general anaesthetic by Parke, Davis and Co. in the late 1950s, but during the initial clinical trials it was discovered that approximately 30% of the patients, as they emerged from anaesthesia, developed psychotic reactions that had a close resemblance to schizophrenia [11]. PCP was soon after withdrawn from further clinical development, but it has received considerable interest as a model compound of schizophrenia. After intravenous administration PCP induces a confusional state characterised by feelings of unreality, changes in body image, profound sense of aloneness or isolation, disorganisation of thoughts, and amnesia [12]. In many subjects negativism and hostility also occur together with hallucinations and repetitive motor behaviour. These symptoms are similar to many of the primary symptoms of schizophrenia [13], and in addition it was found that PCP could produce schizophrenia-like impairments of primary attention, motor function, proprioception, and symbolic and sequential thinking in healthy volunteers [14, 15]. PCP was also administered to schizophrenic patients, and it was found that PCP could re-instate the acute phase of their illness and that the patients could not distinguish the PCP-induced symptoms from their own illness [12, 16]. A peculiar observation was also that whereas healthy volunteers would recover quite rapidly, schizophrenic patients could be affected by PCP for up to several weeks even after a single administration [17, 18]. In recent years a number of double blind studies using formal rating scales have been conducted with ketamine, a PCP-analogue, and these studies have confirmed that PCP-like compounds can mimic both the positive and negative symptoms of schizophrenia in healthy volunteers and in schizophrenic patients, including thought disorder, as well as some aspects of the cognitive deficits [19–23].

Although drugs such as amphetamine and PCP have been extensively used in simulation models of schizophrenia, the recent surge of evidence suggesting that schizophrenia is due to a disturbance of normal brain development [24, 25] has led to a number of novel approaches in trying to mimic a "*schizophrenia-like*" condition. Among these are very early lesions of the ventral hippocampus [26] or the dopamine system [27], early maternal deprivation [28], isolation rearing [29] and interference with normal cell division by prenatal administration of the mitosis inhibitor methylazoxymethanol acetate [30, 31]. Although these models have not been extensively studies so far, they represent a new and possibly important alternative to drug-centred simulation models [32].

Simulation models for anhedonia

Introduction

Anhedonia is the inability to experience pleasure and as such constitutes one of the key symptoms of schizophrenia, belonging to the negative symptoms or psychomotor poverty cluster. As discussed in Ellenbroek and Cools, Animal models, this volume, it may also be a valuable risk factor in the development of schizophrenia. Since anhedonia is usually measured using a rating scale (see Ellenbroek and Cools, Animal models, this volume) in which subjects have to evaluate a number of statements (using either yes or no), a direct translation to animals is not possible. Nevertheless a number of different paradigms have been developed in which aspects of anhedonia appear to be modelled. The general principle behind such models is that if animals are freely increasing a specific behaviour, it must represent a certain rewarding value. For instance when rats are given a free choice between water and a weak sucrose solution, they will show a strong preference for sucrose [33]. Several variations on this theme have been developed over the years, such as lever pressing for food reward or water intake [34, 35]. A special case of positively reinforced behaviour is the intracranial self-stimulation model, in which rats are implanted with an electrode, usually in the medial forebrain bundle. Olds and Millner discovered that rats rapidly learn to press a lever triggering a small electric current through the electrode [36].

In addition to measuring the total intake or the total number of lever presses, additional experiments have been performed to look at the effort an animal is willing to undertake in order to be rewarded. Theoretically, if an animal is less hedonic it would show less effort to obtain reward. A technique often used in this respect is the breaking point on a progressive-ratio schedule [37]. In this paradigm rats are trained to press a lever in order to obtain a reward. Once they have reached a stable performance, the number of lever presses required to obtain reward is increased after each reward using a specific regimen. For instance Loh and colleagues [38] studied the effects of clozapine on cocaine reinforcement using an exponential progression schedule (1, 2, 4, 6, 9, 12, 15, 20, 25, 32, 40, etc.). The breaking point is defined as the point where animals stop pressing the lever for a specific length of time.

Inducing a "schizophrenia-like" condition

In contrast to all other simulation models discussed in this chapter, very few attempts have been made to induce "*schizophrenia-like*" anhedonia in rats. A drug, which induces anhedonia should reduce sucrose intake, lower intracranial self-stimulation and/or decrease the breaking point in a progressive-ratio schedule.

The reducing effects of amphetamine (and related compounds) on food and sucrose intake have been reported several times [39, 40]. This is, however, usually regarded as a general anorexic effect of such drugs and not as a specific anhedonic effect. This is supported by the finding that amphetamine reduced normal feeding and sucrose feeding in a similar fashion [41]. Amphetamine, cocaine and apomorphine generally increase intracranial self stimulation [42], although in some animals reductions have been reported with apomorphine [43]. Using the progressive ratio schedule of reinforcement, amphetamine also seems to lack anhedonic effects, since it leads to increases rather than decreases in breaking point [44, 45]. Apomorphine has been reported to have no effect in this model [44].

The finding that dopamine agonists generally fail to induce anhedonia is not surprising. As discussed above, it is still unclear whether amphetamine can induce negative symptoms in humans or not. Furthermore, antipsychotics (predominantly dopamine antagonists) generally fail to affect negative symptoms such as anhedonia in schizophrenic patients. In fact, human data indicate that antipsychotics may induce anhedonia [46]. Animal data seem to support these findings, since antipsychotics reduce water intake [35], food intake [47] and intracranial self-stimulation [42].

One of the few models for anhedonia in which dopaminergic drugs seem to play a prominent role was published by Carnoy and co-workers [48]. Using an approach somewhat similar to the progressive ratio schedule the authors argued that drugs inducing anhedonia should be more effective on a low reinforcement schedule compared to high reinforcement schedules. The authors found that apomorphine (0.03 mg/kg) was much more effective in reducing food reinforcement when a fixed ratio schedule of 4 or 8 was used (i.e. four or eight lever presses are necessary for one food pellet) than when ratios is 1 or 2 were used. This effect was dose dependently reversed by amisulpiride and sulpiride, whereas pimozide and pipothiazine were also effective (although only one dose reached significance). Haloperidol, chlorpromazine, metoclopramide, fluphenazine and thioridazine were ineffective. One clear disadvantage of this (and most other paradigms) is the fact that antipsychotic drugs may influence performance due to motor deficits. Thus whereas amisulpiride effectively reversed the effects of apomorphine at doses of 0.5 and 1 mg/kg, the inhibitory effects was lost at 2 and 4 mg/kg.

Simulation models for social withdrawal

Introduction

Social withdrawal or asociality is a component of the negative symptoms and it reflects the ability, or rather the inability, of patients to establish normal social relations with other people [49, 50]. Classical antipsychotics are generally considered to be ineffective in treating this symptom (e.g. 50), whereas clozapine appears to have a partial effect [51–53]. The newer antipsychotics may also be effective [54–58], but studies in patients with predominantly negative symptoms remain to be conducted. A recurring problem in evaluating the effects of antipsychotics on negative symptoms is that the drugs themselves may appear to cause negative symptoms due to their side effects. The negative symptoms are therefore often subdivided into primary symptoms that are believed to be fundamental to the disorder, and secondary symptoms that include side-effects as a result of drug treatment and social withdrawal due to positive symptoms and depression (e.g. [59, 60]). A decrease in negative symptoms may therefore reflect a decrease in positive symptoms or changes in the level of side-effects instead of a specific effect on primary symptomatology.

Social withdrawal is probably one of the few symptoms of schizophrenia for which a behavioural correlate in animals can be identified that has a high degree of face validity. Most studies have recorded the number of social encounters or the duration of social contact and have interpreted a decrease in these behaviours as an indicator of asociality. The development and validation of animal models of negative symptoms therefore consists first of inducing a reduction in social behaviour and subsequently by demonstrating that atypical, but not typical antipsychotics, can at least partially reverse these deficits. Animal models of negative symptomatology have received renewed interest within the last couple of years as the focus in the development of new antipsychotic drugs has shifted from drugs lacking EPS to drugs with effect on other symptom groups. The most commonly used species are the monkey and the rat, and negative symptomatology is generally induced by d-amphetamine or PCP, however, studies suggest that some of the new models based on the neurodevelopmental theory of schizophrenia can also mimic this symptom group and these may gain increased importance.

Amphetamine and related drugs

In most primates, d-amphetamine and methamphetamine potently induce social withdrawal and isolation [61–65] although negative findings have also been reported [66]. These effects are in marked contrasts to the effects of d-amphetamine in rats, where even the continuous administration of high dosages for up to 5 days does not affect the level of social interaction [67]. The variable effects of d-amphetamine on social behaviour in different species restricts its usefulness as a model compound for negative symptomatology, because apparently only monkeys are highly sensitive to d-amphetamine and these type of studies are often very demanding.

Several groups have studied the effects of antipsychotic compounds on d-amphetamine induced disruption of social behaviour in monkeys. In this paradigm classical antipsychotics do not reverse the effects of d-amphetamine, whereas clozapine and quetiapine can normalise the behaviour [63, 69, 70]. Other types of compounds have also been tested and it has been shown that adrenergic antagonists, benzodiazepines and opiate antagonists are ineffective in treating the d-amphetamine induced social isolation [63,71]. The ability to alleviate the social withdrawal therefore appears to have some specificity for atypical antipsychotics, suggesting that this model has both face and predictive validity as a model of negative symptoms.

PCP and related drugs

Clinical studies have found that PCP can mimic many aspects of the primary symptomatology of schizophrenia, including the negative symptoms [11, 13, 71, 72], and in primates and rats PCP has been shown to induce social withdrawal [73–77]. In spite of this close correlation between clinical and animal studies only few laboratories have systematically used PCP in models of negative symptoms and these studies have been restricted to rats.

The most commonly used behavioural test for assessing the effects of PCP and other NMDA-antagonists on social behaviour is the rat social interaction test, where pairs of rats are placed in an arena and the duration of social interaction is measured. In this test PCP and the PCP-analogues (+) MK-801 and TCP, and ketamine dose-dependently induce social withdrawal at doses where they also precipitate psychotic reactions in man. The antipsychotic clozapine, remoxipride, risperidone, olanzapine and sertindole have been shown to partially reverse the PCP-induced social isolation after long-term treatment, whereas haloperidol and quetiapine do not affect this parameter consistently. The effects of these compounds correlate well with their clinical profile and it is seen at a clinically relevant dose [78–80]. An interesting aspect is that the effect on the PCP-induced behaviours is more pronounced after long-term treatment compared to short-term treatment in this model, which correlate well with the slow onset of antipsychotic effect seen in clinical trials. Several non-antipsychotic drugs have also been evaluated, including the anxiolytic compounds diazepam and buspirone, the antidepressant citalopram, the analgesic compound methadone, and naloxone, an opioid antagonist, and it was found that these drugs did not reverse the PCP-induced abnormal behaviours [80].

Together these studies suggest that PCP can mimic certain aspects of the negative symptoms in rats and that the effects of PCP can be alleviated by antipsychotic drug treatment, but not by other classes of compounds. This model may therefore have face and predictive validity as a model of the negative symptoms of schizophrenia.

Developmental models

Longitudinal studies of schizophrenic patients indicate that pre-schizophrenics in many cases demonstrate difficulty in establishing normal relations with other people and may avoid contact with their peers at school [81–84]. This has been interpreted as early signs of negative symptoms and has suggested that this group of symptoms may be present very early in schizophrenic patients. In contrast, the positive symptoms appear to develop during early adulthood, and the first acute psychotic episodes normally occur around age 18–25 in humans [85]. For developmental models of schizophrenia it is therefore reasonable to expect deficits in the social behaviour to be present both before and after puberty, whereas behaviours corresponding to aspects of the positive symptoms should only emerge after puberty.

Neonatal ibotenic acid lesion of the ventral hippocampus in the rat has been proposed as an animal model of several aspects of schizophrenia [26]. This lesion produces behavioural abnormalities, such as hyperlocomotion and deficits in prepulse inhibition that present themselves relatively late in development, i.e. after puberty, and some of these abnormalities can be normalised by chronic treatment with antipsychotics. The effects of neonatal hippocampal lesion on social behaviour have been evaluated in a single study with measurement before and after puberty [86]. The rats displayed reduced levels of social interaction at both time points, suggesting that this model could also mimic certain aspects of negative symptomatology. The rats were subsequently treated with clozapine for 3 weeks and although clozapine could normalise the locomotor hyperactivity it did not ameliorate the social interaction deficits. These findings suggest that neonatal hippocampal lesion models some aspects of the negative symptoms, but additional studies are needed to evaluate the predictive validity of this model.

Published data is not available on other developmental models with respect to their ability to model negative symptomatology, but preliminary findings with methylazoxymethanol acetate (MAM) induced developmental deficits suggest that this treatment can induce social withdrawal (Sams-Dodd, unpublished observations). Rats received a single treatment with 20 mg/kg MAM (i.p.) during the gestation period and were tested post-puberty in the social interaction test. Rats that had been treated either on Day 9, 10, 11 or 12 did not display any effects of the treatment, whereas rats treated on Day 13, 15 or 17 demonstrated reduced levels of social interaction. In addition rats treated on Day 17 were hyperactive and had cognitive deficits [87]. These findings suggest that this may be a possible model of schizophrenia, but studies on the ability of antipsychotic drugs to reduce this symptomatology remain to be conducted and are necessary to evaluate the predictive validity of the model.

Simulation models for P_{50} gating

Introduction

The reduction in amplitude of a positive wave in the auditory evoked potential by prior application of the same stimulus is generally referred to as P_{50} gating. This gating is reduced in schizophrenic patients, but also in acute manic patients (Ellenbroek and Cools, Animal models, this volume). Since neither the evoked potential nor the gating appears to be influenced by attentional processes [88], this paradigm lends itself for the translation to animal models

Adler et al. were the first to demonstrate that gating of auditory evoked potentials also occurs in rats [89]. When recorded from the vertex, they observed four different components, two positive (P_{15} and P_{35}) and two negative ones (N_{25} and N_{50}). The authors also showed that Sprague Dawley rats obtained from another breeder showed a different evoked potential (component P_{35} was missing), suggesting that genetic factors may influence the evoked potential. We have also studied the auditory evoked potentials and found similar results, with a strong negative component occurring approximately 50 ms after stimulus presentation [90]. Of these four components only the N_{25} and the N_{50} showed clear signs of gating. The gating of the N_{50}, but not of the N_{25} was reduced by arousal, similar to the P_{50} in humans [91]. From these studies it was concluded that the rat N_{50} most closely parallels the human P_{50}. Miyazato and colleagues, [93] on the other hand, argued that the P_{13} in rats most closely parallels the human P_{50} since both are sleep-state dependent, undergo rapid habituation and are sensitive to scopolamine. As discussed elsewhere [90] the debate is not yet resolved but it should be kept in mind that N_{50} gating is also sleep state dependent [92] and that the P_{13} is insensitive to amphetamine [93].

The effects of amphetamine and related drugs on sensory gating

Adler and his colleagues showed that amphetamine reduces sensory gating in rats [89]. This reduction in sensory gating was due to a reduction in the amplitude of the first evoked potential, with relative little effect on the amplitude of the second potential [94, 95]. This seems to be in partial agreement with the clinical literature, where decreases in the amplitude of the first evoked potential of schizophrenic patients were reported in some studies [96], but not in all.

Relatively few studies have investigated the effects of antipsychotics on the amphetamine-induced disturbance of sensory gating. Haloperidol was found to significantly antagonise the effects of amphetamine [89], an effect also seen with the selective D_1 antagonist SCH 23390 [95]. Although sulpiride was reported to be without effect [95], this may have been due to the relatively low dose used (40 mg/kg), which already produced a non-significant reduction of almost 50%. Although these data seem to support a role for dopamine in the amphetamine induced reduction in sensory gating, the role of noradrenaline seems to be much more prominent. Thus lesions of the noradrenergic system using DSP-4 completely prevented the amphetamine-induced disruption of sensory gating [97]. Likewise, the α_1-adrenergic antagonist phentolamine and the β-adrenergic antagonist timolol significantly attenuated the amphetamine-induced decrease in sensory gating. Surprisingly, it was recently shown that the 5-HT_2 agonist DOI also reversed the effects of amphetamine [98].

Overall the data tend to indicate that the amphetamine-induced decrease in P_{50} gating is more closely related to its noradrenaline- than to its dopamine-releasing properties. Given the fact that a number of atypical antipsychotics are strong α-adrenergic antagonists, such as risperidone, clozapine and quetiapine (see Leysen, this volume), one might expect these atypical drugs to strongly interfere with the amphetamine-induced P_{50} gating disturbance. On the other hand, it was recently shown that the 5-HT_2 antagonist ketanserin reduced sensory gating [98]. Since most atypical antipsychotics also have a strong 5-HT_2 antagonistic component, the net effect of these drugs is difficult to predict.

The effects of PCP and related drugs on P_{50} gating

Like amphetamine, PCP reduces P_{50} gating in rats [89]. Ketamine, however, was found to be without effect on auditory gating in rats [94]. As with amphetamine, this reduction in gating by PCP seems to be due to a reduction in the amplitude of the first P_{50} wave.

In the only study on the pharmacology of the PCP-induced disruption of P_{50} performed so far, haloperidol was found to reverse the disruption [89]. This is in sharp contrast to the effects of PCP on prepulse inhibition (see below), which seem to be insensitive to haloperidol and most other antipsychotics. A possible explanation for this discrepancy may be the additional inhibitory action of PCP on the dopamine transporter [99]. Since the effects of PCP on P_{50} gating were seen at higher doses than the effects on prepulse inhibition, the inhibition of dopamine re-uptake may be more important in the P_{50} gating paradigm. Since ketamine has very little effect on the dopamine re-uptake, this may also explain why this drug does not affect P_{50} gating.

Developmental manipulations and P_{50} gating

As with pharmacological manipulations, very few attempts have been made to affect sensory gating by manipulating animals early in development. Stevens et al. recently showed that 6-OHDA lesions at postnatal day 7 did not affect sensory gating in adult rats, although it did prevent the effects of amphetamine [100]. Isolation rearing reduced sensory gating in Sprague Dawley rats [101], although similar social isolation after weaning had no effect on sensory gating in Wistar rats (DeBruin et al., unpublished data). The effects seen in Sprague Dawley rats could not be reversed by haloperidol treatment, but were sensitive to nicotine pre-treatment. We recently found that a single period of maternal deprivation at postnatal day 9 induced a decrease in sensory gating in adult rats (Ellenbroek et al., unpublished data). So far the effects of antipsychotics on these sensory gating deficits have not been studied.

Simulation models for latent inhibition

Introduction

As discussed in Ellenbroek and Cools, Animal models, this volume, latent inhibition refers to the retarding effect of stimulus pre-exposure upon subsequent stimulus-response learning. This implies that latent inhibition can only be measured in a learning paradigm. As discussed at length in other papers [102, 103] many different learning paradigms have been used to assess latent inhibition in rats, including the conditioned emotional response, the conditioned avoidance response and the conditioned taste aversion paradigm. In humans another paradigm has been used [104]. Essential for the comparison between humans and animals is that the learning paradigm *per se* is unimportant for the process of latent inhibition. In other words the mechanisms involved in latent inhibition should be the same, irrespective of whether a conditioned avoidance response or a conditioned taste aversion response is being used. So far, it is still unclear whether this condition is actually met. In fact Killcross and colleagues have argued that, at least for the effect of amphetamine the learning paradigm is of primary importance [105]. The authors found that the often observed disruption of latent inhibition by amphetamine in rats does not occur when a positively reinforcing paradigm was used. In humans, on the other hand amphetamine does disrupt latent inhibition when using a positively reinforcing paradigm [106]. Nevertheless, a number of the inconsistencies reported in the literature (both in the clinical and in the animal literature) may be due to the differences in learning paradigms used.

Amphetamine and related drugs

Amphetamine has been found to disrupt latent inhibition in virtually all studies reported to date, using the conditioned avoidance response [107], the conditioned emotional response [108] and the conditioned taste aversion paradigm [109]. The only exception known to date is the study by Killcross et al. [106], where a positively reinforcing paradigm was used. It is at present unclear whether other dopamine agonists also disrupt latent inhibition. Feldon and colleagues reported that the D_1 agonists SKF 38393, the D_2 agonist quinpirole and the mixed $D_{1/2}$ agonist apomorphine did not affect latent inhibition in the conditioned emotional paradigm [110]. We have recently shown that, using the conditioned taste aversion paradigm, apomorphine, but not 7-OHDPAT reduced latent inhibition [111].

The amphetamine-induced disruption in latent inhibition is reversed by all antipsychotics tested so far. Thus chlorpromazine [107], haloperidol [112], sertindole [113], clozapine [114] and MDL 100,907 [115] all reverse the effects of amphetamine on latent inhibition. Very few non-antipsychotic drugs have so far been tested on the amphetamine-induced disruption of latent inhibition. Warburton et al. showed that the selective 5-HT_3 antagonist ondansetron reversed the amphetamine induced disruption of LI [112]. Since ondansetron is devoid of antipsychotic activity, this drug represents a false positive.

Phencyclidine and related drugs

The effects of PCP on LI have so far not been studied in any great extent. In an early study it as found that in doses of 1 and 5 mg/kg i.p. PCP did not affect LI using the conditioned suppression paradigm [116]. Recently, using the conditioned taste aversion paradigm, PCP was found to reverse LI [117]. The effects were, however, only seen when PCP was given 20 h before the preexposure and before the test, but not when it was given 15 min before the experiment. So far, the effects of antipsychotics on PCP have not been studied in the latent inhibition paradigm.

Developmental models

Weiner and colleagues were probably the first to point to the importance of rearing conditions in simulation models for schizophrenia. Using the conditioned suppression paradigm, they found that non handling of puppies during the pre-weaning period led to a decrease in LI [118]. When tested at an age of 3 months only males show a reduction in LI. When tested at 16 months of age, however, both males and females were found to show a reduction on LI [119]. The effects of non-handling are attributed to an enhanced "*emotionality*" or stress sensitivity in these animals as compared to handled controls.

In line with this finding it was found that short-term maternal deprivation (MD, a single period of 24 h) shortly after birth also disrupted LI [28]. This procedure also leads to an enhanced stress responsiveness in the offspring [120]. Since repeated maternal deprivation for shorter periods does not affect the HPA axis in the same manner [121] it is not surprising that this manipulation does not affect LI [122]. The effects of antipsychotics in these developmental models have not been investigated so far. Another technique for inducing changes in normal development is the isolation rearing procedure, in which rats are reared in isolation after weaning. This procedure does not affect LI [123].

Summarising, a number of different developmental manipulations have been found to disrupt latent inhibition. So far, however, there have been no attempts to study the pharmacology of these manipulations.

Simulation models for prepulse inhibition (PPI)

Introduction

None of the simulation models discussed so far have been so extensively investigated as the PPI model. This model has gained widespread interest because it can be assessed in humans and animals with almost identical techniques. The only differences being that in humans the eye blink response is recorded, whereas in animals the whole body response is usually measured. As discussed in Ellenbroek and Cools, Animal models, this volume, PPI is reduced in patients with schizophrenia (as well as in several other patient groups).

Although PPI can be observed in several sensory modalities (acoustic, tactile) and can even be seen using cross-modal techniques (i.e. tactile prepulse followed by acoustic startle stimulus), most experiments in animals assess the acoustic startle response. Generally the animals are exposed to a loud acoustic stimulus (in the range of 105 to 120 dB[A]), which involuntarily elicits a startle response. This startle response is reduced when the startle stimulus is preceded by a much weaker stimulus (usually only a few decibels above baseline) which by itself does not elicit an overt behavioural response. The degree of PPI depends both on the intensity of the prepulse (the stronger the prepulse, the stronger the inhibition) and on the interstimulus interval (most effective inhibition with intervals in the range of 50 to 100 ms).

Amphetamine and related drugs

Amphetamine is known to reduce PPI, similar to that seen in schizophrenia [124]. Other dopamine agonists such as apomorphine, 7-OHDPAT and methylphenidate [111, 124, 125] produce the same disruption of PPI. Most pharmacological experiments have, however, been performed with the direct dopamine agonist apomorphine.

The effects of apomorphine on PPI are reversed by all effective antipsychotics, including spiperone, raclopride, haloperidol and quetiapine [126–128]. Moreover, the potency of antipsychotics to block the apomorphine-induced disruption of PPI is well correlated with their clinical potency. The effects of clozapine are more equivocal. Thus Swerdlow et al. found that low doses reversed the effects of apomorphine, whereas high doses had no effect [127]. Varty and Higgins [129] failed to find a reversal by clozapine. A possible explanation for this discrepancy may be the use of different rat strains [130].

So far very few non-antipsychotic drugs have been evaluated in this model. The selective dopamine D_1 antagonist SCH 23390 has been reported to reverse the effects of apomorphine [127, 131] although others have reported no effect [132]. Selective dopamine D_4 antagonists such as CP-293,019, U-101,387 and L-745,870 have been reported to reverse the effects of apomorphine [133]. Although these drugs have not been tested extensively in clinical trails, preliminary data with L-745,870 are not encouraging (see Den Boer and Korf, this volume).

PCP and related drugs

Like dopamine agonists PCP disrupts PPI [135], an effect also seen with other non-competitive NMDA antagonists, such as ketamine and MK801 [134, 135]. Competitive NMDA antagonists, such as NPC 12626 or CGS 19755, on the other hand, do not affect PPI [136].

The PCP effects are not reversed by pre-treatment with classical antipsychotics such as haloperidol [137, 138], nor by raclopride [138, 139]. There is some evidence that the atypical antipsychotic clozapine may reverse the effects of PCP or MK 801 [139], although others have failed to replicate this [129, 138, 140, 141]. Remoxipride [138], olanzapine [142] and quetiapine [143] have also been reported to reverse the effects of PCP. Several non-antipsychotics have also been tested on their ability to reverse the PCP induced disruption of PPI. The selective 5-HT_2 antagonists ritanserin and ketanserin, the selective D_1 antagonist SCH 23390, the selective M1 muscarinic antagonist pirenzepine and the selective $GABA_a$ antagonist pitrazepin all failed to affect the effects of PCP [144]. The only drug found to reverse the effects of PCP on PPI was the selective α_1 antagonist prazosin. Overall, the data suggest that the PCP induced disruption of PPI is resistant to most drugs (including most antipsychotics) and can only be reversed by a few atypical antipsychotics.

Developmental models

Since PPI is such an often used animal model, it is not surprising that many of the consequences of early manipulations have also been evaluated in this model. Thus PPI is disrupted by neonatal hippocampal lesion [145], by neonatal 6-OHDA lesion [27] early maternal deprivation [146] and by isolation rearing [29]. Interestingly, the effects of neonatal hippocampal lesions and of maternal deprivation appear only after puberty, suggesting a face validity with schizophrenia. The effects of isolation rearing strongly depend on the genetic background of the animals. Thus hooded Listar rats appear very sensitive to isolation rearing, whereas only a small disruptive effect was seen in Wistar rats [147, 148]. In hooded Fawn rats an enhancement of PPI was seen after isolation rearing [147].

Relatively few pharmacological studies have been performed with these developmental models. The effects of maternal deprivation could be temporarily reversed by pre-treatment with haloperidol or quetiapine, but other drugs have not been tested [146]. Neither the effects of early postnatal ibotenic acid nor of 6-OHDA treatment have been pharmacologically evaluated. The disruptive effects of isolation rearing can be reversed by haloperidol, raclopride, clozapine, risperidone, olanzapine and quetiapine [29, 129, 149].

Conclusions

The development of animal models for schizophrenia has greatly improved in the last decade for two important reasons. First it was realised that certain psychological and psychophysiological disturbances of schizophrenic patients can be modelled in animals with virtually identical techniques. This has lead to models such as latent inhibition, P_{50} gating and PPI, and the field will undoubtedly grow as we gain more insight into the cognitive deficits schizophrenic patients suffer from.

The second important factor is the increased knowledge on the aetiology of schizophrenia. Although the exact cause (or causes) of the illness is (are) still largely unknown, it has now become clear that schizophrenia is (at least in part) due to a disturbed development of the central nervous system. This has lead to a large number of studies investigating the long-term consequences of, for instance, early ventral hippocampal lesions, isolation rearing and maternal deprivation. So far these manipulations have given us a lot of insight into the behavioural effects of such early manipulations. The overall results are displayed in Table 1.

From this table it is clear where our knowledge is already quite extensive and where gaps are still present. Most of the manipulations have concentrated on PPI and P_{50} gating. Relatively few studies have dealt with the problem of the negative symptoms such as social isolation and especially

Table 1. Summary of the simulation models for schizophrenia. +: indicates some studies reported positive finding (i.e. disruption by the treatment of reversal by antipsychotics); ++: indicates most studies reported positive findings; –: indicates some studies reported negative findings; – –: indicates most studies reported negative findings; 0: no studies known

	Anhedonia	Social isolation	P_{50} gating	Latent inhibition	PPI
Amphetamine	–	+/– [a]	++	++/– [b]	++
Cl. AP	0	–	+	++	++
Atyp AP	0	+	0	++	++
Phencyclidine	–	++	+	+/–	++
Cl. AP	0	– –	+	0	– –
Atyp AP	0	+/– [c]	0	0	+/–
Hippo lesion	0	+	0	0	+
Cl. AP	0	0	0	0	0
Atyp AP	0	0	0	0	0
6OHDA lesion	0	0	–	0	+
Cl. AP	0	0	0	0	0
Atyp AP	0	0	0	0	0
Isolation rearing	0	0	+	–	++
Cl. AP	0	0	0	0	++
Atyp AP	0	0	0	0	+/–
Maternal deprivation	0	0	+	+	+
Cl. AP	0	0	0	0	+
Atyp AP	0	0	0	0	+

[a]: Amphetamine induces social isolation in monkeys, but not in rats.
[b]: The effects of amphetamine on latent inhibition appear dependent upon the paradigm used.
[c]: Atypical antipsychotics seem to partially reverse the effects of phencyclidine.

anhedonia. A second clear gap in our knowledge is the relative lack of pharmacological studies. Thus the effects of antipsychotics on the alterations seen after early ventral hippocampus lesions or maternal deprivation have not been very extensively studied. A positive exception is the isolation rearing model, of which the pharmacology has been extensively studied.

In summary, the last couple of years has led to a large increase in animal model for (aspects) of schizophrenia. Undoubtedly, when more studies have been performed and more pharmacological evaluation has taken place, we will be able to better determine the validity of these models for schizophrenia. It is not unlikely that these models will help us develop completely new pharmacological approaches to this severe psychiatric disorder.

References

1 Connell PH (1958) *Amphetamine psychosis*, Maudsley Monographs 5, Oxford University Press, London
2 Kalant OJ (1973) *The amphetamines: toxicity and addiction*. Brookside monographs of the addiction research foundation, University of Toronto Press, Toronto
3 Angrist B (1994) Amphetamine psychosis: Clinical variants of syndrome. In: AK Cho, DS Segal (eds): *Amphetamine and its analogs. Psychopharmacology, toxicology and abuse*, Academic Press, San Diego 387–414
4 Tatetsu S (1972) Methamphetamine psychosis. In: EH Ellinwood, S Cohen (eds): *Current concepts on amphetamine abuse*, US Gov. Printing office, Washington DC, 159–161
5 Konuna K (1994) Use and abuse of amphetamines in Japan. In: AK Cho, DS Segal (eds): *Amphetamine and its analogs. Psychopharmacology, toxicology and abuse*, Academic Press, San Diego 415–435
6 Lieberman JA, Kane JM, Alvir J (1987) Provocative tests with psychostimulant drugs in schizophrenia. *Psychopharmacology* 91: 415–433
7 Dolan RJ, Fletcher P, Frith CD, Friston KJ, Frackowiak RSJ, Grasby PM (1995) Dopaminergic modulation of impaired cognitive activation in the anterior cingulate cortex in schizophrenia. *Nature* 378: 180–182
8 Cleghorn JM, Szechtman H, Garnett ES, Nahmias C, Brown GM, Kaplan RD, Szechtman B, Franco S (1991) Apomorphine effects on brain metabolism in neuroleptic-naive schizophrenic patients. *Psychiat Res* 40: 135–153
9 Griffith JD, Cavanaugh J, Held J, Oates JA (1972) Dextroamphetamine evaluation of psychotomimetic properties in man. *Arch Gen Psychiatr* 26: 97–100
10 Angrist B, Sathananthan G, Wilk S, Gershon S (1974) Amphetamine psychosis: Behavioural and biochemical aspects. *J Psychiatr Res* 11: 13–23
11 Greifenstein FE, Yoshitake J, DeValut M, Gajewski JE (1958) A Study of 1-aryl cyclo hexyl amine for anesthesia. *Anest Analgesia* 37: 283–294
12 Luby ED, Cohen BD, Rosenbaum G, Gottlieb JS, Kelley R (1959) Study of a new schizophrenomimetic drug – sernyl. *Amer Med Assoc Arch Neurol Psychiatry* 81: 363–369
13 Dominion EF, Luby ED (1978) Abnormal mental states induced by phencyclidine as a model of schizophrenia. In: JO Cole, AM Freedman, AJ Friedhoff (eds): *Psychopathology and psychopharmacology*. The John Hopkins University Press, Baltimore, London 37–50
14 Rosenbaum G, Cohen BD, Luby ED, Gottlieb JS, Yelen D (1959) Comparison of sernyl with other drugs. *Arch Gen Psychiatry* 1: 651–656
15 Cohen BD, Rosenbaum G, Luby ED, Gottlieb JS (1962) Comparison of phencyclidine hydrochloride (sernyl) with other drugs. *Arch Gen Psychiatry* 6: 395–401.
16 Bodi T, Share I, Levy H, Moyer JH (1959) Clinical trials of phencyclidine (sernyl) in patients with psychoneurosis. *Antibiotic Medicine and Clinical Therapy* 6: 79–84
17 Itil T, Keskiner A, Kiremitci N, Holden JMC (1967) Effect of phencyclidine in chronic schizophrenics. *Can Psychiatric Assoc J* 12: 209–212
18 Erard R, Luisada PV and Peele R (1980) The PCP psychosis: prolonged intoxication or drug-precipitated functional illness? *J Psychedelic Drugs* 12: 235–251
19 Krystal, JH, Karper LP, Seibyl JP, Freeman GK, Delaney R, Bremner JD, Heninger GR, Bowers MB, Charney DS (1994) Subanesthetic effects of the noncompetitive NMDA antagonist, ketamine, in humans. *Arch Gen Psychiatry* 51: 199–214
20 Lathi AC, Holocomb HH, Medoff DR, Tamminga CA (1995) Ketamine activates psychosis and alters limbic blood flow in schizophrenia. *Neuroreport* 6: 869–873
21 Harborne GC, Watson FL, Healy DT, Groves L (1996) The effects of sub-anaesthetic doses of ketamine on memory, cognitive performance and subjective experience in healthy volunteers. *J Psychopharmacol* 10: 134–140
22 Malhotra AK, Pinals DA, Weingartner H, Sirocco K, Missar CD, Pickar D, Breier A (1996) NMDA receptor function and human cognition: the effects of ketamine in healthy volunteers. *Neuropsychopharmacology* 14: 301–307
23 Adler CM, Goldberg TE, Malhotra AK, Pickar D, Breier A (1998) Effects of ketamine on thought disorder, working memory and semantic memory in healthy volunteers. In preparation

24 Weinberger DR (1996) On the plausibility of *the neurodevelopmental hypothesis* of schizophrenia. *Neuropsychopharmacology* 14: 1S–11S
25 Pilowsky LS, Kerwin RW, Murray RM (1993) Schizophrenia: A neurodevelopmental perspective. *Neuropsychopharmacology* 9: 83–91
26 Lipska BK, Weinberger DR (1996) Hippocampal damage in the neonatal rat as a model of some aspects of schizophrenia. In: N Kato (ed): *The hippocampus: functions and clinical relevance*. Elsevier Science, Amsterdam, 465–475
27 Schwarzkopf SB, Mitra T, Bruno JP (1992) Sensory gating in rats depleted of dopamine as neonates: Potential relevance to findings in schizophrenic patients. *Biol Psychiatr* 31: 759–773
28 Ellenbroek BA, Cools AR (1996) Maternal separation reduces latent inhibition in the conditioned taste aversion paradigm. *Neurosci Res Comm* 17: 27–33
29 Geyer MA, Wilkinson LS, Humby T, Robbins TW (1994) Isolation rearing of rats produces a deficit in prepulse inhibition of acoustic startle similar to that in schizophrenia. *Biol Psychiatr* 34: 361–372
30 Talamini LM, Koch T, Ter Horst GJ, Korf J (1998) Methylazoxymethanol acetate-induced abnormalities in the entorhinal cortex of the rat; parallels with morphological findings in schizophrenia. *Brain Res* 789: 293–306
31 Moore H, Grace AA (1997) Anatomical changes in limbic structures produced by methylazoxymethanol acetate during brain development are associated with changes in physiological interactions among afferents to nucleus accumbens. *Soc Neurosci Abst* 23, #926.8.
32 Ellenbroek BA, Cools AR (1998) The neurodevelopmental hypothesis of schizophrenia: Clinical evidence and animal models. *Neurosci Res Comm* 22: 127–136
33 Phillips G, Willner P, Muscat R (1991) Reward-dependent suppression or facilitation of consummatory behaviour by raclopride. *Psychopharmacology* 105: 355–360
34 Wise RA (1982) Neuroleptics and operant behavior: The anhedonia hypothesis. *Behav Brain Sci* 5: 39–87
35 Ljunberg T (1987) Blockade by neuroleptics of water intake and operant responding for water in the rat: Anhedonia, motor deficit, or both? *Pharmacol Biochem Behav* 27: 341–350
36 Olds J, Milner P (1954) Positive reinforcement produced by electrical stimulation of septal area and other regions. *J Comp Physiol Psychol* 47: 419–427
37 Van Haaren F (1993) Schedule-controlled behavior: positive reinforcement. In: F van Haaren (ed): *Methods in behavioral pharmacology*. Elsevier, Amsterdam, 81–99
38 Loh EA, Fitch T, Vickers G, Roberts DCS (1992) Clozapine increases breaking points on a progressive-ration schedule reinforced by intravenous cocaine. *Pharmacol Biohem Behav* 42: 559–562
39 Sofia RD, Knobloch LC (1976) Comparative effects of various naturally occurring cannabinoids on food, sucrose and water consumption by rats. *Pharmacol Biochem Behav* 4: 591–599
40 Borsini F, Bendotti C, Samnin R (1985) Salbutamol, d-amphetamine and d-fenfluramine reduce sucrose intake in freely fed rats by acting on different neurochemical mechanisms. *Int J Obes* 9: 277–283
41 Orthen Gambill N (1985) Sucrose intake unaffected by fenfluramine but suppressed by amphetamine administration. *Psychopharmacology* 87: 25–29
42 Wauquier A (1979) Neuroleptics and brain self-stimulation behavior. *Int Rev Neurobiol* 21: 335–403
43 Broekkamp CLE, van Rossum JM (1974) Effects of apomorphine on self-stimulation behavior. *Psychopharmacology* 34: 71–80
44 Poncelet M, Chermat R, Soubrie P, Simon P (1983) The progressive ratio schedule as a model for studying the psychomotor stimulant activity of drugs in the rat. *Psychopharmacology* 80: 184–189
45 Thomas JR (1976) Interaction between hyperbaric air and d-amphetamine effects on performance. *Psychopharmacology* 48: 69–73
46 Ellenbroek BA (1993) Treatment of schizophrenia: A clinical and preclinical evaluation of neuroleptic drugs. *Pharmacol Ther* 57: 1–78
47 Salamone JD, Cousins MS, Maio C, Champion M, Turski T, Kovach J (1996) Different behavioral effects of haloperidol, clozapine and thioridazie in a concurrent lever pressing and feeding procedure. *Psychopharmacology* 125: 105–112

48 Carnoy P, Ravard S, Wemerman B, Soubrie Ph, Simon P (1986) Behavioral deficits induced by low doses of apomorphine in rats: Evidence for a motivational and cognitive dysfunction which discriminates among neuroleptic drugs. *Pharmacol Biochem Behav* 25: 503–509

49 Andreasen NC, Roy MA and Flaum M (1994) Positive and negative symptoms. In: SR Hirsch, DR Weinberger (eds): *Schizophrenia*. Blackwell Science, Oxford, 28–45

50 McLaren S, Cookson JC, Silverstone T (1992) Positive and negative symptoms, depression and social disability in chronic schizophrenia: a comparative trial of bromperidol and fluphenazine decanoates. *Int Clin Psychopharmacol* 7: 67–72

51 Kane J, Honigfeld G, Singer J, Meltzer H (1988) Clozapine for the treatment-resistant schizophrenic: a double-blind comparison with chlorpromazine. *Arch Gen Psychiatry* 49: 789–796

52 Meltzer HY, Alphs LD, Bastani B, Ramirez LF, Kwon K (1991) Clinical efficacy of clozapine in the treatment of schizophrenia. *Pharmacopsychiatry* 24: 44–45

53 Breier A, Buchanan RW, Kirkpatrick B, Davis OR, Irish D, Summerfelt A, Carpenter WT (1994) Effects of clozapine on positive and negative symptoms in outpatients with schizophrenia. *Am J Psychiatry* 151: 20–26

54 Chouinard G, Jones B, Remington G, Bloom D, Addington D, MacEwan GW, Labelle A, Beauclair L, Arnott W (1993) A Canadian multicenter placebo-controlled study of fixed doses of risperidone and haloperidol in the treatment of chronic schizophrenic patients. *J Clin Psychopharmacology* 13: 25–39

55 Grant S, Fitton A (1994) Risperidone. A review of its pharmacology and therapeutic potential in the treatment of schizophrenia. *Drugs* 48: 253–273

56 Van Kammen D, McEnvoy J, Targum S, Kardatzke D, Sebree T, Sertindole Study group (1996) A randomized, controlled, dose-ranging trial of sertindole in patients with schizophrenia. *Psychopharmacology*, 124:168–175

57 Beasley Jr CM, Sanger T, Satterlee W, Tollefson G, Tran P, Hamilton S, Olanzapine HGAP Study Group (1996) Olanzapine vs placebo: results of a double-blind, fixed-dose olanzapine trial. *Psychopharmacology,* 124: 159–167

58 Casey DE (1996) "Seroquel" (quetiapine): preclinical and clinical findings of a new atypical antipsychotic. *Exp Opinion Inv Drugs* 5: 939–957

59 Raskin A, Pelchat R, Sood R, Alphs LD, Levine J (1993) Negative symptoms assessment of chronic schizophrenia patients. *Schiz Bull* 19: 627–635

60 Gerbaldo H, Helisch A, Schneider B, Philipp M, Benkert O (1994) Subtypes of negative symptoms: The primary subtype in schizophrenic and non-schizophrenic patients. *Prog Neuro-Psychopharmacol Biol Psychiatry* 18: 311–320

61 Ellenbroek BA, Willemen APM, Cools AR (1989) Are antagonists of dopamine D_1 receptors drugs that attenuate both positive and negative symptoms of schizophrenia? A pilot study in Java monkeys. *Neuropsychopharmacology* 2: 191–199

62 Scraggs PR, Ridley RM (1979) The effects of dopamine and noradrenaline blockade on amphetamine-induced behavior in the marmoset. *Psychopharmacology* 62: 41–45

63 Schiörring E (1977) Changes in individual and social behavior by amphetamine and related compounds in monkeys and man. In: Ellinwood EH, Kilbey MM (eds) *Cocaine and other stimulants*. Plenum Press, New York, 481–522

64 Miczek KA, Gold LH (1983) d-Amphetamine in squirrel monkeys of different social status: Effects on social and agonistic behavior, locomotion, and stereotypies. *Psychopharmacology* 81: 183–190

65 Nielsen EB, Lyon M, Ellison G (1983) Apparent hallucinations in monkeys during around-the-clock amphetamine for seven to fourteen days. *J Nerv Mental Dis* 171: 222–233

66 Sams-Dodd F, Newman JD (1997) Effects of administration regime on the psychotomimetic properties of d-amphetamine in the squirrel monkey (Saimiri sciureus). *Pharmacol Biochem Behav* 56: 471–480

67 Sams-Dodd F (1998) Effects of continuous d-amphetamine or phencyclidine administration on social behaviour, stereotyped behaviour and locomotor activity in rats. *Neuropsychopharmacology* 19: 18–25

68 Miczek K, Yoshimura H (1982) disruption of primate social behavior by d-amphetamine and cocaine: differential antagonism by antipsychotics. *Psychopharmacology* 76: 163–171

69 Ellenbroek BA, Lubbers LJ Cools AR (1996) Activity of *seroquel* (ICI 204,636) in animal models for atypical properties of antipsychotics: a comparison with clozapine. *Neuropsychopharmacol* 15: 406–416
70 Winlow JT, Miczek KA (1988) Naltrexone blocks amphetamine-induced hyperactivity, but not disruption of social and agonistic behavior in mice and squirrel monkeys. *Psychopharmacology* 96: 493–499
71 Davies BM, Beech HR (1960) The effects of 1-arylcyclohexylamine (sernyl) on twelve normal volunteers. *J Mental Sci* 106: 912–914
72 Siegel RK (1978) Phencyclidine and ketamine intoxication a study of four populations of recreational users. In: RC Peterson, RC Stillman (eds): *National Institute of Drug Abuse Research Monograph #21*. Washington DC, NIH Press, 119–147
73 Schlemmer RF, Jackson, JA, Preston, KL, Bederka JP, Garver DL, Davis JM (1978) Phencyclidine-induced stereotyped behavior in monkeys: antagonism by pimozide. *Eur J Pharmacol* 52: 379–384
74 Russell J, Greenberg B, Segal D (1984) The effects of phencyclidine on spontaneous aggressive behavior in the rat. *Biol Psychiatry* 19: 195–202
75 Steinpreis RE, Sokolowski JD, Papanikolaou A, Salamone JD (1994) The effects of haloperidol and clozapine on PCP- and amphetamine-induced suppression of social behavior in the rat. *Pharmacol Biochem Behav* 47: 579–585
76 Steinpreis RE, Kuppinger HE, Panos JJ, Hollenberg D (1994) Determining the source of PCP-induced social withdrawl in the rat. *Soc Neurosci Abst* 20: 169
77 Sams-Dodd F (1996) Phencyclidine-induced stereotyped behaviour and social isolation in the rat: A possible animal model of schizophrenia. *Behav Pharmacol* 7: 3–23
78 Corbett R, Camacho F, Woods AT, Kerman LL, Fishkin RJ, Brooks K, Dunn RW (1995) Antipsychotic agents antagonize non-competetive N-methyl-d-asparatate antagonist-induced behaviors. *Psychopharmacology* 120: 67–74
79 Sams-Dodd F (1997) Effect of novel antipsychotic drugs on PCP-induced stereotyped behaviour and social isolation in the rat social interaction test. *Behav Pharmacol* 8: 196–215
80 Sams-Dodd F (1998) Effects of diazepam, citalopram, methadone and naloxone on PCP-induced stereotyped behaviour and social isolation in the rat social interaction test. *Neurosci Behav Rev* 23: 287–293
81 Neuchterlein KH (1986) Childhood precursors of adult schizophrenia. *J Child Psychology* 27: 133–144
82 Auerbach JG, Hans S, Marcus J (1993) Neurobehavioral functioning and social behavior of children at risk for schizophrenia. *Israel J Psychiatry Related Science* 30: 40–49
83 Jones P, Rodgers B, Murray R, Marmot M (1994) Child developmental risk factors for adult schizophrenia in the British 1946 birth cohort. *Lancet* 344: 1398–1402
84 Done DJ, Crow TJ, Johnstone EC, Sacker A (1994) Childhood antecendents of schizophrenia and affective illness: social adjustment at ages 7 and 11. *Brit Med J* 309: 699–703
85 Eaton WW, Tien AY, Poeschla BD (1995) Epidemiology of Schizophrenia. In: JA Den Boer, HGM Westenberg, HM van (eds): *Advances in the neurobiology of schizophrenia*. John Wiley and Sons. Ltd, Chichester, 27–57
86 Sams-Dodd F, Lipska BK, Weinberger DK (1997) Neonatal lesions of the rat ventral hippocampus result in hyperlocomotion and deficits in the social behaviour in adulthood. *Psychopharmacology* 132: 303–311
87 Didriksen M, Sams-Dodd F, Arnt J (1999) Cognitive deficits in rats treated prenatally with the mitosis inhibitor methylazoxymethanol (MAM) at different time points during gestation. *Abstract International Congress on Schizophrenia Research; in press*
88 Freedman R, Mirsky, AF (1991) Event related potentials: exogenous components. In: SR Steinhauer, JH Gruzelier, J Zubin (eds): *Handbook of schizophrenia, vol 5, Neuropsychology, psychophysiology and information processing*. Elsevier, Amsterdam, 71–90
89 Adler LE, Rose GM, Freedman R (1986) Neurophysiological studies of sensory gating in rats: effects of amphetamine, phencyclidine and haloperidol. *Biol Psychiatr* 21: 787–798
90 Ellenbroek BA, van Luijtelaar ELJM, Frenken M, Cools AR (1999) Sensory gating in rats: Lack of correlation between auditory evoked potential gating and prepulse inhibition. *Schizophr Bull; in press*
91 Johnson MR, Adler LE (1993) Transient impairment in P_{50} auditory sensory gating induced by a cold-pressor test. *Biol Psychiatr* 33: 380–397

92 Miyazato H, Skinner RD, Reese NB, Mukawa J, Garcia-Rill E (1996) Midlatency auditory evoked potentials and the startle response in the rat. *Neuroscience* 75: 289–300
93 van Luijtelaar ELJM, Miller CAFJ, Coenen AML, Drinkenburg WHIM, Ellenbroek BA (1998) Differential effects of non-REM and REM sleep on sensory gating in rats. *Acta Neurobiol Exp* 58: 263–270
94 DeBruin NMWJ, Ellenbroek BA, Cools AR, Copenen AML, van Luijtelaar ELJM (1999) Differential effects of ketamine on gating of auditory evoked potentials and prepulse inhibition in rats. *Psychopharmacology* 142: 9–17
95 Stevens KE, Fuller LL, Rose GM (1991) Dopaminergic and noradrenergic modulation of amphetamine-induced changes in auditory gating. *Brain Res* 555: 91–98
96 Waldo MC, Adler LE, Freedman R (1988) Defect in auditory sensory gating and their apparent compensation in relatives of schizophrenica. *Schizophr Res* 1: 19–24
97 Adler LE, Pang K, Gerhardt G, Rose GM (1988) Modulation of the gating of auditory evoked potentials by norepinephrine: Pharmacological evidence obtained using a selective neurotoxin. *Biol Psychiatr* 24: 179–190
98 Johnson RG, Stevens KE, Rose GM (1998) 5-Hydroxytryptamine$_2$ receptors modulate auditory filtering in the rat. *J Pharmacol Exp Ther* 285: 643–650
99 Bowyer JF, Spuhler KP, Weiner N (1984) Effects of amphetamine, phencyclidine and related compounds on dopamine release from and uptake into striatal synaptosomes. *J Pharmacol Exp Ther* 229: 671–680
100 Stevens KE, Luthman J, Lindqvist E, Johnson RG, Rose GM (1996) Effects of neonatal dopamine depletion on sensory inhibition in the rat. *Pharmacol Biochem Behav* 53: 817–823
101 Stevens KE, Johnson RG, Rose GM (1997) Rats reared in isolation show schizophrenia-like changes in auditory gating. *Pharmacol Biochem Behav* 58: 1031–1036
102 Lubow RE (1973) Latent inhibition. *Psychol Bull* 79: 398–407
103 Lubow RE (1989) *Latent inhibition and conditioned attention theory.* Cambridge University Press, Cambridge
104 Baruch I, Hemsley D, Gray JA (1988) Differential performance of acute and chronic schizophrenics in a latent inhibition task. *J Nerv Ment Dis* 176: 589–606
105 Killcross AS, Dickinson A, Robbins TW (1994) Amphetamine-induced disruptions of latent inhibition are reinforcer mediated: implications for animal models of schizophrenic attentional dysfunction. *Psychopharmacology* 115: 185–195
106 Gray NS, Pickering AD, Hemsley DR, Dawling S, Gray JA (1992) Abolition of latent inhibition by a single 5 mg dose of d-amphetamine in man. *Psychopharmacology* 107: 425–530
107 Solomon PR, Crider A, Winkelmann JW, Turi A, Kramer RM, Kaplan LJ (1981) Disrupted latent inhibition in the rat with chronic amphetamine or haloperidol-induced supersensitivity: Relationship to schizophrenic attention disorder. *Biol Psychiatr* 16: 519–537
108 Weiner I, Lubow RE, Feldon J (1981) Chronic amphetamine and latent inhibition. *Behav Brain Res* 2: 285–286
109 Ellenbroek BA, Knobbout DK, Cools AR (1997) The role of mesolimbic and nigrostriatal dopamine in latent inhibition as measured with the conditioned taste aversion. *Psychopharmacology* 129: 112–120
110 Feldon J, Shofel A, Weiner I (1991) Latent inhibition is unaffected by direct dopamine agonists. *Pharmacol Biochem Behav* 38: 309–314
111 Ellenbroek BA, Cools AR (1996) Dopamine susceptibility and information processing. In: RJ Beninger, T Palamo, T Archer (eds): *Dopamine disease states*, Editorial CYM, Madrid, 447–462
112 Warburton EC, Joseph MH, Feldon J, Weiner I, Gray JA (1994) Antagonism of amphetamine-induced disruption of latent inhibition in rats by haloperidol and ondansetron: Implications for a possible antipsychotic action of ondansetron. *Psychopharmacology* 114: 657–664
113 Weiner I, Kidron R, Tarrasch R, Arnt J, Feldon J (1994) The effects of the new antipsychotic sertindole, on latent inhibition in rats. *Behav Pharmacol* 5: 119–124
114 Moran PM, Fischer TR Hitchcock JM, Moser PC (1996) Effects of clozapine on latent inhibition in the rat. *Behav Pharmacol* 7: 42–48
115 Moser PC, Moran PM, Frank RA, Kehne JH (1995) Reversal of amphetamine-induced behaviours by MDL 100,907, a selective 5-HT$_{2A}$ antagonist. *Behav Brain Res* 73: 163–167

116 Weiner I, Feldon J (1992) Phencyclidine does not disrupt latent inhibition in rats: Implications for animal models of schizophrenia. *Pharmacol Biochem Behav* 42: 625–631
117 Turgeon SM, Auerbach EA, Heller MA (1998) The delayed effects of phencyclidine (PCP) disrupt latent inhibition in a conditioned taste aversion paradigm. *Pharmacol Biochem Behav* 60: 553–558
118 Weiner I, Schnabel I, Lubow RE, Feldon J (1985) The effects of early handling on latent inhibition in male and female rats. *Dev Psychobiol* 18: 291–298
119 Shalev U, Feldon J, Weiner I (1998) Gender- and age-dependent differences in latent inhibition following pre-weaning non-handling: implications for a neurodevelopmental animal model of schizophrenia. *Int J Dev Neurosci* 16: 279–288
120 Vazquez DM, van Oers H, Levine S, Akil H (1996) Regulation of glucocorticoid and mineralocorticoid receptor mRNAs in the hippocampus of the maternally deprived infant rat. *Brain Res* 731: 79–90
121 Anisman H, Zaharia MD, Meaney MJ, Merali Z (1998) Do early-life events permanently alter behavioral and hormonal responses to stressors? *Int J Dev Neurosci* 16: 149–164
122 Lehmann J, Stöhr T, Schüller J, Domeney A, Heidbreder C, Feldon J (1998) Long-term effects of repeated maternal separation on three different latent inhibition paradigms. *Pharmacol Biochem Behav* 59: 873–882
123 Wilkinson LS, Killcross SS, Humby T, Hall FS, Geyer MA, Robbins TW (1994) Social isolation in the rat produces developmentally specific deficits in prepulse inhibition of the acoustic startle response without disrupting latent inhibition. *Neuropsychopharmacol* 10: 61–72
124 Mansbach RS, Geyer MA, Braff DL (1988) Dopaminergic stimulation disrupts sensorimotor gating in the rat. *Psychopharmacology* 94: 507–514
125 Caine SB, Geyer MA, Swerdlow NS (1995) Effects of D_3/D_2 dopamine receptor agonists and antagonists on prepulse inhibition of acoustic startle in the rat. *Neuropsychopharmacol* 12: 139–145
126 Swerdlow NR, Braff DL, Taaid N, Geyer MA (1994) Assessing the validity of an animal model of deficient sensorimotor gating in schizophrenic patients. *Arch Gen Psychiatr* 51: 149–154
127 Swerdlow NR, Keith VA, Braff DL, Geyer MA (1991) The effects of spiperone, raclopride, SCH 23390 and clozapine on apomorphine-inhibition of sensorimotor gating of the startle response in the rat. *J Pharmacol Exp Ther* 256: 530–536
128 Swerdlow NR, Zisook D, Taaid N (1994) Seroquel (ICI 204,636) restores prepulse inhibition of acoustic startle in apomorphine-treated rats: Similarities to clozapine. *Psychopharmacology* 114: 675–678
129 Varty GB, Higgins GA (1995) Examination of drug-induced and isolation-induced disruptions of prepulse inhibition as models to screen antipsychotic drugs. *Psychopharmacology* 122: 15–26
130 Swerdlow N, Varty GB, Geyer MA (1998) Discrepant findings of clozapine effects on prepulse inhibition of startle: Is it the route or the rat? *Neuropsychopharmacol* 18: 50–56
131 Hoffman DC, Donovan H (1994) D_1 and D_2 dopamine receptor antagonism reverse prepulse inhibition deficits in an animal model of schizophrenia. *Psychopharmacology* 115: 447–453
132 Schwarzkopf SB, Bruno JP, Mitra T (1993) Effects of haloperidol and SCH 23390 on acoustic startle and prepulse inhibition under basal and stimulated conditions. *Prog Neuropsychopharmacol Biol Psychiatr* 17: 1023–1036
133 Mansbach RS, Brooks EW, Sanner MA, Zorn SH (1998) Selective dopamine D_4 receptor antagonists reverse apomorphine-induced blockade of prepulse inhibition. *Psychopharmacology* 135: 194–200
134 Mansbach RS, Geyer MA (1989) Effects of phencyclidine and phencyclidine biologs on sensorimotor gating in the rat. *Neuropsychopharmacol* 2: 299–308
135 Mansbach RS, Geyer MA (1991) Parametric determinants in pre-stimulus modification of acoustic startle: Interaction with ketamine. *Psychopharmacology* 105: 162–168
136 Mansbach RS (1991) Effects of NMDA receptor ligands on sensorimotor gating in the rat. *Eruop J Pharmacol* 202: 61–66
137 Keith VA, Mansbach RS, Geyer MA (1991) Failure of haloperidol to block the effects of phencyclidine and dizolcipine on prepulse inhibition of startle. *Biol Psychiatr* 30: 557–566

138 Johansson C, Jackson DM, Svensson L (1994) The atypical antipsychotic, remoxipride, blocks phencyclidine-induced disruption of prepulse inhibition in the rat. *Psychopharmacology* 116: 437–442
139 Bakshi VP, Swerdlow NR, Geyer MA (1994) Clozapine antagonizes phencyclidine-induced deficits in sensorimotor gating of the startle response. *J Pharmacol Exp Ther* 271: 787–794
140 Hoffman DC, Donovan H, Casella JV (1993) The effects of haloperidol and clozapine on the disruption of sensorimotor gating induced by the noncompetitive glutamate antagonist MK 801. *Psychopharmacology* 111: 339–344
141 Wiley JL (1994) Clozapine's effects on phencyclidine-induced disruption of prepulse inhibition of the acoustic startle response. *Pharmacol Biochem Behav* 49: 1025–1028
142 Bakshi VP, Geyer MA (1995) Antagonism of phencyclidine-induced deficits in prepulse inhibition by the putative atypical antipsychotic olanzapine. *Psychopharmacol* 122: 198–201
143 Swerdlow NR, Bakshi VP, Geyer MA (1996) Seroquel restores sensorimotor gating in phencyclidine-treated rats. *J Pharmacol Exp Ther* 279: 1290–1299
144 Bakshi VP, Geyer MA (1997) Phencyclidine-induced deficits in prepulse inhibition of startle are blocked by prazosin, an alpha-1 noradrenergic antagonist. *J Pharmacol Exp Ther* 283: 666–674
145 Lipska BK, Swerdlow NR, Geyer MA, Jaskiw GE, Raff DL (1995) Neonatal excitotoxic hippocampal damage in rats causes post-pubertal changes in prepulse inhibition of startle and its disruption by apomorphine. *Psychopharmacology* 122: 35–43
146 Ellenbroek BA, van den Kroonenberg PTJM, Cools AR (1998) The effects of an early stressful life-event on sensorimotor gating in adult rats. *Schizophr Res* 30: 251–260
147 Hall FS, Huang S, Fong G (1997) Effects of isolation-rearing on acoustic startle and pre-pulse inhibition in Wistar and Fawn Hooded rats. *Ann NY Acad Sci* 8: 542–544
148 Domeney A, Feldon J (1998) The disruption of prepulse inhibition by social isolation in the Wistar rats: How robust is the effect? *Pharmacol Biochem Behav* 59: 883–890
149 Bakshi VP, Swerdlow NR, Braff DL, Geyer MA (1998) Reversal of isolation rearing-induced deficits in prepulse inhibition by seroquel and olanzapine. *Biol Psychiatr* 43: 436–445

The clinical evaluation of atypical antipsychotics

Atypical Antipsychotics
ed. by B.A. Ellenbroek and A.R. Cools

Clozapine: the first atypical antipsychotic

Dieter Naber, Christian Haasen and Christian Perro

Universitäts-Krankenhaus Eppendorf, Klinik für Psychiatrie und Psychotherapie, Martinistrasse 52, D-20246 Hamburg, Germany

Introduction

Clozapine was synthesised in 1958, and first clinical trials were carried out in the 1960s. These trials already showed that the typical motor side-effects did not occur under clozapine treatment. Although the antipsychotic effect was recognised early, the manufacturer was reluctant to propose the introduction of clozapine as an antipsychotic agent, as it did not meet the "psychopharmacologic dogma" that antipsychotic effect could not be expected without extrapyramidal motor effect [1]. In 1972, clozapine was introduced in Austria, Switzerland, and Germany, within the following 5 years in 30 other countries. More than 100000 schizophrenic patients had been treated with clozapine, antipsychotic effect and tolerance were shown in 13 double-blind controlled studies [2, among others]. The rapid increase in the distribution of clozapine dramatically stopped in 1974, when 16 patients developed agranulocytosis under clozapine treatment and eight of them died [3]. In many countries clozapine was withdrawn from the market, while in the German speaking countries, due to the intervention of several renowned psychiatrists, it was not withdrawn and since then is prescribed under precautionary restrictions. Pharmacological and clinical research on clozapine increased after Kane et al. [4] were able to prove the special effect of clozapine on treatment-resistant schizophrenics. That study led to the (re-)introduction of clozapine in most countries.

Clozapine is an atypical antipsychotic not only due to the pharmacology and clinical effect, but also due to the impressionable history [5, 6]. The large interest in clozapine is characterised by multiple review articles on the pharmacological and clinical effect [7–13], as well as 40 double-blind controlled studies and numerous open and case studies.

Indications

The risk of agranulocytosis forces a concise evaluation of risks and benefits for the indication for treatment with clozapine. Since the introduction into the US market in 1992, a world-wide restriction of the indication "only for the treatment of acute and chronic forms of schizophrenia" was implemented. For the treatment with clozapine the following criteria also have to be fulfilled:

1) normal white blood cell count before beginning treatment;
2) potential for regular haematological controls;
3) insufficient effect or tolerance of other antipsychotics.

In Germany, the treatment with clozapine can be carried out if the physician has answered all the above and has agreed (with signature) to carry out the responsibility for meeting the above criteria.

Treatment of non-schizophrenics with clozapine has been reported in many open studies as well as case reports, and has been practised world-wide [14]. In general, a treatment attempt is indicated for all patients with a paranoid-hallucinatory syndrome or psychotic symptoms, when typical antipsychotics did not bring sufficient results or were not tolerated. These indications, which are practised in many clinics yet not officially eligible, include, for example, delusional depression, manias, and organic psychosis. Especially for Parkinson patients, who developed a pharmacotoxic psychosis under dopaminomimetics, clozapine is clearly more effective than typical antipsychotics [15]. Furthermore, movement disorders such as Chorea Huntington [16], torticollis spasmodicus or tremor [17] are indications for clozapine treatment. Since these are not eligible indications for clozapine, treatment is therefore an individual evaluation on a case-by-case basis, where the physician carefully evaluates all risks and benefits of such a treatment.

Contraindications

Clozapine may not be prescribed:

1) when a hypersensitivity to clozapine exists,
2) for patients who have reacted to any antipsychotic or other drug with leucopenia or agranulocytosis,
3) for patients with haematological disorders, especially when white blood cells are affected.

Furthermore, clozapine should not be prescribed together with tricyclic depot-antipsychotics or other drugs, which may cause haematological disorders.

Switching from typical antipsychotic to clozapine

When switching from conventional antipsychotics to clozapine, usually no rush is necessary. Patients are usually continued on their typical antipsychotic when beginning with clozapine. While the clozapine dose is slowly increased, the typical antipsychotic is then gradually reduced and after 1–2 weeks stopped. Some clinics end treatment with the typical antipsychotic before beginning with clozapine. Even if this leads to no complications among some patients, the risk of psychotic decompensation or suicidal ideation should however be avoided if possible with the overlapping dosage regimen.

If tolerated well, clozapine can be increased as follows (even if clozapine was only discontinued for a short period, this regimen should be followed): 12.5 mg on day 1, 25–50 mg on day 2–4, 50–100 mg on day 5–7, 100–200 mg on day 8–14, 200–400 mg on day 15–21, 400–600 mg on day 22–28. If side-effects appear, which may be due to the anticholinergic effect of clozapine (i.e. hypotension, fatigue, obstipation, delirium), the dose increase should occur even slower: out of 52 patients, where clozapine treatment (above regimen) was discontinued due to side-effects, 44 patients (85%) tolerated a clozapine dose of 225–165 mg after a 1–2 week clozapine-free period under a dose increase twice as slow as above. Only eight patients (15%) showed massive side-effects even under the slower regimen, forcing discontinuation of clozapine [18].

Controlled prescription

To discover haematological effects in time, guidelines differ worldwide. In Germany, weekly haematological controls are necessary in the first 18 weeks of treatment, thereafter on a monthly basis, as long as treatment with clozapine is continued. A rapid fall of white blood cells or the occurrence of cold-like symptoms, i.e. fever, cold shivers, sore throat, inflammation of mucous membrane of the mouth or disturbed wound healing, should lead to an immediate haematological control, as these can be symptoms of agranulocytosis. Haematological controls should occur twice a week if two consecutive haematological controls show a decrease of white blood cells of about $3000/mm^3$ or if the neutrophile granulocyte count lies between $1500–2000/mm^3$.

A white blood cell count of less than $3000/mm^3$ or neutrophile granulocyte count less than $1500/mm^3$ should lead to a discontinuation of clozapine. Furthermore, a discontinuation is recommended if an increase of the eosinophile granulocyte count above $3000/mm^3$ or a decrease of the thrombocyte count below $50\,000/mm^3$ occurs.

Dosage

Similar as with typical antipsychotics, the optimal dose varies from individual to individual and therefore calls for a slow increase so as to find the best dose in relation to remission of psychotic symptoms and tolerance. There seems to be great regional or transatlantic differences: while in German speaking countries the daily clozapine dose lies between 200 and 250 mg [11, 18], in Denmark a daily dose between 300 and 400 mg [19, 20] and in Sweden between 400 and 500 mg [36] is common. In Great Britain the average daily dose for treatment resistant patients lies between 400 and 450 mg [21, 22]. From a European viewpoint, a dose between 600 and 900 mg is seldom necessary and usually poorly tolerated in the long-run. In the USA, treatment with clozapine is restricted to the seriously ill and chronic patients due to the high costs compared to typical antipsychotics, leading to a higher negative selection than in Europe. This may be the reason for the higher daily dose in general in the USA of 400 to 800 mg [4, 23–25], while a lower dose of 250–450 mg has only become more common in recent years [13]. Out-patients, especially those after successful rehabilitation or again vocationally active, should receive a low dose if possible. For many patients 100 to 200 mg are sufficient for relapse prevention. If given as one dose in the evening, the sedation can be a welcomed side-effect and the often experienced early morning fatigue is tolerable. In the German speaking countries [18, 26] as well as in Great Britain [21] a single dose of 50 mg per day has been shown to be sufficiently effective.

In earlier studies of the 1970s, no correlation between plasma levels and antipsychotic effect was found ([27] among others). Of three US studies on treatment-resistant patients on a relatively high dose of 300 to 900 mg, only one [28] showed a significant correlation between plasma levels and reduction of psychotic symptoms. Another result, a significant remission of symptoms starting at a clozapine plasma level of 350 ng/ml, was reproduced in part [29]. A previous study [23] showed no relationship between clozapine dose, steady-state plasma concentration and successful antipsychotic treatment.

Numerous studies agree on the fact that successful treatment cannot be expected before a 4- to 6-week treatment period, among "treatment resistant" schizophrenics even up to 12–24 weeks are necessary to evaluate wanted and unwanted effects [25]. A continuous improvement especially of schizophrenic negative symptoms can be seen up to 6–12 months with some patients [30], although one study saw little clinical gain in prolonging exposure to clozapine beyond 8 weeks if no response is seen [31].

Positron-emission-tomography

The pharmacological and clinical speciality of clozapine was shown among others in studies using positron-emission-tomography (PET) and selective radioligands, measuring D_1- and D_2-receptor occupancy in the basal ganglia of schizophrenic patients. While those under typical antipsychotic treatment showed a D_2-receptor occupancy of 70–90%, under clozapine treatment it was only 18–80%, without evidence for a critical degree of D_2-receptor occupancy required to sustain clozapine's therapeutic effects [32]. Those patients with acute extrapyramidal motor side-effects had a significantly higher occupancy than those without motor side-effects [33].

These PET results, measured on 17 patients receiving typical antipsychotics and five receiving clozapine, were replicated in a larger sample by the same Swedish group [34]. Seventeen clozapine patients, treated with 125–600 mg/day, again showed a D_2-receptor occupancy of 20–67%, for the D_1-receptor the relatively high occupancy of 36–59% (under typical antipsychotics 0–44%). The 5-HT_2-receptor occupancy even under a low clozapine dose was very high (84–94%). Although the clozapine plasma level varied greatly (105–2121 ng/ml), the D_2-receptor occupancy was low or below 60% for all patients and did not correlate with the plasma level or the dose. This study also shows that careful and slow "titration" of the individual clozapine dosage cannot be replaced by plasma level controls.

Antipsychotic effect

In about 25 double blind controlled studies clozapine was compared with typical antipsychotics such as haloperidol, levomepromazine, and perphenazine. In about half of these studies clozapine was superior to the other antipsychotics, in the other half of the studies the antipsychotic effect was evaluated to be equal. Out of 13 studies comparing clozapine to chlorpromazine, six came out in favour of clozapine, seven showed no difference [8–10, 12, 13]. For so-called "treatment resistant" schizophrenics who showed insufficient remission or severe side-effects under typical antipsychotics, the advantage of clozapine is unmistakable. In now eight double-blind controlled studies clozapine was more effective than chlorpromazine, haloperidol, and fluphenazine [12, 13, 35].

The numerous retrospective studies from the German speaking and Scandinavian countries also agree that 40–60% of treatment resistant schizophrenics show a clinically relevant improvement, with in part impressive results with respect to variables such as independent living or vocational situation [18, 20, 36, 37]. These results were also documented in Great Britain [21, 22] and in the USA [25, 30]. The remission of schizophrenic symptoms is not restricted to positive symptoms, even negative symptoms showed greater remission than under typical antipsychotics, shown in numerous open studies, but also in controlled studies over 6–12 weeks i.e. with a significant decrease of the anhedonia BPRS-factor [4, 23, 24, 38]. One more recent study, however, showed superior efficacy for positive symptoms but not for negative symptoms in patients with a deficit syndrome [39]. A US study showing a decrease of involuntary measures such as constraint by 90% and isolation by 85% [40], correlates with the clinical experience in German speaking countries.

The efficacy of clozapine for relapse prevention has not been proven in a double-blind controlled study, yet six retrospective and six prospective open studies agree on a significant reduction of rehospitalization [13]. Two German studies showed that clozapine compared to previous typical antipsychotic treatment reduced the number of hospitalisations within a 2-year period from 1.1 ± 1.3 to 0.6 ± 1.0 and the in-patient days from 87 ± 96 to 42 ± 47 [18]. Similar results were presented by Klimke et al. [26], showing a reduction of the yearly relapse rate from 0.48 ± 0.66 to 0.21 ± 0.30 after switching to clozapine. The patient with the greatest success under clozapine compared to typical antipsychotics has the diagnosis of paranoid schizophrenia, subchronic to chronic course and strong extrapyramidal motor side-effects under typical antipsychotics [25].

Clozapine and risperidone have been compared in two double-blind controlled studies. Klieser et al. [41] reported similar efficacy for both drugs in chronic schizophrenic patients. However, subjects were not categorised as treatment-resistant and the number of patients was too low to adequately test for a differential effect between the two drugs. The other double-blind study, comparing 6.4 mg risperidone with 291 mg clozapine in 86 chronic schizophrenic patients who were resistant to or intolerant of conventional neuroleptics, also did not reveal a significant difference: 67% of the risperidone group and 65% of the clozapine group had a reduction of 20% or more in total PANSS [42]. In contrast, there are numerous open cross-over studies showing that risperidone is effective only in 0–15% of clozapine non-responders [43–46], but clozapine improved 40–80% of risperidone non-responders [43, 44, 47]. Although one cross-over study by Daniel et al. [48] on 20 therapy-resistant patients did not find a significant difference between both atypicals, both open comparisons with a higher number of subjects indicated that clozapine had better efficacy than risperidone [49, 50]. The only double-blind controlled comparison between clozapine and zotepine (150–450 mg/day each) in 50 therapy-resistant patients did not reveal any significant difference, both drugs induced "a relevant improvement" in 52% of patients [51]. For patients who did not tolerate or did not respond to clozapine, 18 of 45 (40%) or 6 of 16 (38%) responded with at least a 20% reduction in PANSS total score under olanzapine treatment [52]. However, there are also patients who do not respond to olanzapine, but improve under clozapine. That was the case for 11 of 21 patients (52%) in the study by Conley et al. [42]. The double-blind study compared 15–25 mg olanzapine and 200–600 mg clozapine over 18 weeks in 180 patients (Beuzen et al., in press). 107 patients completed the study (olanzapine 60%, clozapine 59%), the rates of discontinuation due to adverse events were lower for olanzapine than for clozapine (4.4% vs 15.6%, $p = 0.013$). There was no significant difference regarding efficacy, 60% of olanzapine and 54% of clozapine patients improved for at least 20% in PANSS total score. Further studies comparing atypicals will however be needed to be able to select the right (atypical) antipsychotic for each subgroup of psychotic disorders.

Side-effects

About 60–70% of all schizophrenics treated with clozapine experience one or more side-effects. Most often EEG-alterations, fatigue, increase of liver enzymes and postural hypotension are seen, while another typical side-effect of clozapine is a sometimes strong hypersalivation. The sedation of clozapine sometimes is seen as a wanted effect, while other side-effects do not last very long and are of little consequence. Especially the side-effects due to the cholinergic component (fatigue, hypotension, obstipation up to bowel obstruction, and confusion up to delirious states) fade away within 1–2 weeks for most patients despite a dose increase. Increase in liver enzymes, fever and leucocytosis are also often phenomena of the first 2 weeks and seldom necessitate discontinuation of clozapine. A strong correlation to the clozapine dose can be seen with the following side-effects: EEG-alterations or epileptic seizures, fatigue, tachycardia and hypersalivation. The clinical relevance of EEG-alterations necessitates a special evaluation of benefits and risks [53] and was the main reason for clozapine dose reduction in the Munich study, where the incidence of epileptic seizures was much lower (0.2%) than in other studies [18]. A delayed increase in clozapine dose or a reduction of the dose is necessary in about 10–15% of the patients. Serious side-effects, which lead to clozapine discontinuation, occur in 6–9% of the cases [18–20, 36]. Only one study out of Great Britain showed a significantly higher rate of serious side-effects, with 13% of an extremely negatively selected sample of schizophrenics discontinuing treatment due to side-effects [22]. Out-patient treatment shows a different profile of relevant side-effects. Most common reasons for reduction or discontinuation are weight gain and sedation.

If dose reduction does not alleviate side-effects or leads to an increase in psychotic symptoms, other pharmacological interventions are possible, which have not been evaluated in controlled studies, but have been recommended in reviews and case studies: postural hypotension can be treated with sympathomimetics, extreme hypersalivation with the peripheral anticholinergic agent pirenzepine. metoclopramide or similar drugs can alleviate nausea or vomiting, beta-blockers can be used against tachycardia, but the hypotensive effect may limit their use. EEG-alterations or epileptic seizures should be compensated with phenytoin, because carbamazapine's potential haematological effects limit their concurrent use with clozapine or warrant an 18 week longer

Table 1. Prevalence of side-effects under clozapine [10–12, 18, 36]

	Clinically relevant	Reason for discontinuation
EEG-alterations	20–40	0.5
fatigue	15–40	1.5
leucocytosis	15–40	–
increase of liver enzymes	10–20	1
postural hypotension	5–20	1.5
weight gain	8–20	2
tachycardia	5–20	0.5
hypersalivation	2–30	1
fever	2–20	1
nausea/vomiting	2–20	0.5
obstipation/bowel obstruction	5–15	0.5
ECG–alterations	2–13	2
confusion/delirious states	2–5	1
seizures	1–4	0.5
dermatological	1–2	–

period of haematological controls. The treatment of sedation with low-dose stimulants, such as sometimes propagated in the USA, is only necessary in a few cases.

When comparing side-effects of clozapine and typical antipsychotics, the most important aspect is the absence of motor side-effects. With respect to early dyskinesia, dystonia, Parkinsonism, and rigor, there exists general agreement that these symptoms do not appear with clozapine, or only in extremely seldom cases. Akathisia has been shown in two US studies, yet with small sample sizes [38, 54], to appear as often as with typical antipsychotics. However these results are contradicted by experiences in Germany [18] and Scandinavia [36, 37]. Early US studies [4, 30] as well as a new US study agree with European studies that patients suffering from akathisia under typical antipsychotics experience a highly significant improvement within 3–12 weeks after switching to clozapine. Those patients, who did not suffer from akathisia under typical antipsychotics, will also not experience it under clozapine [55].

The malignant neuroleptic syndrome, with a deadly course in 20% of cases, may also occur under clozapine treatment [13, 56]. A critical view of the reported cases shows great variance in the inclusion criteria. A well-known side-effect of clozapine is a benign reversible hyperthermia, which occurs more often than under typical antipsychotics. High fever combined with autonomous nervous symptoms, but without rigor, should not automatically be seen as a malignant neuroleptic syndrome.

Overdose, intoxication

An overdose or intoxication with a dose of 2000 mg clozapine leads to a mortality of 12%, according to the manufacturer. The reason of death is usually cardiac failure or aspiration pneumonia. There are, however, reports of patients, who after an intoxication with 10000 mg clozapine recuperated without complications. For adult patients, who have never consumed clozapine, a dose of 400 mg can already lead to coma or death.

A specific antidote for an intoxication with clozapine is not available. Besides an immediate and repeated gastric lavage within the first 6 h after consumption, physostigmine can be used to treat anticholinergic effects and intravenous diazepam or diphenylhydantoin against seizures.

Compliance, subjective effect, quality of life

Most studies agree on a relatively high compliance for schizophrenics receiving long-term treatment with clozapine. For typical antipsychotics compliance lies at about 20–50%, for clozapine depending on length of treatment and sample population between 50–70% [21], 57% [35], 68% [19], 86% [55], 87% [18] and about 90% [25].

This clinically important difference is probably due to better tolerance, as well as lack of motor side-effects. Furthermore many schizophrenics under long-term treatment with a typical antipsychotic report affective and cognitive deficits, which are difficult to show objectively. Typical complaints such as anhedonia and lack of drive, difficult to separate from negative symptoms or extrapyramidal side-effects, have long been known and labelled "pharmacogenic depression, akinetic depression, or neuroleptic-induced deficit syndrome". Clinical experience, that the subjective effect of clozapine differs greatly from that of typical antipsychotics, was verified by a study on 40 patients each [57]. Despite the negative selection – clozapine patients had reacted to typical antipsychotics with treatment resistance or severe side-effects – well-being was described as significantly greater in all five sub-factors of a questionnaire developed to measure subjective well-being under neuroleptic drugs.

Quality of life of schizophrenic patients under neuroleptic treatment was scientifically neglected for a long time. In the first study on that issue, Meltzer et al. [30] showed in an open study in 38 chronic patients that their quality of life increased significantly within 6 months of clozapine treatment. Recently, a double-blind controlled study comparing haloperidol and clozapine, both in rather high dosages, confirmed this result. Within 1 year of treatment, compliance as well as quality of life were significantly better under therapy with the atypical neuroleptic [85].

Clozapine and tardive dyskinesia

There is no doubt that clozapine causes less extrapyramidal motor symptoms. Mostly academic interest has been focused on the question of whether a clozapine monotherapy can cause tardive dyskinesia. Of more clinical interest is the effect of clozapine in the treatment of already manifest tardive dyskinesia. Most publications, open studies or case reports, are contradictory and have methodological deficits such as small sample size, low clozapine dose or short observation period. The range goes from no difference to complete remission [58]. Clinical reports have determined a significant improvement in about 40–50% [22, 59].

Lieberman et al. [58] treated 30 schizophrenics with a clozapine dose of 500 to 900 mg daily over 3 years, showing an extremely diverse individual reaction, without being able to define clinical variables for a success. The severity of tardive dyskinesia and a dystonic symptomatology correlated weakly while dose did not correlate with an improvement. Similar results were shown by Tamminga et al. [60], who treated 32 schizophrenics for 1 year either with 300 mg clozapine (n = 19) or 29 mg haloperidol (n = 13). A significant difference in favour of clozapine was shown, yet resulting no earlier than after 4 months.

Combination of clozapine with typical antipsychotics and interaction with other psychopharmacologic agents

If clozapine tolerance is limited due to side-effects or the tolerated dose is insufficiently effective, then clozapine may be combined with low-dose typical antipsychotics. The underlying concept is a summation of antipsychotic potency with low side-effects due to the different side-effect profiles. Phenothiazines and tricyclic antipsychotics also bear the risk of leucopenia or agranulocytosis, therefore butyrophenones should be used [11, 18, 61]. A combination with a tricyclic depot-antipsychotic is contra-indicated due to the higher risk of leucopenia or agranulocytosis and because of the poor potential of titration in the case of such a side-effect. For patients with a schizoaffective disorder, clozapine should be combined with lithium or antidepressants with as low a dose as possible. A higher side-effect risk is known up to date only for antidepressants: the combined anticholinergic effect can lead to delirious states. Due to the higher risk of leucopenia a combination of clozapine with carbamazepine is only indicated, when lithium or valproate have not shown sufficient effect. Very anxious patients often receive clozapine combined with benzodiazepines. Some reports [11, 62] speak of a higher risk of respiratory depression or circulatory collapse, yet this could not be confirmed by a study with a large sample size [18]. However, a combination of clozapine and benzodiazepines is usually only necessary, if at all, at the beginning of treatment and should lead over to a clozapine monotherapy. Sedation, anxiolysis and better sleep can also be managed by a respective dose and an appropriate distribution of the daily dose of clozapine. In Germany, clozapine treatment is combined with other psychoactive agents among 70% of clozapine patients [61]. In Denmark, only 40% receive a clozapine monotherapy, 35% a combination with other antipsychotics, 28% with benzodiazepines and 11% with antidepressants, without a higher side-effect rate [19, 20].

Of special importance for pharmacokinetics and plasma level of clozapine is the combination with selective serotonin reuptake inhibitors (SSRIs). In a systematic study on 10 to 16 patients each, plasma levels of clozapine and the primary metabolite norclozapine increased by 60% under paroxetine, 30% under fluoxetine and 20% under sertraline [63]. Even greater is the reported increase under fluvoxamine, a report on three patients with a clozapine plasma level increase up to 1600 to 3200 ng/ml – an eight-fold increase [64]. These findings have stimulated discussion on the possibility of SSRI-augmentation of clozapine treatment, yet a double-blind study showed no difference between adjunctive fluoxetine or placebo [65]. Although reduced tolerance or an increase in side-effects was seldom reported, the clozapine dose should be kept low when combining with SSRIs, and plasma levels should be controlled. As the underlying mechanism responsible for the higher concentration either a competitive blockade of hepatic microsomal oxydase or a reduced binding of serum proteins is being discussed.

Rebound-psychosis?

In a few case reports a rapid deterioration of psychopathology was reported after discontinuation of clozapine. This sudden renewed appearance of psychotic symptoms was seen not only as a "pure" discontinuation effect, but as a specific "rebound"-psychosis under clozapine withdrawal [10, 12, 13, 66]. The hypothesis is controversial; it could also be an effect of sedation wearing off. A rebound psychosis could possibly be explained with a higher sensitivity of dopaminergic receptors.

Prevalence and treatment of agranulocytosis

The occurrence of haematological disorders, especially agranulocytosis, is the most feared complication of clozapine treatment. However, it should be kept in mind that leucopenia and agranulocytosis also occur under other tricyclic antipsychotics (and antidepressants). A higher risk under clozapine compared to typical antipsychotics is presumed, yet has not been proven [84]. Agranulocytosis is understood to be a decrease of neutrophile granulocytes below $500/mm^3$. Granulocytopenia is a decrease under 1500 granulocytes/mm^3 in peripheral blood. The definition of leucopenia, however, is not uniform, the cut-off lying between 3000–4000 leucocytes/mm^3.

Due to restrictive regulations especially in the USA, allowing clozapine prescription only after haematological controls (every week even after the period of 18 weeks), new data on leucopenia and agranulocytosis is available [67]: out of 11 555 patients, agranulocytosis occurred in 73 cases, two died. The cumulative incidence is 0.8% for the first year, 0.9% for 1.5 years. 23 patients developed their agranulocytosis within the first 2 months, 61 patients within the first 3 months and 70 within the first 6 months. This confirms European experiences, where 85% of agranulocytosis cases occur in the first 18 weeks.

Agranulocytosis developed on average within 29 ± 23 days, half of the patients already showed a decrease of leucocytes 4 weeks prior to agranulocytosis. Yet 16 patients still had more than 3500 leucocytes/mm^3 1 week before developing agranulocytosis, another six patients developed their agranulocytosis in less than 2 weeks. In Great Britain, where clozapine prescription is as strongly regulated as in the USA, incidence of agranulocytosis is much lower. Of 2337 clozapine patients only 74 (3.2%) developed neutropenia, only 11 (0.4%) agranulocytosis and one of these died [21]. The data from Denmark is similar [19]: although not as accurate, the risk of agranulocytosis was determined to be 0.3%, without any cases of death. Whether the higher incidence in the USA is due to more accurate evaluation or genetic factors has yet to be evaluated.

After discontinuation of clozapine the blood count normalises in general within 2–4 weeks. The prognosis of agranulocytosis is better if treated with haematopoetic growth factors such as the granulocyte-macrophage colony-stimulating-factor (GM-CSF) or the granulocyte colony-stimulating-factor (G-CSF). Information by the company Sandoz on 43 patients shows that the increase of neutrophile granulocytes, which without treatment commences after 15 days, under GM-CSF or G-CSF treatment already starts after 8 days. The much lower mortality for agranulocytosis today may be due to the rapid treatment with haematopoetic growth factors [68].

Suicide attempts and suicides under clozapine

The risk of suicide among schizophrenics is 20-fold higher, 9–13% of all schizophrenics commit suicide. Meltzer and Okayla [69] examined suicidal behaviour for 88 schizophrenics before and after 2 years of clozapine treatment. Under typical antipsychotics before clozapine treatment 22 (25%) attempted suicide with a "low risk" (n = 17) or "high risk" (n = 6). Within the 2 years of clozapine treatment none attempted a "high risk" suicide, and only three patients attempted a "low risk" suicide. Clozapine therefore reduced the quantity of suicide attempts by 85%, as well as the severity of them. Another study examining the suicide rate in Texas over a 6-year period found a risk reduction from 63.1 suicides per 100000 patients with schizophrenia or schizoaffective disorder to 12.7 suicides per 100000 patients treated with clozapine [70].

Similar data can be found in the "Clozapine National Registry", showing that of the 102000 patients treated with clozapine in the USA until 1995, only 39 (0.038%) committed suicide. Adjusted by length of clozapine treatment, the suicide rate is 0.1 to 0.2% per year. This is a much lower rate than the expected rate according to US and Scandinavian studies.

Cognitive functions under clozapine

Most trials document improvement, but on some cognitive functions, the clozapine effect is controversial. Classen and Laux [71] found no significant difference between 150–500 mg clozapine, 10–30 mg haloperidol and 5–20 mg flupenthixol with respect to sensomotor capabilities and other cognitive functions, however found a tendency in some tests in favour of clozapine. Yet another study showed an improvement of numerous cognitive functions for treatment resistant schizophrenics after a 6-week treatment period with clozapine. In some tests after 6 months of clozapine treatment further significant improvements were found [72]. Another study showed a significant remission of positive and negative symptoms, but no change in the cognitive deficits of attention, memory and problem solving, and even a deterioration in some memory tests, probably due to the anticholinergic properties of clozapine [73]. In this research group further studies on treatment resistant and non-resistant schizophrenics showed that clozapine led to an improvement in speed dependent properties such as speech fluidity, reaction time and attention, yet a deterioration in properties such as visual memory.

Similar results were found in a study comparing a 10-week treatment period between clozapine and haloperidol in an open study over 1 year [74]: some tests (speech fluidity, visuomotor speed) showed differences in favour of clozapine, however due more to a deterioration in the haloperidol group. Long-term evaluation led to significant improvement in visuomotor and attention tests, while six tests measuring memory function showed stable results.

Prediction of clozapine effect through molecular biological techniques

There have been several attempts to predict the individual clozapine effect with respect to antipsychotic effect, side-effects, especially agranulocytosis, using molecular biological techniques. These attempts have not been fruitful with respect to agranulocytosis. The discovery of the dopamine D_4-receptor with high affinity to clozapine [75] stimulated research, yet initial positive findings could not be confirmed by later studies with large sample sizes: Neither the polymorphism on the dopamine D_4-receptor-gene [76, 77] nor on the 5-HT_{2A}-receptor-gene [78] are related to the antipsychotic effect or the tolerance of clozapine. Clinical experience also contrasts the expectation of genetic factors determining the individual reaction of clozapine, as effect and tolerance may vary in one person in different treatments within a 2- to 5-year period.

Pharmacoeconomics

Studies on pharmacoeconomic aspects or cost-effectiveness of clozapine treatment are surveyed by Morris et al. [79]. Due to the higher cost of the medication as well as the more intense monitoring of clozapine patients including haematologic controls, out-patient treatment is significantly more expensive than with typical antipsychotics. Costs of in-patient treatment, on the other hand, are much lower due to higher compliance and lower rate of rehospitalization. Two US studies showed a savings per patient of $ 20 000–41 500 per year. A recent study by Meltzer et al. [80] on 37 clozapine patients over at least 2 years showed a decrease in costs of 23%. A similar result was shown by Reid et al. [81] on 311 treatment resistant schizophrenics, where clozapine treatment significantly reduced the number of in-patient days with a savings of $ 33 000 to $ 50 000 per patient per year.

Not so extensive is the cost reduction in a British study [82], coming up with a savings per year for a treatment resistant schizophrenic of 91 £. However, the study also found that clozapine treatment resulted in a gain of 6 years without significant disabilities. Only one Swedish study showed a different result with respect to costs [83]: the observed reduction of in-patient costs was more than compensated by the increase of out-patient costs, resulting in a net increase of costs of 10% compared to typical antipsychotics. However, the decrease in psychotic symptoms and improvement in social competency might be worth the increase in costs. Detailed studies which also include the indirect non-medical costs (unemployment, social welfare, etc.) are still missing.

Outlook

In the discussion on benefits and risks of a treatment with clozapine often the danger of agranulocytosis is emphasised, while the much higher risk of tardive dyskinesia for typical antipsychotics is seldomly mentioned. Often clozapine is used as the antipsychotic of last choice, leading to an extremely negative selection of patients treated with clozapine. From the point of view of the patient and in the interest of his quality of life, this is not justifiable with respect to an antipsychotic effect at least comparable to typical antipsychotics, but with significantly better tolerance (no relevant extrapyramidal, less affective and cognitive side-effects). The much lower rate of rehospitalization and lower suicide rate as well as an improved treatment of agranulocytosis should be considered more strongly.

For many years, clozapine was the only atypical neuroleptic. Now, with the arrival of other drugs such as risperidone, olanzapine, sertindole, amisulpride, quetiapine, and ziprasidone, comparisons between clozapine and these compounds are urgently needed. All these drugs have different pharmacological profiles, possibly also different antipsychotic efficacy, and certainly different side-effect profiles. At present, the psychiatrists still do not have enough data to decide which atypical neuroleptic is the "right" drug for the individual patient.

References

1 Stille G, Hippius H (1971) Kritische Stellungnahme zum Begriff der Neuroleptika (anhand von pharmakologischen und klinischen Befunden mit Clozapin). *Pharmakopsychiat* 4: 182–191
2 Angst J, Bente D, Berner P, Heimann H, Helmchen H, Hippius H (1971) Das klinische Wirkungsbild von Clozapin (Untersuchung mit dem Amp-System). *Pharmakopsychiat* 4: 201–211
3 Amsler H, Teerenhovi L, Barth E, Harjula K, Voupio P (1977) Agranulocytosis in patients treated with clozapine. A study of the Finnish epidemic. *Acta Psychiatr Scand* 56: 241–248
4 Kane J, Honigfeld G, Singer J, Meltzer H, Clozapine Study Group (1988) Clozapine for the treatment-resistant schizophrenic. A double-blind comparison with chlorpromazine. *Arch Gen Psychiatry* 45: 789–796
5 Stille G, Fischer-Cornelssen K (1988) Die Entwicklung von Clozapin (Leponex) – ein Mysterium? In: OK Linde (ed.) *Pharmako-Psychiatrie im Wandel der Zeit: Erlebnisse und Ergebnisse*. Tilia-Verlag, Klingenmünster, 339–348
6 Hippius H (1989) The history of clozapine. *Psychopharmacol* 99: 53–55
7 Ereshefsky L, Watanabe MD, Tran-Johnson TK (1989) Clozapine an atypical antipsychotic agent. *Clin Pharmacol* 8: 691–709

8 Fitton A, Heel R (1990) Clozapine: a review of its pharmacological properties and therapeutic use in schizophrenia. *Drugs* 40: 722–747
9 Baldessarini R, Frankenburg F (1991) Clozapine: a novel antipsychotic agent. *N Engl J Med* 324: 746–754
10 Safferman A, Lieberman J, Kane J, Szymansky S, Kinon B (1991) Update on the clinical efficacy and side-effects of clozapine. *Schizophr Bull* 17: 247–261
11 Klimke A, Klieser E (1995) Das atypische Neuroleptikum (Leponex R) – aktueller Kenntnisstand und neuere klinische Aspekte. *Fortschr Neurol Psychiat* 63: 173–193
12 Wagstaff AJ, Bryson HM (1995) Clozapine – a review of its pharmacological properties and therapeutic use in patients with schizophrenia who are unresponsive to or intolerant of classical antipsychotic agents. *CNS Drugs* 4: 370–400
13 Buchanan R (1995) Clozapine: efficacy and safety. *Schizophr Bull* 21: 579–591
14 Young CR, Longhurst JG, Bowers MB, Mazure CM (1997) The expanding indications for clozapine. *Experim Clin Psychopharmacol* 5: 216–234
15 Wolters ECH, Hurwitz TA, Mak E (1990) Clozapine in the treatment of Parkinsonian patients with dopaminomimetic psychosis. *Neurology* 40: 832–834
16 Bonucelli U, Ceravolo R, Maremmani C, Nuti A, Rossi G, Muratorio A (1994) Clozapine in Huntington's chorea. *Neurology* 44: 821–823
17 Pakkenberg H, Pakkenberg B (1986) Clozapine in the treatment of tremor. *Acta Neurol Scand* 73: 295–297
18 Naber D, Holzbach R, Perro C, Hippius H (1992) Clinical management of clozapine patients in relation to efficacy and side-effects. *Br J Psychiatry* 160 (suppl 17): 54–59
19 Peacock K, Gerlach J (1994) Clozapine treatment in Denmark: concomitant psychotropic medication and hematologic monitoring in a system with liberal usage practices. *J Clin Psychiatry* 55: 44–49
20 Povlsen UJ, Nording U, Fog R, Gerlach J (1985) Tolerability and therapeutic effect of clozapine. *Acta Psychiatr Scand* 71: 176–185
21 Hirsch S, Puri B (1993) Clozapine: progress in treating refractory schizophrenia. *Br Med J* 306: 1427–1428
22 Clozapine Study Group (1993) The safety and efficacy of clozapine in severe treatment-resistant schizophrenic patients in the UK. *Br J Psychiatry* 163: 150–154
23 Pickar D, Owen R, Litman R, Konicki P, Gutierrez R, Rapaport M (1992) Clinical and biological response to clozapine in patients with schizophrenia crossover comparison with fluphenazine. *Arch Gen Psychiatry* 49: 345–353
24 Breier A, Buchanan R, Kirkpatrick B, Davis O, Irish D, Summerfeldt A, Carpenter W (1994) Effects of clozapine on positive and negative symptoms in outpatients with schizophrenia. *Am J Psychiatry* 151: 20–26
25 Lieberman J, Safferman A, Pollack S, Szymanski S, Johns C, Howard A, Kronig M, Bookstein P, Kane J (1994) Clinical effects of clozapine in chronic schizophrenia response to treatment and predictors of outcome. *Am J Psychiatry* 151: 1744–1752
26 Klimke A, Klieser E, Lemmer W (1995) Clozapin in der Rezidivprophylaxe. In: D Naber, F Müller-Spahn (eds) *Clozapin. Pharmakologie und Klinik eines atypischen Neuroleptikums*. Springer, Berlin Heidelberg London Tokyo, 81–92
27 Ackenheil M, Braeu H (1976) Antipsychotische Wirksamkeit im Verhältnis zum Plasmaspiegel von Clozapin. *Arzneimittelforschung/Drug Res* 26: 1156–1158
28 Perry PJ, Miller DD, Arndt SV et al. (1991) Clozapine and norclozapine plasma concentrations and clinical response of treatment-refractory schizophrenic patients. *Am J Psychiatry* 148: 231–235
29 Kronig M, Munne R, Szymanski S, Safferman A, Pollack S, Cooper S, Kane J, Lieberman J (1995) Plasma clozapine levels and clinical response for treatment-refractory schizophrenic patients. *Am J Psychiatry* 152: 179–182
30 Meltzer H, Burnett S, Bastani B, Ramirez L (1990) Effects of six months of clozapine treatment on the quality of life of chronic schizophrenic patients. *Hosp Comm Psychiatry* 41: 892–897
31 Conley RR, Carpenter WT, Tamminga CA (1997) Time to clozapine response in a standardized trial. *Am J Psychiatry* 154: 1243–1247
32 Pickar D, Su T-P, Weinberger DR, Coppola R, Malhotra AK, Knable MB, Lee KS, Gorey J, Bartko JJ, Breier A, Hsiao J (1996) Individual variation in D2 dopamine receptor occupancy in clozapine-treated patients. *Am J Psychiatry* 153: 1571–1578

33 Farde L, Nordström A, Wiesel F-A, Pauli S, Halldin C, Sedvall G (1992) PET analysis of central D1- and D2-dopamine receptor occupancy in patients treated with classical neuroleptics and clozapine: relation to extrapyramidal side-effects. *Arch Gen Psychiatry* 49: 538–544
34 Nordström A-L, Farde L, Nyberg S, Karlsson P, Halldin C, Sedvall G (1995) D1, D2, and 5-HT2 receptor occupancy in relation to clozapine serum concentration: a PET study of schizophrenic patients. *Am J Psychiatry* 152: 1444–1449
35 Rosenheck R, Cramer J, Xu W, Thomas J, Henderson W, Frisman L, Fye C, Charney D (1997) A comparison of clozapine and haloperidol in hospitalized patients with refractory schizophrenia. *N Engl J Med* 337: 809–815
36 Lindström L-H (1988) The effect of long-term treatment with clozapine in schizophrenia: A retrospective study in 96 patients treated with clozapine for up to 13 years. *Acta Psychiatr Scand* 77: 524–529
37 Gerlach J, Jorgensen EO, Peacock L (1989) Long-term experience with clozapine in Denmark: research and clinical practice. *Psychopharmacol* 99: 92–96
38 Claghorn J, Honigfeld G, Abuzzahab F, Wang R, Steinbook R, Tuason V, Klerman G (1987) The risks and benefits of clozapine vs. chlorpromazine. *J Clin Psychopharmacol* 7: 377–384
39 Buchanan RW, Breier A, Kirkpatrick B, Ball P, Carpenter WT (1998) Positive and negative symptom response to clozapine in schizophrenic patients with and without the deficit syndrome. *Am J Psychiatry* 155: 751–760
40 Mallya A, Roos P, Roebuck-Colgan K (1992) Restraint, seclusion and clozapine. *J Clin Psychiatry* 53: 395–397
41 Klieser E, Lehmann E, Kinzler E, Wurthmann C, Heinrich K (1995) Randomized, double-blind, controlled trial of risperidone vs. clozapine in patients with chronic schizophrenia. *J Clin Psychopharmacol* 15 (suppl 1): 45–51
42 Bondolfi G, Dufour H, Patris M, May JP, Billeter U, Eap CB, Baumann P (1998) Risperidone vs clozapine in treatment-resistant chronic schizophrenia: a randomized double-blind study. *Am J Psychiatry* 155: 499–504
43 Buckley P, Buchanan R, Schulz S, Tamminga C (1996) Catching up on schizophrenia. The Fifth International Congress on Schizophrenia Research Warm Springs, Va, April 8–12, 1995. *Arch Gen Psychiatry* 53: 456–462
44 Pajonk F, Naber D, Hippius H (1997) Alternativen zum Clozapin? Klinische Erfahrungen mit Risperidon. In: D Naber, F Müller-Spahn (eds): *Clozapin. Pharmakologie und Klinik eines atypischen Neuroleptikums*. Springer, Heidelberg, 89–104
45 Still D, Dorson P, Crismon M, Pousson C (1996) Effects of Switching Inpatients With Treatment-Resistant Schizophrenia From Clozapine to Risperidone. *Psychiat Serv* 47: 1382–1384
46 Lacey R, Preskorn S, Jerkovich G (1995) Is risperidone a substitute for clozapine patients who do not respond to neuroleptics? [Letter]. *Am J Psychiatry* 152: 1401
47 Cavallaro C, Cordoba C, Smeraldi E (1995) A pilot, open study on the treatment of refractory schizophrenia with risperidone and clozapine. *Human Psychopharmacol* 10: 231–234
48 Daniel DG, Goldberg TE, Weinberger DR, Kleinman JE, Pickar D, Lubick LJ, Williams TS (1996) Different side-effect profiles of risperidone and clozapine in 20 outpatients with schizophrenia or schizoaffectiv disorder: a pilot study. *Am J Psychiatry* 153: 417–419
49 Lindenmayer J, Alexander A, Park M, Smith R, Apergi F-S, Czobor P (1997) Psychpathological and neuropsychological profile of clozapine vs. risperidone in refractory schizophrenics. *Schizophr Res* 24: 195
50 Flynn S, MacEwan G, Altman S, Kopola LC, Fredrikson DH, Smith GN, Honer WG (1998) An Open Comparison of Clozapine and Risperidone in Treatment-Resistant Schizophrenia. *Pharmacopsychiat* 31: 25–29
51 Meyer-Lindenberg A, Gruppe H, Bauer U, Lis S, Krieger S, Gallhofer B (1997) Improvement of cognitive function in schizophrenic patients receiving clozapine or zotepine: results from a double-blind study. *Pharmacopsychiat* 30: 35–42
52 Tran P, Shamir E, Poyorovski M, Lokshin P, Weizer N, Dorfman P, Mark M, Bikett M, Ben-Assayag E, Shoshani D, Wimmer P, Dossenbach M (1997) Olanzapine in the treatment of patients who failed to respond to or tolerate clozapine. *Psychopharmacol Bull* 33: 599
53 Treves IA, Neufeld MY (1996) EEG abnormalities in clozapine treated schizophrenic patients. *Eur Neuropsychopharmacol* 6: 93–94
54 Cohen BM, Keck PE, Satlin A, Cole JO (1991) Prevalence and severity of akathisia in patients on clozapine. *Biol Psychiatry* 163: 1215–1219

55 Safferman A, Lieberman J, Pollack S, Kane J (1993) Akathisia and clozapine treatment. *J Clin Psychopharmacol* 13: 286–287
56 Sachdev P, Kruk J, KneeboneM, Kissane D (1995) Clozapine-induced neuroleptic malignant syndrome: review and report of new cases. *J Clin Psychopharmacol* 15: 365–371
57 Naber D (1995) A self-rating to measure subjective effects of neurolpetic drugs, relationships to objective psychopathology, quality of life and other clinical variables. *Int Clin Psychopharmacol* 10 (suppl 3): 133–138
58 Lieberman JA, Saltz BL, Johns CA, Pollak S, Borenstein M, Kane J (1991) The effects of clozapine on tardive dyskinesia. *Br J Psychiatry* 158: 503–510
59 Naber D, Leppig M, Grohmann R, Hippius H (1989) Efficacy and adverse effects of clozapine in the treatment of schizophrenia and tardive dyskinesia – a retrospective study of 387 patients. *Psychopharmacol* 99: 73–76
60 Tamminga C, Thaker G, Moran M, Kakigi T, Gao X (1994) Clozapine in tardive dyskinesia: Observations from human and animal model studies. *J Clin Psychiatry* 55 (suppl B): 102–106
61 Gaebel W, Klimke A, Klieser E (1994) Kombination von Clozapin mit anderen Psychopharmaka. In: D Naber, F Müller-Spahn (eds): *Clozapin. Pharmakologie und Klinik eines atypischen Neuroleptikums*. Springer, Berlin Heidelberg London Tokyo, 43–58
62 Sassim N, Grohmann R (1988) Adverse drug reactions with clozapine and simultaneous application of benzodiazepines. *Pharmacopsychiat* 21: 306–307
63 Centorrino F, Baldessarini R, Kando J, Frankenburg F, Volpicelli S, Puopolo P, Flood J (1994) Serum concentrations of clozapine and its major metabolites: effects of cotreatment with fluoxetine or valproate. *Am J Psychiatry* 151: 123–125
64 Hiemke C, Weigmann H, Härtter S, Dahmen N, Wetzel H, Müller H (1994) Elevated levels of clozapine in serum after addition of fluvoxamine. *J Clin Psychopharmacol* 14: 279–281
65 Buchanan RW, Kirkpatrick B, Bryant N, Ball P, Breier A (1996) Fluoxetine augmentation of clozapine treatment in patients with schizophrenia. *Am J Psychiatry* 153: 1625–1627
66 Shiovitz TM, Welke TL, Tigel PD, Anand R, Hartman RD, Stramek JJ, Kurtz NM, Cutler NR (1998) Cholinergic rebound and rapid onset psychosis following abrupt clozapine withdrawal. *Schizophr Bull* 22: 591–595
67 Alvir J, Lieberman J, Safferman Z, Schwimmer J, Schaaf JA (1993) Clozapine- induced agranulocytosis. Incidence and risk factors in the United States. *N Engl J Med* 329: 161–167
68 Young CR, Bowers MB, Mazure CM (1998) Management of the adverse effects of clozapine. *Schizophr Bull* 24: 381–390
69 Meltzer H, Okayli G (1995) Reduction of suicidality during clozapine treatment of neuroleptic resistant schizophrenia: Impact on risk-benefit assessment. *Am J Psychiatry* 152: 183–190
70 Reid WH, Mason M, Hogan T (1998) Suicide prevention effects associated with clozapine therapy in schizophrenia and schizoaffective disorder. *Psychiatr Serv* 49: 1029–1033
71 Classen W, Laux G (1988) Sensorimotor and cognitive performance of schizophrenic inpatients treated with haloperidol, flupenthixol, or clozapine. *Pharmacopsychiat* 21: 295–297
72 Hagger C, Buckley P, Kenny J, Friedman L, Ubogy D, Meltzer H (1993) Inprovement in cognitive functions and psychiatric symptoms in treatment-refractory schizophrenic patients receiving clozapine. *Biol Psychiatr* 34: 702–712
73 Goldberg T, Greenberg R, Griffin S, Gold J, Kleinman J, Pickar D, Schulz S, Weinberger D (1993) The effects of clozapine on cognition and psychiatric symptoms in patients with schizophrenia. *Br J Psychiatry* 162: 43–48
74 Buchanan R, Holstein C, Breier A (1994) The comparative efficacy and long-term effect of clozapine treatment on neuropsychological test performance. *Biol Psychiatry* 36: 717–725
75 Van Tol H, Bunzow J, Guan H, Ohara K, Bunzow JR, Civelli O, Kennedy J, Seeman P, Niznik HB, Jovanovic V (1991). Cloning of the gene for a human dopamine D4 receptor with high affinity for the antipsychotic clozapine. *Nature* 350: 610–614
76 Rao PA, Pickar D, Gejman PV, Ram A, Gershon ES, Gelernter J (1994) Allelic variation in the D4 dopamine receptor (DRD4) gene does not predict response to clozapine. *Arch Gen Psychiatry* 51: 912–917
77 Rietschel M, Naber D, Oberländer H, Holzbach R, Fimmers R, Eggermann K, Möller HJ, Propping P, Nöthen MM (1996) Efficacy and side-effects of clozapine testing for association with allelic variation in the dopamine D4 receptor gene. *Neuropsychopharm* 15: 491–496
78 Nöthen MM, Rietschel M, Erdmann J, Oberländer H, Möller HJ, Naber D, Propping P (1995) Genetic variation of the 5-HT2A-receptor and response to clozapine. *Lancet* 346: 908–909

79 Morris S, Hogan T, McGuire A (1998) The cost-effectiveness of clozapine. *Clin Drug Invest* 15: 137–152
80 Meltzer H, Cola P, Way L, Thompson P, Bastani B, Davies M, Snitz B (1993) Cost effectiveness of clozapine in neuroleptic-resistant schizophrenia. *Am J Psychiatry* 150: 1630–1638
81 Reid W, Mason M, Toprac M (1994) Savings in hospital bed-days related to treatment with clozapine. *Hosp Commun Psychiatry* 45: 261–264
82 Davies LM, Drummond MF (1993) Assessment of costs and benefits of drug therapy for treatment-resistant schizophrenia in the United Kingdom. *Br J Psychiatry* 162: 38–42
83 Jonsson D, Walinder J (1995) Cost-effectiveness of clozapine treatment in therapy-refractory schizophrenia. *Acta Psychiatr Scand* 92: 199–201
84 Grohmann R, Schmidt LG, Spiess-Kiefer C, Rüther E (1989) Agranulocytosis and significant leucopenia with neuroleptic drugs: results from the AMÜP program. *Psychopharmacol* 99: 109–112
85 Rosenheck R, Cramer J, Xu W, Thomas J, Henderson W, Frisman L, Fye C, Charney D (1997) A comparison of clozapine and haloperidol in hospitalized patients with refractory schizophrenia. *New Engl J Med* 337: 809–815

Atypical Antipsychotics
ed. by B.A. Ellenbroek and A.R. Cools

Dopamine receptor subtypes and schizophrenia: a clinical perspective

Johan A. Den Boer and Jakob Korf

Department of Biological Psychiatry, University of Groningen, P.O. Box 30001, NL-9700 RB Groningen, The Netherlands

Introduction

The pathogenesis of schizophrenia is not known, but several causative factor have been proposed, such as the existence of a genetic defect [1], prenatal infections with viruses [2], structural abnormalities in the brain [3, 4], receptor dysfunctions in many neurotransmission or transduction systems [5, 6]. Concerning the latter the dopaminergic system has been implicated in schizophrenia for more than four decades. Whereas in early studies the metabolism of dopamine (DA) was studied, in the last decade the emphasis has been on dopamine receptors and transduction mechanisms. A major lead in the DA-approach has been the fact that clinically effective antipsychotics in schizophrenia appear to exert anti-DA-ergic activity, either by inhibiting subtypes of DA-receptors, or by decreasing metabolism or other aspects of neurotransmission of cerebral DA-containing neurons. These pharmacological properties led to the proposal of an increased DA-activity in the limbic system in schizophrenia [7–10].

Where initially only the D_1 and the D_2 DA-receptor subtypes were distinguished, at present these types consist of two or three subtypes, respectively. These receptors were delineated on the basis of their binding profiles *in vitro*, behavioural effects and, more recently, by the induction of immediate early genes such as the Fos protein. The latter are the consequence of intracellular transduction mechanisms and provide a novel way to characterise regional and/or receptor mediation *in vivo* in experimental animals.

The possible importance of each of the subtypes in the possible pathogenesis and in the action of antipsychotic medication will be reviewed here. The hypothesis that the classical neuroleptics block D_2 receptors was supported by preclinical research, both *in vitro* and *in vivo*, only. More recently imaging of patients with positron emission tomography (PET) or single photon emission tomography (SPECT) with receptor specific ligands have proved more directly that blockade (or occupancy) of D_2 receptors during optimal medication is a prerequisite for both therapeutic efficacy and extrapyramidal side-effects (EPS) in patients treated with classical antipsychotic drugs (e.g. [11–15]). However, several studies have also demonstrated that maximal D_2 receptor occupancy does not guarantee therapeutic efficacy [16, 17], indicating that (a subgroup) of patients with schizophrenia is not determined by aberrations of the DA-neurotransmission that may become normalised by antipsychotic medication. It is widely accepted that the propensity towards EPS of the classical antipsychotics is a consequence of high DA D_2 receptor occupancy in the nigrostriatal system, as shown with PET and SPECT studies [18, 19]. Some antipsychotics, most often indexed as atypical, such as remoxipride and risperidone show high D_2 receptor occupancy concomitant with little EPS [20], suggesting that other neuronal systems attenuate these symptoms. Perhaps additional blockade of serotonin receptors may explain the lack of EPS during risperidone treatment, thus broadening the therapeutic window at relatively high doses. It should, however, be mentioned that risperidone can induce EPS at high dosages. Concerning remoxipride little can be said about possible alternative actions of the drug. The wide acceptance of atypical antipsychotics with a broad ("rich") pharmacological profile (such as clozapine, olanzapine, ziprasidone and quetiapine) shows that less D_2 receptor blockade – thus reducing risks of EPS – does not necessarily mean inferior therapeutic efficacy [18, 19, 21, 22].

In contrast to classical neuroleptics the prototype of the atypical antipsychotic clozapine has affinity for the DA D_1, D_3, D_4 and D_5 receptors, as well for the $5HT_{2/3}$, $\alpha_{1/2}$-adrenergic and H_1-histamine receptors [23–27]. These data provide strong evidence that the therapeutic effects of atypical antipsychotics with a broad pharmacological receptor binding profile and transduction response should not necessarily be attributed to its action at D_2-receptors. Based on similarities in structure and pharmacological profile DA receptors has been divided into two families: the D_1-like receptor family, including D_1 and D_5 receptor, and the D_2-like receptor family, including the D_2, D_3 and D_4-like receptors. In this chapter we will review the possible involvement of specific D_1, D_5, D_2, D_3, and D_4 receptor subtypes in the action of atypical antipsychotic drugs and in the pathogenesis of schizophrenia and summarise the clinical studies which have been performed with selective DA receptors a/antagonists.

The D_1 receptor family

D_1 Receptors in schizophrenia

The D_1 receptor-family consists of the D_1 and the D_5 receptor. Like the D_2-receptor, the dopamine D_1 receptor belongs to the family of G protein-coupled receptors. D_1 receptors are positively coupled to cyclic-AMP generating transduction mechanism and *in vivo* agonists of this receptor can induce Fos-protein in several brain areas, including basal ganglia, cerebral cortex and in most of the other locations where also the D_1-receptor has been found. It has also been shown that blockade of D_1 receptors, without previous activation is not sufficient to induce c-fos expression. So, the prefrontal induction of FOS seen with clozapine cannot be attributed to D_1-blockade [28, 29]. In virtually all brain areas the density of the D_1 receptor (Bmax) in the rat is at least more than five times that of receptors of the D_2 family.

The exact nucleotide sequence of the corresponding gene has been identified [30, 31]. D_1-like receptors are highly localised in superficial and deep layers of the prefrontal cortex, the caudate-putamen, nucleus accumbens, olfactory tubercle and the substantia nigra pars reticulata of the rat brain [32, 33]. In view of the relationship between frontal lobe functions such as "working memory" and D_1 receptors, D_1 receptor mediated neurotransmission may be important for the pathophysiology of schizophrenia [34].

Since the majority of dopaminergic cells do not express the D_1 receptor mRNA, the D_1 receptor is considered to be a postsynaptic receptor [35]. A presynaptic localisation was demonstrated in the amygdala and the substantia nigra [36].

The abundance of D_1 receptor mRNA is much higher than observed for the D_5 receptor [37]. D_5 mRNA has been shown in the hippocampus, the parafascicular nucleus of the thalamus and the prefrontal cortex. The D_5 receptor has been primarily identified as an autoreceptor [38].

The possible involvement of the D_1 receptor in schizophrenia has been studied in several genetic studies using different research methodologies. Sobell and co-workers [39] failed to find mutations in the DA receptor D_1 gene locus in patients with schizophrenia and bipolar disorder. Family-based linkage studies investigating markers at the D_1 receptor gene were also negative for schizophrenia [40, 41]. Using another method Cichon and co-workers found no changes in the D_1 receptor gene, suggesting that this receptor may not be commonly involved in schizophrenia. More recent studies failed to find sequence changes [42] or other indications pointing to mutations in the D_1 gene [43] in schizophrenia.

Post mortem studies revealed no changes in the cellular expression of D_1 receptor genes in the caudate nucleus [44] in both untreated and neuroleptic-treated schizophrenic patients, indicating that chronic neuroleptic treatment does not modify D_1 receptor gene expression in the caudate nucleus.

In view of the accumulating evidence that the prefrontal cortex might be dysfunctional in schizophrenia, Knable et al. [46] reported significant elevation of the binding of the D_1 receptor antagonist [^{3}H]-SCH 23390 in the intermediate layer of the prefrontal cortex. In addition, there was a trend towards a higher binding in the cingulate cortex. These findings may, however, implicate that increases in D_1 receptor density in schizophrenic patients may be the consequence of neuroleptic treatment, although increased receptor density that might exist as a feature of psychotic illness could not be excluded.

D_1 receptor blockade is not a prerequisite for antipsychotic activity, since many effective antipsychotics compounds have little or no D_1 affinity. Clozapine, however, has considerable affinity for D_1 receptors, and it has been suggested that the atypical profile might in part be related to these D_1 blocking properties. A 40–60% receptor occupancy of D_1 receptors has been found during treatment with clozapine, whereas remoxipride, raclopride and haloperidol did not induce D_1 receptor occupancy [18]. These findings prompted investigations about the antipsychotic efficacy of selective D_1 receptor antagonists.

DA D_1 receptor antagonists in the treatment of schizophrenia

The *in vivo* affinities of both D_2-, and D_1 antagonists like SCH 39166, exhibited a high correlation with their activities in the conditioned avoidance response test in the rat [46]. Based upon these and other animal models, blockade of D_1-receptors was hypothesised to be of therapeutic value in the treatment of positive symptoms of schizophrenia, but also negative symptoms were hypothesised to be related to D_1 receptors [47]. The latter is supported by animal experiments, as the prototypical D_1-antagonist SCH 23390 is able to antagonise D-amphetamine induced social isolation in Java monkeys [48]. SCH 23390 was reported to be ineffective in one open label study in schizophrenic patients, but further studies with this compound have been cancelled [49].

In vitro and preclinical studies in different species have shown that SCH 39166 is also a highly selective D_1 antagonist, with a preclinical profile of an antipsychotic agent with a low propensity to induce EPS [50–52].

Two pilot studies investigated the effects of SCH39166 in positive and negative symptoms in schizophrenia. Den Boer and co-workers [53] found no effect on positive symptoms but reported a significant treatment effect on negative symptoms assessed with the negative subscale of the PANSS in a small open pilot study (Fig. 1).

Using a similar design Karlsson and co-workers [54] could not find a reduction in positive symptoms, but this group did not study the effects on negative symptomatology.

In a PET study in volunteers it was shown that [^{11}C] SCH 39166 in a dose of 100 mg induced a 70% D_1 receptor occupancy, which is considered sufficient for obtaining an antipsychotic response [55].

Several reasons may account for the observed lack of antipsychotic efficacy in schizophrenic patients. First, it is possible that the dosage was too low. Second, it is conceivable that the patient sample selected for this clinical study, consisting of a population with mixed positive and negative symptoms, did not exhibit the target symptoms for a D_1 antagonist. It is conceivable that schizophrenic patients with predominant negative symptoms would show a more favourable response to this drug.

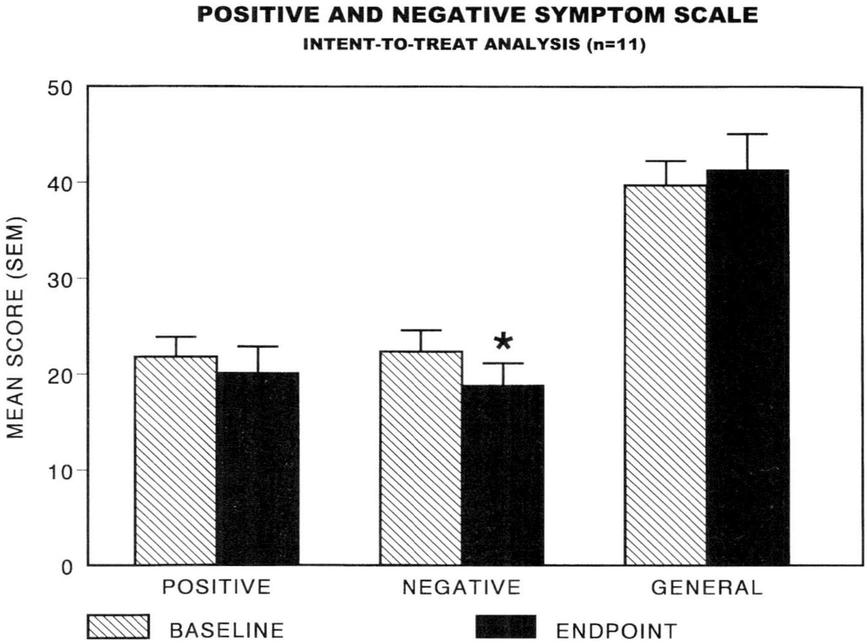

Figure 1. Effects on total PANSS score and positive- and negative subscale of the D_1 receptor antagonists SCH 39166 (* = $p < 0.05$). Reprinted with permission from den Boer et al. (1995).

The recently developed D_1 receptor-antagonist NN 01-0687, a benzazepine with very low affinity for other neurotransmitter receptors, was found to reduce psychotic symptomatology in an open label study [56]. Further placebo-controlled studies with this compound are warranted. An unequivocal conclusion about the efficacy of D_1 antagonists, based upon the published studies is premature.

Regardless of these methodological considerations, these preliminary findings question the validity of the hypothesis that D_1 receptors are involved in the pathogenesis of schizophrenia. In addition, based upon these findings, it is unlikely that antagonism of D_1 receptors can explain the antipsychotic effects of other atypical antipsychotics.

In a recent PET study in which D_1 and D_2 receptors were labelled by [^{11}C] SCH 23390 and [^{11}C]N-methylspiperone respectively, no evidence was found for differences in D_2 receptor binding in the striatum between healthy controls and drug free schizophrenic patients [57]. However, the mean values of D_1 receptor binding in the prefrontal cortex were significantly lower in the patients compared to healthy controls. This reduced D_1 receptor binding in schizophrenic patients was positively correlated to the presence of negative symptoms and a poor performance on the Wisconsin Card Sorting Test. These findings indicate that instead of D_1 receptor antagonists, D_1 receptor *agonists* could be effective in treating negative symptoms in schizophrenia.

The interest in D_1 receptors as potential targets for antipsychotic activity was prompted by studies which indicated that clozapine in clinically effective dosages occupied D_1 receptors to a greater extent than other antipsychotics. The effects of chronic treatment with clozapine on the D_1 receptor are, however, equivocal. In a recent study, chronic treatment with haloperidol, clozapine or raclopride failed to alter [^{3}H] SCH 23390 binding to D_1-like receptors in any brain region indicating that the antipsychotic efficacy is not mediated *via* this receptor [58].

Upregulation of D_1 receptors in the caudate putamen was found after chronic treatment with clozapine, whereas Lidow and Goldman-Rakic [59] reported downregulation of D_1 receptors in medial prefrontal and temporal cortices of monkeys after chronic treatment with clozapine, haloperidol or remoxipride. In an extension of their earlier study the same group examined the effects on the D_1 and D_5 receptor of chronic treatment (6 months) with olanzapine, remoxipride, molindole, pimozide, risperidone and the D_2 antagonist tiapride which lacks antipsychotic activity [60]. All tested compounds induced a downregulation of both the D_1 and D_5 receptor mRNA in the primate prefrontal cortex, whereas no changes were found in neostriatal areas. Interestingly, the downregulation of D_1 and D_5 receptors appeared not to be confined to clinically active antipsychotics, since also tiapride (which lacks antipsychotic activity) had the same effect. The observed downregulation may thus be related to D_2 blockade irrespective of clinical efficacy. If a reduced density of D_1 receptors is involved in the pathogenesis of schizophrenia then a further reduction of D_1 function in the prefrontal cortex as a consequence of chronic antipsychotic treatment might critically further impair the function of the prefrontal cortex leading to a worsening of cognitive functions.

Again, these findings suggest that future development of D_1 selective antipsychotics should aim at designing compounds that stimulate and do not antagonise the prefrontal D_1 receptor.

Taken together, based upon genetic, neuroimaging, autoradiographic and treatment studies a primary role for D_1 receptors in the pathogenesis of schizophrenia appears unlikely, although the effects of D_2 antagonists on D_1 receptor-downregulation suggest that D_1 agonists could be clinically effective. The recently discovered subtyping of D_1 receptors in D_{1A}, D_{1B}, D_{1C} and D_{1D} receptors [61] may in the future allow for a better understanding of D_1-like mediated events.

Interestingly, recent studies in monkeys have shown that D_1 receptors are present in the foetal cerebral wall even prior to the arrival of dopaminergic innervation. D_1 receptors therefore probably play a significant role during formation of the cerebral cortex [62].

Although the role of D_1 receptors in schizophrenia is not apparent, it is tempting to speculate that at a very early stage during development of the brain, discrete abnormalities in D_1 receptors may hamper the formation of cortical tissue leading to a predisposition towards the development of psychosis.

The D_2 receptor family

D_2 receptor in schizophrenia

The localisation of D_2 receptors has often been confined to the basal ganglia, the septum and the tubero-infundubular regions of the brain, although a widespread innervation of dopaminergic neurons in men to several cortical and posterior brain regions have been described. More recently, D_2 receptors in areas such as the hippocampus and amygdala has been reported. D_2 receptors are often negatively coupled to cyclic AMP generating transduction mechanism. *In vivo* both agonists and antagonists of this receptor can induce Fos-protein in several brain areas, including ventral and dorsal parts of the basal ganglia, where a relatively high D_2-receptor density has been found (e.g. [28, 63–67] and references therein).

Despite the clinical efficacy of classical neuroleptics, it has been difficult to reconcile the notion that D_2 receptor blockade in the striatum modulates psychosis, with data showing disturbances in cortical function and structure in schizophrenia [67, 68].

Using PET, several conflicting reports were published suggesting involvement or non-involvement of the D_2 receptor in schizophrenia. One group reported increased number of D_2 receptors in drug-free schizophrenics [69], although other groups have failed to replicate this [18, 79]. This discrepancy was probably related to different selectivity-profile for the ligands used; Wong and co-workers for instance used a ligand with high affinity for the D_4 receptor [71].

Post mortem studies suggested an increase in D_2 or D_2-like (see below) receptor-density in schizophrenics [72, 73], but this could be due to upregulation caused by prior antipsychotic treatment. Recent studies have not been able to replicate this but identified disruptions in the modular and laminar organisation of D_2 receptors in temporal cortex [74]. Quantitative receptor autoradiography for D_2 receptor binding with [^{125}I]epidepride in *post mortem* tissue of schizophrenic patients revealed that D_2 receptor concentration was decreased in superficial laminae, and abnormal concentrations of D_2 receptors were observed in granular layer IV.

In view of the relationship between neuropathology in temporal cortex in schizophrenia and positive symptoms [75], it is tempting to speculate that blockade of D_2 receptors may normalise the altered synaptic organisation in the temporal cortex and thus contribute to a reduction of psychosis.

D_3 receptors in schizophrenia

The distribution of D_3 receptors in human brain is different from the pattern of distribution of the D_1 and D_2 receptors. Quantitative autoradiographic studies showed the highest densities of D_3 receptors in the ventral striatum, nucleus accumbens, the neostriatum, olfactory tubercle, cerebral cortex and cerebellar cortex, and to a lesser extent in the substantia nigra [76, 77]. This regional distribution is consistent with D_3 receptor mRNA studies in the rat and human brain [78, 79]. *In vivo* studies suggest that in the substantia nigra the D_3 receptor acts as a DA synthesis modulating autoreceptor [80]. In addition, D_3 receptors are possibly involved in the control of locomotor activity [81], body temperature [82] and cocaine self-administration [83].

Postsynaptic D_3 receptors are found in higher concentrations in the targets of the mesolimbic DA system and in the limbic loop, which makes them likely candidates for mediating antipsychotic action, for these brain areas have been implicated in the regulation of affect and cognition. In line with this notion is the recent findings that D_3 receptor-deficient mice showed an anxiolytic profile in the elevated plus maze [84]. In addition, the localisation in the cerebellum also suggests a role in the control of behaviour [85].

It is also conceivable that D_3 receptor agonists might be effective antipsychotics, by presynaptically inhibiting ventral striatal DA release.

Several groups have reported the existence of D_3 polymorphism resulting in a serine-glycine substitution in the N-terminus of the receptor [86]. In a recent study, Shaikh and co-workers [87] reported a significant association between the D_3 Ser_9 allele and the Ser_9/Ser_9 genotype in 133 schizophrenic patients. Interestingly, they also found that the presence of this Ser_9/Ser_9 genotype was significantly more frequently present in non-responders to clozapine. A recent study, however, could not replicate the involvement of this genotype in schizophrenia. Malhotra and colleagues [88] determined D_3 Ser_9Gly genotypes in 58 schizophrenics and found that 1) Ser_9 is not preferentially transmitted in schizophrenia, and 2) could not replicate the previously reported association between this genotype and clozapine response.

Quantitative autoradiography in *post mortem* tissue of schizophrenic patients revealed 45 to 56% elevations in the number of D_3 receptors in rostral and caudal basal ganglia and ventral forebrain compared to controls [73].

Interestingly, schizophrenic patients free of antipsychotics at time of death showed twice as many D_3 receptors compared to controls. Patients receiving antipsychotics showed no difference in D_3 receptor density which may suggest that there exists a disease related increase in D_3 receptors which is normalised by antipsychotic treatment. Therefore, the likely site of antipsychotic action could be the D_3 receptor. This is, however, not supported by a recent *in vitro* receptor autoradiography study, which showed that chronic treatment with haloperidol, clozapine, raclopride or SCH 23390 failed to alter [^{3}H]7-OH-DPAT binding to D_3 receptors [58]. This lack of changes in binding could, however, be explained by the fact that the D_3 receptor has another regulatory mechanism compared to other DA receptor subtypes (for discussion, see [58]).

Treatment studies with selective $DA_{2/3}$ receptor antagonists

Sulpiride and remoxipride

Of the DA-selective compounds, the benzamides form a distinct chemical class, characterised by a high selectivity for $D_{2/3}$ receptors. Within this class of compounds, sulpiride has been the most extensively investigated. In animal experiments sulpiride shows a DA-blocking pharmacological profile: it inhibits apomorphine induced climbing behaviour in the rat, causes an increase in plasma prolactin and increases DA-turnover in striatal and mesolimbic systems. In certain respects however, sulpiride differs form classical neuroleptics in that it induces virtually no catalepsy, does inhibit stereotyped behaviour induced by apomorphine when administered in very high doses only, and causes no inhibition of DA-stimulated adenylate cyclase. The latter is interpreted as evidence for the hypothesis that sulpiride blocks D_2 receptors and not D_1 receptors. However, animal studies have shown that the separation between effects in models for antipsychotic effects and extrapyramidal side-effects is much less than previously thought [89]. In addition, there is some evidence that in low dosages sulpiride might induce presynaptic receptor blockade as well [90, 91]. Moreover, sulpiride, like other benzamides, appeared to have virtually no effect on other receptor systems suggesting the induction of only a limited number of autonomic side-effects. Sulpiride has been demonstrated to be effective in acute as well as in chronic schizophrenic patients, and to be equipotent as compared to classical neuroleptics like chlorpromazine and haloperidol [92, 93]. Since sulpiride shows a relatively low affinity for DA-receptors in the nigrostriatal systems, it was postulated that this compound (like clozapine) would induce few EPS. However, this could not be confirmed in double-blind studies with schizophrenic patients. Several clinical studies have suggested that sulpiride is not less likely to induce EPS as compared to haloperidol, indicating that a selective D_2 antagonist may act as an antipsychotic with the motor side-effect profile of a typical neuroleptic [94, 93]. These findings indicate that it is questionable whether sulpiride is correctly classified as an atypical anti-psychotic.

In a double-blind study, Petit et al. [95] investigated the effects of sulpiride on negative symptoms of chronic schizophrenic patients, comparing normal *versus* low-dosage of this compound. It was found that only the low-dose group improved significantly as reflected specifically by a reduction in negative symptoms. These preliminary results, may be related to an interaction of sulpiride with presynaptically located DA-receptor systems.

The substituted benzamide remoxipride shares many of the properties of sulpiride. The results of animal experiments with remoxipride suggested that this compound causes a preferential blockade of the mesolimbic DA-receptors [96]. Subsequently, it was found that DA-stimulated adenylate cyclase activity, which is mediated by D_1-receptors, is not blocked by remoxipride, suggesting that remoxipride acts selectively on $D_{2/3}$-receptors. In addition it was suggested that remoxipride has a preferential action in extrastriatal (e.g. mesolimbic) DA-ergic neuronal systems [97]. How this regional selectivity of remoxipride is accomplished is not altogether clear. It has been suggested that there exist two different isoforms of DA D_2 receptors: D_{2A} and D_{2B} receptors. There is electrophysiological evidence indicating that the relative density of these two isoforms may differ across brain regions (for references see [98]). A recent *in vitro* study showed that D_2 receptors in the ventral and dorsal hippocampus differ from those in the striatum, suggesting that this might in part explain the selectivity of atypical antipsychotics for these receptors in the limbic system [99].

In novel investigations in which the affinity of different antipsychotics to human DA D_{2A}, D_{2B}, and D_3 receptors was studied, it was found that remoxipride displayed a two- to threefold higher affinity for D_{2B} receptors than for the D_{2A} receptors [100].

The functional limbic selectivity of remoxipride is also supported by biochemical data. When DA receptors are occupied by either an agonist or antagonist, and the second messenger systems are inhibited or activated, the activity of Fos is increased. This increase can be measured as c-Fos-like immunoreactivity. In a recent study it was found that remoxipride and clozapine, unlike typical neuroleptics like haloperidol, have selective effects in different parts of the limbic system (e.g. prefrontal cortex, parts of the nucleus accumbens, lateral septal nucleus), whereas very little effect was noted in the basal ganglia after acute administration of remoxipride or clozapine to rats [101]. Another explanation for the atypical clinical profile of remoxipride which has been suggested is the demonstration that remoxipride may act as a dopamine autoreceptor agonist, in addition to its postsynaptic antagonistic properties [102].

Several open (see [103] for a review) as well as controlled studies with a variable duration have been performed showing that remoxipride has similar antipsychotic efficacy as traditional neuroleptics like haloperidol [104–107], thioridazine [108], chlorpromazine [109], concurrently with a reduced propensity for the induction of EPS. Since remoxipride was withdrawn from the market several years ago, we will not fully review the clinical data.

DA autoreceptor agonists

Another way of reducing DA neurotransmission, apart from blocking postsynaptic D_2 receptors, is through modulation of DA autoreceptors. It has been shown that DA autoreceptor agonists inhibit synthesis and release of DA as well as the firing rate of central DA neurons [110]. DA-autoreceptor agonists are assumed to be devoid of EPS since autoreceptor stimulation is supposed to reduce dopaminergic tone rather than abruptly diminishing dopaminergic output, as seen by conventional antipsychotics. Tamminga et al. [111] showed the potential of antipsychotic effect of an apomorphine derivative N-propylnorapomorphine. This compound has, in addition to affinity to the dopamine autoreceptor, high affinity to the D_3 receptor, predominantly postsynaptically localised in mesolimbic brain structures.

Experimental DA autoreceptor agonists which have been investigated to some extent in schizophrenia include terguride, an ergot autoreceptor agonist, talipexole (B-HT 920), which has a high affinity for D_2 receptors and agonistic effects on the autoreceptor, roxindole (EMD 49980) which possesses a more pronounced effect on presynaptic than on postsynaptic D_2 receptors, and OPC-4392 which acts as an agonist at DA autoreceptors and as antagonist at postsynaptic dopamine receptors. Roxindole is also a 5-HT_{1A} agonist with 5-HT uptake inhibiting properties [112, 113].

Preliminary studies with talipexole in small numbers of schizophrenic patients were discouraging, since hardly any antipsychotic effects were found [114].

Roxindole, which possesses a somewhat greater selectivity for DA autoreceptors than talipexole [115], was investigated in five open label studies.

The first study, in which seven patients were treated, did not reveal any improvement in BPRS scores [116]. In the second study [117], 12 acute ill schizophrenic patients with predominantly paranoid symptoms were included. Only in four patients was a clinically relevant improvement (reduction of $>50\%$ on the BPRS) found.

Interestingly, some improvement of patients with predominant negative symptoms was reported in two small open label studies [113, 118].

More recently, Wetzel and co-workers [119] reported a lack of effect on positive symptoms and a small but clinically relevant improvement in total score of the Scale for the Assessment of Negative Symptoms in two small open label studies.

Taken together these findings suggest absence of clear antipsychotic efficacy of roxindole. The effects on negative symptoms do merit further research in double blind studies. In view of the pharmacological profile of roxindole, which in addition to being a DA autoreceptor agonist also inhibits 5-HT uptake, displays 5-HT_{1A}, 5-HT_{1B} agonistic activity and acts as a 5-HT_{2A} antagonist [120], it is likely to be the case that the effects on negative symptoms are not exclusively related to the interaction with DA autoreceptors but are mediated by the serotonergic effects. In line with its pharmacological profile roxindole might possess antidepressant and anxiolytic properties [120, 115].

In sum, the experiences with DA autoreceptor agonists like talipexole, pramipexole, support the view that DA autoreceptor agonists are not effective antipsychotics. The preliminary findings with roxindole suggesting moderate efficacy in negative symptoms may be ascribed to its affinity for 5-HT receptor subtypes.

OPC-4392 has only been investigated in one small open study comprising 11 schizophrenic patients. Preliminary results indicate that positive symptoms are hardly affected, whereas more promising results were obtained with respect to negative symptoms [121].

The successor of talipexole is pramipexole (SND 919). Pramipexole is a $D_{2,3}$ receptor agonist which also modest affinity for the D_4 receptor [122, 123]. Preclinical and clinical studies suggested a potential role in schizophrenia, Parkinson's disease and possibly anxiety disorders [115, 124, 125]. Pramipexole is thought to act as a preferential D_2 agonist only in intact dopaminergic system. In cases of degeneration of presynaptic fibres (like Parkinson's disease) it acts as a postsynaptic D_2 agonist.

In schizophrenia, the use of D_2 agonists like pramipexole could be an alternative way to reduce dopaminergic transmission and thus ameliorate positive symptoms. In corticofrontal areas where D_2 receptors are postsynaptically located, pramipexole might stimulate dopaminergic transmission and thus lead to therapeutic effects in negative symptoms.

A 4-week open label study has been performed in 37 schizophrenic patients, yielding inconsistent and no convincing antipsychotic effects [126].

In a preliminary open study in 15 schizophrenic patients pramipexole was given to haloperidol treated patients [127]. A mean decrease in the positive subscale of the PANSS was found of 9.7%, whereas the negative subscale showed a reduction of 24.2%. Although preliminary in nature, these findings are in accordance with the hypothesis that addition of a $D_{2/3}$ agonist to ongoing haloperidol therapy is able to stimulate corticofrontal postsynaptic $D_{2/3}$ receptors, mimicking enhanced dopaminergic transmission in this area.

Based upon the hypothesis that hyperdopaminergic function can be reduced by administering a DA autoreceptor agonist (with effect on positive symptoms) and hypofunctioning of corticofrontal areas could be enhanced by postsynaptic $D_{2/3}$ agonists (with effects on negative symptoms) a series of combined agents has been synthesised [128]. CI-1007 is a DA autoreceptor agonist and a partial $D_{2/3}$ agonist that is currently under development for the treatment of schizophrenia [129].

Partial D_2 agonists

To the best of our knowledge only two compounds with the profile of a partial D_2-agonist which have been tested in schizophrenia: SDZ HDC 912 and terguride.

The rationale for developing compounds with a partial agonistic activity is that they have a dual action, depending on the functional state of the DA system. During increased dopaminergic activity which according to the DA hypothesis is coupled to schizophrenia, they act as DA antagonists, whereas they may act as agonists in situations in which there is a reduced dopaminergic function. SDZ HDC 912 is such a partial D_2 agonist and animal models suggested an antipsychotic profile [130, 131].

In an open 4-week study in schizophrenic patients it was found that SDZ HDC 912 showed good antipsychotic efficacy in most patients, but in a subsequent double-blind study *versus* haloperidol these results could not be confirmed, EPS being similar in the two treatment conditions [132]. Irrespective of these results the concept of partial D_2 agonists seems worthy of further investigation, since one might hypothesise that in the treatment of negative symptoms these drugs might be effective, for in the case of a reduced dopaminergic transmission these agents would act a DA agonists. In an open study in 11 schizophrenic patients terguride showed a marked reduction in negative symptoms as measured with the scale for the assessment of negative symptoms [133].

The $D_{2/3}$ antagonist amisulpiride

A large body of evidence suggests that the substituted benzamide amisulpiride act as a specific DA receptor antagonist with high affinity for D_2 and D_3 receptors (and virtually none for D_1, D_4 and D_5 and 5-HT receptor subtypes) displaying a degree of limbic selectivity [134]. At low doses amisulpiride has preferential effects on D_2/D_3 autoreceptors, thus controlling the release and synthesis of DA. The alleged selectivity of amisulpiride for the limbic dopaminergic system is supported by the fact that there is as greater abundance of D_3 than D_2 receptors in limbic *versus* striatal regions [135], and also by its selectivity for DA autoreceptors which are of the D_3 subtype [136].

The combination of several neurochemical properties, selectivity for D_3 and to a lesser extent for D_2 receptors, its limbic selectivity and its preferential affinity at low doses for presynaptic DA autoreceptors suggest that amisulpiride at low doses increased DA transmission and could be effective in negative symptoms of schizophrenia. At higher doses amisulpiride blocks postsynaptic DA $D_{2/3}$ receptors and thus reduces dopaminergic transmission leading to antipsychotic efficacy in productive schizophrenia [134, 137].

Clinical studies with amisulpiride in schizophrenia

At least five double-blind studies have been conducted comparing amisulpiride with either haloperidol or flupenthixol in acute schizophrenia with florid psychotic symptomatology [138–142]. All studies showed that amisulpiride showed comparable antipsychotic efficacy as the reference drug. At doses between 800–1200 mg/day a somewhat higher incidence of EPS was found [138], dose levels of 440 and 800 mg/day are nowadays considered the optimal regimen. In these dosages amisulpiride also has a reduced propensity for the induction of EPS compared to classical neuroleptics and thus fulfills the criteria for an atypical antipsychotic.

In two of the studies (for a review see [143]) a significant difference favouring amisulpiride was observed on negative symptoms as measured with the negative subscale of the PANSS. Given the high intensity of positive symptoms in the patient samples it is conceivable that these effects can be ascribed to a reduction in secondary negative symptomatology.

In order to allow a better understanding of the effects of amisulpiride on primary negative symptoms (or deficit symptoms) three placebo controlled double-blind studies have been carried out in chronic schizophrenic patients with a predominance of negative symptoms (see Table 1).

In view of the established efficacy of clozapine, risperidone and olanzapine in the treatment of schizophrenia, comparative studies of amisulpride against other atypical antipsychotics are warranted, and such studies are ongoing. In a recent European multicentre study amisulpiride 800 mg/day was compared with risperidone 8mg/day in acute schizophrenia [145]. This study showed similar efficacy of risperidone and amisulpiride in reducing

Table 1. Clinical studies showing efficacy on negative symptoms with amisulpiride in deficit schizophrenia

Author	Design	Duration	No. patients	Dose regimen
Boyer et al. 1995 [146]	DB, parallel group, 3 arms	6 weeks (6 weeks placebo run-in for neuroleptic pretreated patients) SANS > 75	104 (70 AMI)	AMI at 100, 300 mg/day; placebo: oral; twice a day
Paillère-Martinot et al. 1995 [147]	DB, parallel group, 2 arms	6 weeks SANS > 55	27 (14 AMI)	AMI at 50–100 mg/day; placebo; oral; once a day
Loo et al. 1997 [148]	DB, parallel group, 3 arms	6 months (extension 12 months) SANS > 60	141 (69 AMI)	AMI at 100 mg/day; placebo; oral; once a day

AMI = amisulpiride; SANS = Schedule for the Assessment of Negative Symptoms; DB = double-blind; inclusion criteria according to DSM-IIIR.

positive symptoms of schizophrenia. Both antipsychotics showed a reduction in the negative subscale of the PANSS, although in this patient sample it was difficult to disentangle secondary and primary negative symptoms.

To ensure the predominance of negative symptoms a minimum score on the Scale for the Assessment of Negative Symptoms (SANS) [145] was required (see Table 1). In addition, other scales measuring global psychopathology, anxiety symptoms and depression were used together with scales for the measurement of Parkinsonism.

The results of these studies showed that amisulpiride at a low dose range between 50 and 300 mg/day is effective in reducing primary negative symptoms of schizophrenia. The results of these studies confirm that the clinical effects of amisulpiride in patients with predominant negative symptoms could not be ascribed to a reduction in Parkinsonism, improvement of positive symptoms or reductions in depression-scores.

Theoretical implications

With conventional neuroleptics a DA D_2 receptor occupancy of 70–80% is considered an optimal interval for the treatment of positive symptomatology [149], whereas D_2 receptor occupancy of 85% has been associated with increased risk of EPS [18]. In a recent PET study it was shown that high doses of amisulpiride (630–910 mg/day) results in a D_2 receptor occupancy of 70–80% which is consistent with the dose range found to be effective in reducing positive symptoms [150]. Higher dose levels (up to 1107 mg/day) led to D_2 receptor occupancy of 85% and were associated with increased EPS. Low doses (50–100 mg/day) of amisulpiride resulted in only a 4–26% D_2 occupancy, suggesting that the effect on negative symptoms which was observed in this dose-range is not mediated *via* D_2 receptors, but could be mediated *via* the D_3 receptor.

The fact that a $D_{2/3}$ receptor antagonist is effective in reducing positive and negative symptoms challenges the view that a high degree of 5-HT_{2A} receptor occupancy characterises atypical antipsychotics. Using PET and [^{18} F]-setoperone, a radioligand with high affinity for cortical 5-HT_{2A} receptors, it was found that in contrast to clozapine and chlorpromazine, amisulpiride lacks a significant *in vivo* interaction with the 5-HT_{2A} receptor [151]. Thus, these findings are in accordance with the hypothesis that the effects of amisulpiride on negative symptoms are related to a low striatal D_2 receptor occupancy, independent of an action on 5-HT_{2A} receptors.

Finally, the observation that amisulpiride only has very low affinity for DA D_1, D_4 and D_5 receptors suggests that interaction with these receptors is not an absolute requirement for therapeutic efficacy in schizophrenia.

D_3 selective compounds

Several D_3 antagonists have been described (see Table 2) such as (+)-AJ 76; (+)-UH 232 [152]; (+)-S-14297 [153,154] and nafadotride [155], but these agents have only a 5–20 fold selectivity for D_3 vs D_2 receptors.

The pharmacological profile of recently developed more selective D_3 antagonists like PNU 99194A [156] and PD 152255 [157] suggest potential antipsychotic activity.

None of the mentioned agents has been tested in schizophrenia and therefore the role of highly selective D_3 antagonists in the treatment of schizophrenia remains to be elucidated.

Table 2. Examples of some old and new dopaminergic agents

1. *Antipsychotics with selective dopamine receptor blockade*		
	D_1 receptor antagonists	
		SCH 23390
		SCH 39166
		SDZ PSD 958
		NNC 01-0687
		NNC 01-756
	D_2, D_3 receptor antagonists	
		sulpiride
		amisulpride
		remoxipride
		raclopride
	Selective D_3 receptor antagonists	
		AJ 76
		UH 232
		S-14297
		Nafadotride
		PNU 99194
		PD 152255
	Selective D_3 agonists	
		PD 128907
		piribedil
	D_4 receptor antagonists	
		U-101387
		L-745,879
		GMC 1072
		GMC 1078
	D_4 selective agonist	
		PD 168077
2. *DA autoreceptor agonists*		
		pramipexole (SND 919)
		talipexole (B-HT 920)
		roxindole (EMD 49980)
		OPC-4392
3. *Partial D_2 agonists*		
		SDZ HDC 912
		Terguride

D_4 receptors

Using polyclonal antibodies, D_4 receptors in rat brain were localised in frontal and parietal cortex, hippocampus, globus pallidus and thalamus [158, 159]. In human brain D_4 receptor mRNA expression was found in frontal cortex, amygdala, thalamus, hypothalamus, cerebellum, entorhinal cortex, pituitary the dentate gyrus and CA2 regions of the hippocampus [160, 161].

A very interesting recent finding has been the discovery that the D_4 receptor can be activated not only by DA but also by adrenaline and noradrenaline, suggesting that this receptor could play a role in signalling between catecholamine systems [162, 163]. In view of the fact that the hippocampus is rich in noradrenergic innervation this could be the region where noradrenaline activates the D_4 receptor.

Another intriguing feature of D_4 receptors is that several polymorphic variants of this receptor have been found (for review see [164]). If these variants were functionally different and involved in the pathogenesis of schizophrenia this might explain 1) differences in the vulnerability for schizophrenia, and 2) the variability in clozapine response in treatment-refractory schizophrenic patients.

Several genetic-linkage analyses and association studies, however, failed to establish a link between the D_4 receptors and schizophrenia [165, 166], although this does not exclude the possibility that certain polymorphic variants of the D_4 receptor gene may increase susceptibility for schizophrenia.

In two studies in which responders and non-responders to clozapine were genotyped for expression of the D_4 repeat alleles, no association of the clozapine response with any D_4-allele was found [167, 168]. Thus, the variability in clinical response to clozapine could not be explained by the polymorphic variability of the D_4 receptor.

D_4 receptor density in schizophrenia

Four groups have reported an increased density of D_4 receptors in the striatum of schizophrenics [169–172]. Because no specific ligand was available at the time these studies were done, the D_4-like sites were calculated by subtracting the density of $[^3H]$ raclopride (binds to D_2 and D_3 receptors) from the density of $[^3H]$ nemonapride (binds to D_2, D_3 and D_4 receptors). This indirect estimation of the density of D_4 receptors has raised considerable debate. The lack of a pharmacological profile of these alleged D_4 receptors has led to the use of the term "D_4-like" receptors, which are not necessarily the same as D_4 receptors [173]. Moreover, two recent *post mortem* studies failed to detect significant levels of D_4 mRNA in the striatum [174, 175], whereas Roberts and co-workers [176] failed to find differences in D_4 mRNA expression between schizophrenics and controls, raising the possibility that the previously reported upregulation of D_4 could be due to another DA receptor. A recent study also found evidence for decreased mRNA expression of D_3 and D_4 receptors in the orbitofrontal cortex in schizophrenic patients, which is in accordance with the hypothesis of prefrontal hypodopaminergic neurotransmission in schizophrenia [175].

It is conceivable that these methodological problems will be solved by using highly selective radioligands for the D_4 receptor which have recently become available [177].

Preliminary findings, however, with D_4 selective [^{3}H]-ligands indicated hardly detectable D_4 receptors in human control or schizophrenia striata [178] suggesting that the previously reported upregulation of D_4 receptors could represent altered D_2-like receptors [179].

Finally, the possibility that the reported upregulation of D_4 receptors in schizophrenia is the result of prior antipsychotic treatment cannot be excluded, as chronic treatment with raclopride and clozapine has been shown to lead to a significant increase in D_4-like receptors in the caudate-putamen of the rat [58].

In search of selective D_4 receptor antagonists

The D_4 receptor has received much attention since the discovery that clozapine displays a 10-fold higher affinity to the D_4 compared to D_2 and D_3 receptors, suggesting that the unique clinical profile of clozapine could be mediated through D_4 instead of D_2 [180].

The first selective D_4 antagonist which has been tested in a sample of schizophrenic patients is L-745,870, a compound with a 2000-fold selectivity for the D_4 receptor compared to other DA receptor subtypes. Thirty-eight schizophrenic patients were included in a double-blind study of 4 weeks with L-745,870 vs placebo [181]. No antipsychotic effects were observed. In contrast, there was a consistent mild worsening of measures on several psychometric scales raising the possibility that L-745,870 was mildly psychotogenic. This preliminary study does not support the contention that antagonism of the D_4 receptor alone is sufficient to induce antipsychotic efficacy and questions the rationale for further development of D_4 antagonists [182]. Whether the psychotogenic properties of L-745,870 would call for treatment with D_4 *agonists* is unclear. So far, only one D_4 agonist has been developed [183], and this compound has not yet been tested in the clinic.

Other D_4 antagonists with a high degree of selectivity include U-101387 [184], RBI-257 [185], GMC 1072 and GMC 1078 which possess a 70–140-fold selectivity for D_4 compared to D_2 [186]. These new compounds have not yet been tested in schizophrenia.

In summary, the lack of a relationship between genetic alterations of the D_4 gene and either the response to clozapine or the development of schizophrenia, combined with the lack of efficacy of the first clinically tested selective D_4 antagonist in schizophrenia call into question the rationale for developing a specific D_4 antagonist. Still, these receptor-specific compounds hold great promise for our understanding of the function of the D_4 receptor *in vivo*, even in the absence of clinical efficacy.

Epilogue

The DA hypothesis of schizophrenia in its oversimplified "classical" form suggesting overactive dopaminergic pathways as the cornerstone of the pathophysiology underwent considerable refinement over the past years. We are now aware of the fact that the alleged overexpression of D_2 receptors described in the 1980s is due to a combination of different receptor belonging to the D_2-receptor family. It has also been shown that the D_1- and D_2 receptor family show a regional distribution in different areas of the brain. D_1 receptors are found in prefrontal cortex and caudate putamen, D_5 receptors in prefrontal cortex and hippocampus, D_2 receptors in the medial temporal lobe structures and dorsal striatum, D_3 receptors in the ventral striatum and its efferents, and D_4 receptors widely dispersed in cortical areas. This regionally specific expression of different receptor subtypes relates to differential involvement in behavioural, cognitive and affective dysfunctions important in schizophrenia. Increased understanding of the functional significance of this regional distribution will enhance the development of a more "rational" psychopharmacology for schizophrenia.

References

1 McGue M, Gottesman II (1991) The genetic epidemiology of schizophrenia and the design of linkage studies. *Eur Arch Psychiatry Clin Neurosci* 240: 174–181
2 McGrath JJ, Pemberton MR, Welham JL, Murray RM (1994) Schizophrenia and the influenza epidemics of 1954, 1957 and 1959: a Southern Hemisphere study. *Schizophr Res* 14: 1–8
3 Supprian T, Hofmann E, Warmuth-Metz M, Franzek E, Becker T (1997) MRI T2 relaxation times of brain regions in schizophrenic patients and control subjects. *Psychiatry Res* 75: 173–182
4 Sullivan EV, Lim KO, Mathalon D, Marsh L, Beal DM, Harris D, Hoff, AL, Faustman WO, Pfefferbaum A (1998) A profile of cortical gray matter volume deficits characteristic of schizophrenia. *Cereb Cortex* 8: 117–124
5 Lee T, Seeman P (1980) Elevation of brain neuroleptic/dopamine receptors in schizophrenia. *Am J Psychiatry* 137: 191–197
6 Seeman P, Niznik HB, Guan H-C, Booth G, Ulpian C (1989) Link between D_1 and D_2 dopamine receptors is reduced in schizophrenia and Huntington diseased brain. *Proc Natl Acad Sci* 86: 10156–10160
7 Haracz JL (1982) The dopamine hypothesis. An overview of studies with schizophrenic patients. *Schizophr Bull* 8: 438–469

8 Carlton PL, Manowitz P (1984) Dopamine and schizophrenia, an analysis of the theory. *Neurosci Biobehav Rev* 8: 137–151
9 Davis KL, Kahn RS, Ko G, Davidson M (1991) Dopamine in schizophrenia, a review and reconceptualization. *Am J Psychiatry* 148: 1474–1486
10 Korf J (1996) Dopamine hypothesen bij schizofrenie. In: Den Boer JA, Vanden den Bosch RJ (eds): *Leerboek Schizofrenie, een neurobiologische benadering*. De Tijdstroom, Utrecht, 128–142
11 Farde L, Hall H, Ehrin E, Sedvall G (1986) Quantitative analysis of D_2 dopamine receptor binding in the living human brain by PET. *Science* 231: 258–261
12 Smith M, Wolf AP, Brodie JD, Arnett CD, Barouche F, Shiue C-Y, Fowler JS, Russel JAG, MacGregor RR, Wolkin A et al. (1988) Serial [^{18}F] N-methylspiroperidol PET studies to measure changes in antipsychotic drug D_2 receptor occupancy in schizophrenic patients. *Biological Psychiatry* 23: 653–663
13 Baron JC, Martinot JL, Cambon H, Boulenger JP, Poirier MF, Caillard V, Blin J, Huret JD, Loc'h C, Maziere B (1989) Striatal dopamine receptor occupancy during and following withdrawal from neuroleptic treatment: correlative evaluation by positron emission tomography and plasma prolactin levels. *Psychopharmacology* 99: 463–472
14 Louwerens JW, Buddingh JA, Zijlstra S, Pruim J, Korf J, Paans AMJ, Vaalburg W, Slooff CJ (1993) Dopamine(D_2)-receptor occupancy in clozapine-treated patients as measured by positron emission tomography using 18 FESP. In: Brunello N, Mendelwicz J, Racagni G (eds): *New generation of antipsychotic drugs: Novel mechanisms of action*. Karger, Basel, 130–135
15 Klemm E, Grünwald F, Kasper S, Menzel C, Broich K, Danos P, Reichmann K, Krappel C, Rieker O, Briele B et al. (1996) [^{123}I] IBZM SPECT for imaging of striatal D_2 dopamine receptors in 56 schizophrenic patients taking various neuroleptics. *Am J Psychiatry* 153: 183–190
16 Coppens HJ, Slooff CJ, Paans AMJ, Wiegman T, Vaalburg W, Korf J (1991) High central D_2-dopamine occupancy as assessed with positron emission tomography in medicated but therapy-resistant schizophrenic patients. *Bil Psychiatry* 29: 629–634
17 Wolkin A, Barouche F, Wolf AP (1989) Dopamine blockade and clinical response: evidence for two biological subgroups of schizophrenia. *Am J Psychiatry* 46: 905–908
18 Farde L, Nordström AL, Wiesel FA, Pauli S, Halldin C, Sedvall G (1992) Positron emission tomographic analysis of central D_1 and D_2 dopamine receptor occupancy in patients treated with classical neuroleptics and clozapine. Relation to extrapyramidal side-effects. *Arch Gen Psychiatry* 49: 538–544
19 Scherer J, Tatsch K, Schwarz J, Oertel WH, Konjarczyk M, Albus M (1994) D_2-dopamine receptor occupancy differs between patients with and without extrapyramidal side-effects. Acta Psychiatr Scand 90: 266–268
20 Busatto GF, Pilowsky LS, Costa DC, Ell PJ, Verhoeff NPLG, Kerwin RW (1995) Dopamine D_2 receptor blockade *in vivo* with the novel antipsychotics risperidone and remoxipride – an ^{123}I-IBZM single photon emission tomography (SPET) study. *Psychopharmacology* 117: 55–61
21 Küfferle B, Tauscher J, Asenbaum S, Vesely C, Podreka I, Brücke T, Kasper S (1997) IBZM SPECT imaging of striatal dopamine-2 receptors in psychotic patients treated with the novel antipsychotic substance quetiapine in comparison to clozapine and haloperidol. *Psychopharmacology* 133: 323–328
22 Bench CJ, Lammertsma AA, Dolan RJ, Grasby PM, Warrington SJ, Gunn K, Cuddigan M, Turton DJ, Osman S, Frackowiak RSJ (1993) Dose dependent occupancy of central dopamine D_2 receptors by the novel neuroleptic CP-88,059-01: a study using positron emission tomography and ^{11}C-raclopride. *Psychopharmacology* 112: 308–314
23 Sokoloff P, Giros MP, Martres ML, Bouthenet ML, Schwartz JC (1990) Molecular cloning and characterization of a novel dopamine receptor (D_3) as a target for neuroleptics. *Nature* 347: 146–151
24 Van Tol HHM, Bunzow JR, Guan HC, Sunahara RK, Seeman P, Niznik HB (1991) Cloning of the gene for a human dopamine D_4 receptor with high affinity for the antipsychotic clozapine. *Nature* 350: 610–614
25 Sunahara RK, Guan HC, O'Dowd BF, Seeman P, Laurier LG, Ng G (1991) Cloning of the gene for a human dopamine D_5 receptor with higher affinity for dopamine than D_1. *Nature* 350: 614–619

26 Coward DM, Imperato A, Urwyler S (1989) Biochemical and behavioural properties of clozapine. *Psychopharmacology* 99: S6–S12
27 Bymaster FP, Calligaro DO, Falcone JF, Marsh RD, Moore NA, Tye NC, Seeman P, and Wong DT (1996) Radioreceptor binding profile of atypical antipsychotic olanzapine. *Neuropsychopharmacology* 14: 87–96
28 Robertson GS, Fibiger HC (1992) Neuroleptics increase C-FOS expression in the forebrain: contrasting effects of haloperidol and clozapine. *Neuroscience* 46: 315–328
29 Deutch AY, Duman RS (1996) The effects of antipsychotic drugs on Fos protein exression in the prefrontal cortex: cellular localization and pharmacological characterization. *Neuroscience* 70: 377–389
30 Dearry A, Gingrich JA, Falardeau P, Fremeau RT Jr, Bates MD, Caron MG (1990) Molecular cloning and expression of the gene for a human D_1 dopamine receptor. *Nature* 347: 72–76
31 Zhou QY, Grandy DK, Thambi L, Kushner JA, Van Tol HH, Cone R, Pribnow D, Salon-Bunzow JR, Civelli O (1990) Cloning and expression of human and rat D_1 dopamine receptors. *Nature* 347: 76–80
32 Dawson TM, Gehlert DR, McCabe RT, Barnett A, Wamsley JK (1986) D_1 dopamine receptors in the rat brain: a quantitative autoradiographic analysis. *J Neurosci* 6: 2352–2365
33 Lidow MS, Goldman-Rakic PS, Rakic P (1991) Distribution of dopaminergic receptors in the primate cerebral cortex: quantitative autoradiographic analysis using [^{3}H] raclopride, [^{3}H] spiperone and [^{3}H] SCH 23390. *Neuroscience* 40: 657–671
34 Goldman-Rakic PS (1991) Prefrontal cortical dysfunction in schizophrenia: the relevance of working memory. In: B Carrol (ed): *Psychopathology and the brain*. Raven Press, New York, 1–23
35 Weiner DM, Levey AI, Sunahara RK, Niznik HB, O'Dowd BF, Seeman P, Brann MR (1991) D_1 and D_2 dopamine receptor mRNA in rat brain. *Proc Natl Acad Sci USA* 88: 1859–1863
36 Cameron DL, Williams JT (1993) Dopamine D_1 receptors facilitate transmitter release. *Nature* 366: 344–347
37 Jensen AA, Pedersen UB, Din N, Andersen PH (1996) The dopamine D_1 receptor family: structural and functional aspects. *Recent advances in brain dopaminergic systems* 24: 163–169
38 Pedersen UB, Norby B, Jensen AA, Schiodt M, Hansen A, Suhr-Jessen P, Scheideler M, Thastrup O, Andersen PH (1994) Characteristics of stably expressed human dopamine D1a and D1b receptors: atypical behavior of the dopamine D1b receptor. *Eur J Pharmacol* 267: 85–93
39 Sobell JL, Heston LL, Sommer SS (1993) Novel association approach for determining the genetic predisposition to schizophrenia: case control resource and testing of a candidate gene. *Am J Med Genet* 48: 28–35
40 Jensen S, Plaetke R, Holik J, Hoff M, Myles-Worsley M, Leppert M, Coon H,Vest K, Freedman R, Waldo M et al. (1993) Linkage analysis of schizophrenia: the D_1 dopamine receptor gene and several flanking DNA markers. *Hum Hered* 43: 58–62
41 Coon H, Byerley W, Holik J, Hoff M, Myles-Worsley M, Lannfelt L, Sokoloff P, Schwartz JC, Waldo M, Freedman R et al. (1993) Linkage analysis of schizophrenia with five dopamine receptor genes in nine pedigrees. *Am J Hum Genet* 52: 327–334
42 Liu Q, Sobell JL, Heston LL, Sommer SS (1995) Screening the dopamine D_1 receptor gene in 131 schizophrenics and eight alcoholics: identification of polymorphisms but lack of functionally significant sequence changes. *Am J Med Gen* 60: 165–171
43 Cichon S, Nöthen MM, Stöber G, Schroers R, Albus M, Maier W, Rietschel M, Körner J, Weigelt B, Franzek E et al. (1996) Systematic screening for mutations in the 5′-regulatory region of the human dopamine D_1 receptor (DRD1) gene in patients with schizophrenia and bipolar affective disorder. *Am J Med Gen* 67: 424–428
44 Harrington KA, Augood SJ, Faull RLM, McKenna PJ, Emson PC (1995) Dopamine D_1 receptor, D_2 receptor, proenkephalin A and substance P gene expression in the caudate nucleus of control and schizophrenic tissue: a quantitative cellular in situ hybridisation study. *Mol Brain Res* 33: 333–342
45 Knable MB, Hyde TM, Murray AM, Herman MM, Kleinman JE (1996) A postmortem study of frontal cortical dopamine D_1 receptors in schizophrenics, psychiatric controls, and normal controls. *Biol Psychiatry* 40: 1191–1199

46 McQuade RD, Duffy RA, Coffin VL, Barnett A (1992) *In vivo* binding to dopamine receptors, a correlate of potential antipsychotic activity. *Eur J Pharmacol* 215: 29–34
47 Lynch MR (1992) Schizophrenia and the D_1 receptor, focus on negative symptoms. *Prog Neuro-psychopharmacol and Biol Psychiat* 16: 797–832
48 Ellenbroek BA, Willemen APM, Cools AR (1989) Are antagonists of dopamine D_1 receptors drugs that attenuate both positive and negative symptoms of schizophrenia? A pilot study in java monkeys. *Neuropsychopharmacol* 2: 191–199
49 Gessa GL, Canu A, Del Zompo M, Burrai C, Serra G (1990) Lack of acute antipsychotic effect of SCH 23390, a selective dopamine D_1 receptor antagonist. *Lancet* 337: 854–855
50 Barnett A, Chipkin RE, Crosby G, Fox J (1988) The profile of the new D_1 selective benzonaphthazepine SCH 39166 in four different tests suggests that it has low probability of producing extrapyramidal effects. *Psychopharmacology* 96: 238 (Abstract 14.41.04).
51 Chipkin RE, Lorio LC, MqQuade RD, Berger JG, Barnett A (1988) Pharmacological profile of SCH 39166, a dopamine D_1 selective benzophthazepine with potential antipsychotic activity. *J Pharmacol Exp Ther* 247: 1093–1102
52 Tice MAB, Hashemi T, Taylor LA, Duffy RA, McQuade RD (1994) Characterization of the binding of SCH 39166 to the five cloned dopamine receptor subtypes. *Pharmacol Biochem Behav* 49: 567–571
53 Den Boer JA, Van Megen HJGM, Fleischhacker WW, Louwerens JW, Slaap BR, Westenberg HGM, Burrows GD, Srivastava ON (1995) Differential effects of the D_1-DA receptor antagonist SCH 39166 on positive and negative symptoms of schizophrenia. *Psychopharmacology* 121: 317–322
54 Karlsson P, Smith L, Farde L, Harnryd C, Sedvall G, Wiesel FA (1995) Lack of apparent antipsychotic effect of the D_1-dopamine receptor antagonist SCH 39166 in acutely ill schizophrenic patients. *Psychopharmacology* 121: 309–316
55 Karlsson P, Sedvall G, Halldin C, Swahn CG, Farde L (1995) Evaluation of SCH 39166 as PET ligand for central D_1 dopamine receptor binding and occupancy in man. *Psychopharmacology* 121: 300–308
56 Karle J, Clemmesen L, Hansen L, Andersen M, Andersen J, Fensbo C, Sloth-Nielsen M, Skrumsager BK, Lublin H, Gerlach J (1995) NNC 01-0687, a selective dopamine D_1 receptor antagonist, in the treatment of schizophrenia. *Psychopharmacology* 121: 328–329
57 Okubo Y, Suhara T, Suzuki K, Kobayashi K, Inoue O, Terasaki O, Someya Y, Sassa T, Sudo Y, Matsushima E et al. (1997) Decreased prefrontal dopamine D_1 receptors in schizophrenia revealed by PET. *Nature* 385: 634–636
58 Tarazi FI, Florijn WJ, Creese I (1997) Differential regulation of dopamine receptors after chronic typical and atypical antipsychotic drug treatment. *Neuroscience* 78: 985–996
59 Lidow MS, Goldman-Rakic PS (1994) A common action of clozapine, haloperidol, and remoxipride on D_1- and D_2-dopaminergic receptors in the primate cerebral cortex. *Proc Natl Acad Sci USA* 91: 4353–4356
60 Lidow MS, Elsworth JD, Goldman-Rakic PS (1997) Downregulation of the D_1 and D_5 dopamine receptors in the primate prefrontal cortex by chronic treatment with antipsychotic drugs. *J Pharmacol Exp Ther* 281: 597–603
61 Niznik HB, Liu F, Sugamori KS, Cardinaud B, Vernier P (1998) Expansion of the dopamine D_1 receptor gene family: defining molecular, pharmacological, and functional criteria for D1A, D1B, D1C, and D1D receptors. *Advances in Pharmacology* 42: 404–408
62 Wang F, Bergson C, Howard RL, Lidow MS (1997) Differential expression of D_1 and D_5 dopamine receptors in the fetal primate cerebral wall. *Cerebral Cortex* 7: 711–721
63 Sebens JB, Koch T, TerHorst GJ, Korf J (1995) Differential Fos-protein induction in rat forebrain regions after acute and long-term haloperidol and clozapine treatment. *Europ J Pharmacol* 273: 175–182
64 Sebens JB, Koch T, Korf J (1996). Lack of cross tolerance between haloperidol and clozapine towards Fos-protein induction in rat forebrain regions. *Europ J Pharmacol* 315: 269–275
65 Sebens JB, Koch T, Korf J (1998). Rat regional expression of Fos-protein and cross tolerance with clozapine studies with acute and long-term treatment of olanzapine. *Europ J Pharmacol; in press*
66 Robertson GS, Fibiger HC (1996) Effects of olanzapine on regional C-Fos expression in rat forebrain. *Neuropsychopharmacology* 14: 105–110

67 Shapiro RM (1993) Regional neuropathology in schizophrenia: where are we? Where are we going? *Schizophrenia Res* 10: 187–239
68 Pearlson GD, Petty RG, Ross CA, Tien AY (1996) Schizophrenia: a disease of heteromodal association cortex. *Neuropsychopharmacology* 14: 1–18
69 Wong DF, Wagner HN, Tune LE, Dannals RF, Pearlson GD, Links JM, Tamminga CA, Broussole EP, Ravert HT, Wilson AA et al. (1986) Positron emission tomography reveals elevated D_2 dopamine receptors in drug-naive schizophrenics. *Science* 234: 1558–1563
70 Martinot JL, Peron-Magnan P, Huret JD, Mazoyer B, Baron JC, Boulenger JP, Loch C, Maziere B, Caillard V, Loo H et al. (1990) Striatal D_2 dopaminergic receptors assessed with positron emission tomography and [^{76}Br]bromospiperone in untreated schizophrenic patients. *Am J Psychiatr* 147: 44–50
71 Joyce JN, Meador-Woodruff JH (1997) Linking the family of D_2 receptors to neuronal circuits in human brain: insights into schizophrenia. *Neuropsychopharmacology* 16: 375–384
72 Seeman P, Bzowej NH, Guan HC, Bergeron C, Reynolds GP, Bird ED, Riederer P, Jellinger K, Tourtellote WW (1987) Human brain D_1 and D_2 dopamine receptors in schizophrenia, Alzheimer's, Parkinson's and Huntington's disease. *Neuropsychopharmacology* 1: 5–15
73 Gurevich EV, Bordelon Y, Shapiro RM, Arnold SE, Gur RE, Joyce JN (1997) Mesolimbic dopamine D_3 receptors and use of antipsychotics in patients with schizophrenia. *Arch Gen Psychiatry* 54: 225–232
74 Goldsmith SK, Shapiro RM, Joyce JN (1997) Disrupted pattern of D_2 dopamine receptors in the temporal lobe in schizophrenia. *Arch Gen Psychiatry* 54: 649–658
75 Joyce JN (1993) The dopamine hypothesis of schizophrenia: limbic interactions with serotonin and norepinephrine. *Psychopharmacology* 112: S16–S34
76 Herroelen L, De Backer JP, Wilczak N, Flamez A, Vauquelin G, De Keyser J (1994) Autoradiographic distribution of D_3-type dopamine receptors in human brain using [^{3}H]7-hydroxy-*N*,*N*-di-*n*-propyl-2-aminotetralin. *Brain Res* 648: 222–228
77 Hall H, Halldin C, Dijkstra D, Wikström H, Wise LD, Pugsley TA, Sokoloff P, Pauli S, Farde L, Sedvall G (1996) Autoradiographic localisation of D_3-dopamine receptors in the human brain using the selective D_3-dopamine receptor antagonist (+)-[^{3}H]PD 128907. *Psychopharmacology* 128: 240–247
78 Lévesque D, Diaz J, Pilon C, Martres MP, Giros B, Souil E, Schott D, Morgat JL, Schwartz JC, Sokoloff P (1992) Identification, characterization, and localization of the dopamine D_3 receptor in rat brain using 7-(^{3}H)hydroxy-*N*,*N*-di-*n*-propyl-2-aminotetralin. *Proc Natl Acad Sci* 89: 8155–8159
79 Landwehrmeyer B, Mengod G, Palacios JM (1993) Dopamine D_3 receptor mRNA and binding sites in human brain. *Mol Brain Res* 18: 187–192
80 Aretha CW, Sinha A, Galloway MP (1995) Dopamine D_3-preferring ligands act at synthesis modulating autoreceptors. *J Pharmacol Exp Ther* 274: 609–613
81 Millan MJ, Gressier H, Brocco M (1997) The dopamine D_3 receptor antagonist, (+)-S 14297, blocks the cataleptic properties of haloperidol in rats. *Eur J Pharmacol* 321: R7–R9
82 Millan MJ, Audinot V, Rivet J-M, Gobert A, Vian J, Prost J-F, Spedding M, Peglion J-L (1994) S 14297, a novel selective ligand at cloned human dopamine D_3 receptors, blocks 7-OH-DPAT-induced hypothermia in rats. *Eur J Pharmacol* 260: R3–R5
83 Caine SB, Koob GF (1993) Modulation of cocaine self-administration in the rat through D_3 dopamine receptors. *Science* 260: 1814–1816
84 Steiner H, Fuchs S, Accili D (1997) D_3 dopamine receptor-deficient mouse: evidence for reduced anxiety. *Physiol Behav* 63: 137–141
85 Barik S, de Beaurepaire R (1996) Evidence for a functional role of the dopamine D_3 receptors in the cerebellum. *Brain Res* 737: 347–350
86 Lannfelt L, Sokoloff P, Martres MP, Pilon C, Jonsson E, Sedvall G, Schwartz JC (1992) Amino-acid substitution in the dopamine D_3 receptor as a useful polymorphism for investigating psychiatric disorders. *Psychiatr Genet* 2: 249–256
87 Shaikh S, Collier DA, Sham PC, Ball D, Aitchison K, Vallada H, Smith I, Gill M, Kerwin RW (1996) Allelic association between a Ser-9-Gly polymorphism in the dopamine D_3 receptor gene and schizophrenia. *Hum Genet* 97: 714–719

88 Malhotra AK, Goldman D, Buchanan RW, Rooney W, Clifton A, Kosmidis MH, Breier A, Pickar D (1998) The dopamine D_3 receptor (DRD3) Ser_9Gly polymorphism and schizophrenia: a haplotype relative risk study and association with clozapine response. *Molecular Psychiatry* 3: 72–75

89 Ögren SO, Florvall L, Hall H, Magnusson O, Ångeby-Møller K (1990) Neuropharmacological and behavioral properties of remoxipride in the rat. *Acta Psychiat Scand* 82: 21–26

90 Kendler KS, Bracha HS, Davis KL (1982) Dopamine autoreceptor and postsynaptic receptor blocking potency of neuroleptics. *Eur J Pharmacol* 79: 217–223

91 Worms P (1982) Behavioral pharmacology of the benzamides as compared to standard neuroleptics. In: Stanley M, Rotrosen J (eds): *The benzamides, pharmacology, neurobiology and clinical aspects.* Raven Press, New York

92 Bratfos O, Haug JO (1979). Comparison of sulpiride and chlorpromazine in psychoses, a double-blind multicentre study. *Acta Psychiatr Scand* 60: 1–9

93 Gerlach J, Behnke K, Heltberg J, Munk-Andersen E, Nielsen H (1985) Supliride and haloperidol in schizophrenia, a double-blind cross-over study of therapeutic effect, side-effects and plasma concentrations. *Br J Psychiatry* 147: 283–288

94 Harnryd C, Bjerkenstedt L, Bjork K, Gullberg B, Oxenstierna G, Sedvall G, Wiesel FA, Wik G, Asberg-Wistedt A (1984) Clinical evaluation of sulpiride in schizophrenic patients. A double blind comparison with chlorpromazine. *Acta Psychiatr Scand* 311: 7–30

95 Petit M, Zann M, Lesieur P (1987) The effect of sulpride on negative symptoms of schizophrenia. *Br J Psychiatry* 150: 270–271

96 Ögren SO, Hall H, Köhler C, Magnussen O, Lindbom L-O, Ångeby-Møller K, Florvall L (1984) Remoxipride, a new potential antipsychotic compound with selective antidopaminergic actions in the rat brain. *Eur J Pharmacol* 102: 459–474

97 Köhler C, Hall, H, Magnusson O, Gustafsson K (1990) Biochemical pharmacology of the atypical neuroleptic remoxipride. *Acta Psych Scand Suppl* 358: 27–36

98 Deutch AY, Moghaddam B, Innis RB, Krystal JH Aghajanian GK, Bunney BS, Charney DS (1991) Mechanism of action of atypical neuroleptic drugs. *Schizophrenia Res* 4: 121–156

99 Bruinink A, Bischoff S (1993). Dopamine D_2 receptors are unevely distributed in the rat hippocampus and are modulated differently in the striatum. *Eur J Pharmacol* 245: 157–164

100 Malmberg A, Jackson DM, Eriksson A, Mohell N (1993) Unique binding characteristics of antipsychotic agents interacting with human dopamine D2A, D2B and D3 receptors. *Mol Pharmacol* 43: 749–754

101 Deutch AY, McLee M, Iadarola MJ (1992) Regionally specific affects of atypical antipsychotic drugs on striatal fos expression: the nucleus accumbens shell as a locus of antipsychotic action. *Molecular and Cellular Neurosciences* 3: 332–341

102 Ahlenius S, Ericson E, Wijkström A (1993) Stimulation of brain dopamine autoreceptors by remoxipride administration in reserpine-treated male rats. *J Pharm Pharmacol* 45: 237–239

103 Den Boer JA, Verhoeven WMA, Westenberg HGM (1987) Remoxipride, a novel neuroleptic in the treatment of schizophrenia, *Psychopharmacol Bull* 23: 206–210

104 Ahlfors UG, Rimon R, Appelberg B, Hagert U, Harma P, Katila H (1990). Remoxipride and haloperidol in schizophrenia, a double blind multicentre study. *Acta Psychiatrica Scandinavica* 82: 99–104

105 Den Boer JA, Ravelli DP, Huisman J, Ohrvik J, Verhoeven WMA, Westenberg HGM (1990). Double blind comparative study of remoxipride and haloperidol in acute schizophrenic patients. *Psychopharmacology* 102: 76–84

106 Hebenstreit GF, Laux G, Schubert H, Beckmann H, Amman J, Bunse J, Eikmeier G, Geretsegger Ch, Kanitz RD, Kanzow WTh, et al. (1991) Double-blind multicentre study with remoxipride controlled release and immediate release formulations and haloperidol in schizophrenic patients. Abstract Biological Psychiatry, 5th World Congress, Florence, Italy, 29 (suppl), 0-11-02

107 Ashwood TJ, Hallstrom C, King DJ, Livingston MG, McCreadie RG (1992) An open study of remoxipride in the long-term treatment of schizophrenia. *J Psychopharmacol* 6: 519–525

108 McCreadie RG, Todd M, Livingston M, Eccleston D, Watt JAG, Herrington RN (1990) A double-blind comparative study of remoxipride and thioridazine in the acute phase of schizophrenia. *Acta Psych Scand* 82: 136–138

109 Chouinard G (1990) A placebo-controlled clinical trial of remoxipride and chlorpromazine in newly admitted schizophrenic patients with acute exacerbation. *Acta Psychiatrica Scandinavica* (Suppl 358) 82: 111–120

110 Clark D, Hjorth S, Carlsson A. (1985) Dopamine receptor agonists, mechanisms underlying autoreceptor selectivity. I. Review of the evidence. *J Neural Transm.* 62: 1–52

111 Tamminga CA, Gotts MD, Thaker GK, Alphs LD, Foster NL (1986) Dopamine agonist treatment of schizophrenia with N-propylnorapomorphine. *Arch Gen Psychiatry* 43: 398–402

112 Seyfried CA, Greiner HE, Haase AF (1989) Biochemical and functional studies on EMD 49980, a potent, selectively presynaptic D-2 dopamine agonist with actions on serotonin systems. *Eur J Pharmacol* 160: 31–41

113 Wiedemann K, Krieg JC, Loycke A, Holsboer F (1992) In: Meltzer HY (ed): *Novel dopamine autoreceptor agonists B-HT 920 and EMD 49980 in the treatment of patients with schizophrenia. Novel Antipsychotic Drugs,* Raven Press, New York, 91–98

114 Wiedemann K, Benkert O, Holsboer F (1990) B-HT 920- a novel dopamine autoreceptor agonist in the treatment of patients with schizophrenia. *Pharmacopsychiatry* 23: 50–55

115 Bartoszyk GD (1998) Anxiolytic effects of dopamine receptor ligands: I. Involvement of dopamine autoreceptors. *Life Sci* 62: 649–663

116 Wetzel HA, Hilbert O, Grunder G, Benkert O (1992) Roxindole, a dopamine autoreceptor agonist in the treatment of patients with schizophrenia. *Am J Psychiatry; in press*

117 Klimke, A, Klieser E (1991) Antipsychotic efficacy of the dopaminergic autoreceptor agonist EMD 49980 (roxindole). *Pharmacopsychiatry* 24: 107–112

118 Kasper S, Fuger J, Zinner HJ, Bäuml J, Möller HJ (1992) Early clinical results with the neuroleptic roxindole (EMD 49980) in the treatment of schizophrenia- an open study. *Eur Neuropsychopharmacol* 2: 91–95

119 Wetzel H, Hillert A, Gründer G, Benkert O (1994) Roxindole, a dopamine autoreceptor agonist, in the treatment of positive and negative schizophrenic symptoms. *Am J Psychiatry* 151: 1499–1502

120 Maj J, Kolodziejczyk K, Rogóz Z, Skuza G (1997) Roxindole, a dopamine autoreceptor agonist with a potential antidepressant activity. II. Effects on the 5-hydroxytryptamine system. *Pharmacopsychiat* 30: 55–61

121 Gerbaldo H, Demisch L, Lehmann CO, Bochnik J (1988) The effect of OPC-4392, a partial dopamine receptor agonist, on negative symptoms, results of an open study. *Pharmacopsychiatry* 21: 387–388

122 Mierau J, Schingnitz G (1992) Biochemical and pharmacological studies on pramipexole, a potent and selective dopamine D_2 receptor agonist. *Eur J Pharmacol* 215: 161–170

123 Mierau J, Schneider FJ, Ensinger HA, Chio CL, Lajiness ME, Huff RN (1995) Pramipexole binding and activation of cloned and expressed dopamine D_2, D_3 and D_4 receptors. *Eur J Pharmacol* 290: 29–36

124 Camacho-Ochoa M, Walker EL, Evans DL, Piercey MF (1995) Rat brain binding sites for pramipexole, a clinically useful D_3-preferring dopamine agonist. *Neuroscience Letters* 196: 97–100

125 Guttman M (1997) Double-blind comparison of pramipexole and bromocriptine treatment with placebo in advanced Parkinson's disease. *Neurology* 49: 1060–1065

126 Wetzel H, Benkert O (1993) Dopamine autoreceptor agonists in the treatment of schizophrenic disorders. *Prog Neuropsychopharmacol and Biol Psychiat* 17: 525–540

127 Kasper S, Barnas C, Heiden A, Volz HP, Laakmann G, Zeit H, Pfolz H (1997) Pramipexole as adjunct to haloperidol in schizophrenia safety and efficacy. *Eur Neuropsychopharmacol* 7: 65–70

128 Oshiro Y, Sato S, Kurahashi N, Tanaka T, Kikuchi T, Tottori K, Uwahodo Y, Nishi T (1998) Novel antipsychotic agents with dopamine autoreceptor agonist properties: synthesis and pharmacology of 7-[4-(4-phenyl-1-piperazinyl)butoxy]-3,4-dihydro-2(1H)-quinolinone derivatives. *J Med Chem* 41: 658–667

129 Sramek JJ, Eldon MA, Posvar E, Feng MR, Jhee SS, Hourani J, Sedman AJ, Cutler NR (1998) Initial safety, tolerability pharmacodynamics, and pharmacokinetics of CI-1007 in patients with schizophrenia. *Psychopharmacol Bull* 34: 93–99

130 Coward DM, Dixon K, Enz A, Shearman S, Urwyler S, White T, Karobath M (1989) Partial brain dopamine D_2 agonists in the treatment of schizophrenia. *Psychopharmacology Bull* 25: 292–297

131 Coward DM, Dixon K, Urwyler S, White TG, Enz A, Karobath M, Shearman G (1990) Partial dopamine agonists and atypical neuroleptic properties of the amino-ergolines SDZ 208-911 and SDZ 208 912. *J Pharmacol Exp Ther* 252: 279–285
132 Naber D, Gaussares C, Moeglen JM, Tremmel P, Bailey PE and the SDZ HDC 912 Collaborative Study Group (1992) In: Meltzer HY (ed): Efficacy and tolerability of SDZ HDC 912, A partial Dopamine D_2 Agonist in the treatment of Schizophrenia. *Novel Antipsychotic Drugs*, Raven Press, New York, 99–107
133 Olbrich R, Schanz H (1988) The effect of the partial dopamine agonist terguride on negative symptoms in schizophrenia. *Pharmacopsychiatry* 21: 389–390
134 Schoemaker H, Claustre Y, Fage D, Rouquier L, Chergui K, Curet O, Oblin A, Gonon F, Carter C, Benavides J et al. (1997) Neurochemical characteristics of amisulpride, an atypical dopamine D_2/D_3 receptor antagonist with both presynaptic and limbic selectivity. *J Pharmacol Exp Ther* 280: 83–97
135 Sokoloff P, Martres MP, Giros B, Bouthenet ML, Schwartz JC (1992) The third dopamine receptor (D_3) as a novel target for antipsychotics. *Biochem Pharmacol* 43: 659–666
136 Meller E, Bohmaker K, Goldstein M, Basham DA (1993) Evidence that striatal synthesis-inhibiting autoreceptors are dopamine D_3 receptors. *Eur J Pharmacol* 249: R5–R6
137 Perrault GH, Depoortere R, Morel E, Sanger DJ, Scatton B (1997) Psychopharmacological profile of amisulpride: an antipsychotic drug with presynaptic D_2/D_3 dopamine receptor antagonist activity and limbic selectivity. *J Pharmacol Exp Ther* 280: 73–82
138 Costa e-Silva JA (1990) A comparative double-blind trial of amisulpride *vs* haloperidol in the treatment of acute psychotic disorders. *Ann Psychiatr* 5: 71–78
139 Delcker A, Schoon ML, Ockowski B, Gaertner HJ (1990) Amisulpride *vs* haloperidol in treatment of schizophrenic patients – results of a double-blind study. *Pharmacopsychiatry* 23: 125–130
140 Pichot P, Boyer P (1988) A double-blind, controlled, multicenter trial of amisulpride *vs* high dose haloperidol in acute psychotic disorders. *Ann Psychiatr* 3: 326–332
141 Hillert A, Philip M, Gattaz WF, Sauer H, Adler G, Wetzel H, Benkert O (1994) Amisulpride *vs* flupentixol in the treatment of schizophrenia with predominant positive symptomatology. *Neuropsychopharmcology* 10: 31S
142 Möller HJ, Boyer P, Fleurot O, Rein W (1997) Improvement of acute exacerbations of schizophrenia with amisulpride: a comparison with haloperidol. *Psychopharmacology* 132: 396–401
143 Coukell AJ, Spencer CM, Benfield P (1996) Amisulpride. A review of its pharmacodynamic and pharmacokinetic properties and therapeutic efficacy in the management of schizophrenia. *CNS Drugs* 6: 237–256
144 Bech P, Fleurot O, Turjanski S (1997) Amisulpride *vs* risperidone in the treatment of acute schizophrenia. 6th World Congres Biological Psychiatry, Nice
145 Andreasen NC (1983) The scale for the assessment of negative symptoms (SANS). University of Iowa, Iowa City
146 Boyer P, Lecrubier Y, Puech AJ, Dewailly J, Aubin F (1995) Treatment of negative symptoms in schizophrenia with amisulpride. *Br J Psychiatry* 166: 68–72
147 Paillère-Martinot ML, Lecrubier Y, Martinot JL, Aubin F (1995) Improvement of some schizophrenic deficit symptoms with low doses of amisulpride. *Am J Psychiatry* 152: 130–134
148 Loo H, Poirier-Littre MF, Théron M, Rein W, Fleurot O (1997) Amisulpride *vs* placebo in the medium-term treatment of the negative symptoms of schizophrenia. *Br J Psychiatry* 170: 18–22
149 Farde L, Nordström AL, Karlsson P, Halldin C, Sedvall G (1995) Positron emission tomography studies on dopamine receptors in schizophrenia. *Clin Neuropharmacol* 18: S121–S129
150 Martinot JL, Paillère-Martinot ML, Poirier MF, Dao-Castellana MH, Loc'h C, Mazière B (1996) In vivo characteristics of dopamine D_2 receptor occupancy by amisulpride in schizophrenia. *Psychopharmacology* 124: 154–158
151 Trichard C, Paillère-Martinot ML, Attar-Levy D, Recassens C, Monnet F, Martinot JL (1998) Binding of antipsychotic drugs to cortical $5\text{-}HT_{2A}$ receptors: a PET study of chlorpromazine, clozapine, and amisulpride in schizophrenic patients. *Am J Psychiatry* 155: 505–508

152 Svensson K, Johansson AM, Magnusson T, Carlsson A (1986) (+)-AJ 76 and (+)-UH 232: Central stimulants acting as preferential dopamine autoreceptor antagonists. *Naunyn-Schmiedeberg's Arch Pharmacol* 334: 234–245
153 Gobert A, Rivet JM, Audinot V, Cistarelli L, Spedding M, Vian J, Peglion JL, Millan MJ (1995) Functional correlates of dopamine D3 receptor activation in the rat *in vivo* and their modulation by the selective antagonist, (+)-S 14297: II. Both D_2 and „silent“ D_3 autoreceptors control synthesis and release in mesolimbic, mesocortical and nigrostriatal pathways. *J Pharmacol Exp Ther* 275: 899–913
154 Millan MJ, Audinot V, Melon C, Newman-Tancredi A (1995) Evidence that dopamine D_3 receptors participate in clozapine-induced hypothermia. *Eur J Pharmacol* 280: 225–229
155 Sautel F, Griffon N, Sokoloff P, Schwartz JC, Launay C, Simon P, Costentin J, Schoenfelder A, Garrido F, Mann A et al. (1995) Nafadotride, a potent preferential dopamine D_3 receptor antagonist, activates locomotion in rodents. *J Pharmacol Exp Ther* 275: 1239–1246
156 Gendreau PL, Petitto JM, Schnauss R, Frantz KJ, Van Hartesveldt C, Gariépy J-L, Lewis MH (1997) Effects of the putative dopamine D_3 receptor antagonist PNU 99194A on motor behavior and emotional reactivity in C57BL/6J mice. *Eur J Pharmacol* 337: 147–155
157 Corbin AE, Pugsley TA, Akunne HC, Whetzel SZ, Zoski KT, Georgic LM, Nelson CB, Wright JL, Wise LD, Heffner TG (1998) Pharmacological characterization of PD 152255, a novel dimeric benzimidazole dopamine D_3 antagonist. *Pharmacol Biochem Behav* 59: 487–493
158 Ariano MA, Wang J, Noblett KL, Larson ER, Sibley DR (1997) Cellular distribution of the rat D_4 dopamine receptor protein in the CNS using anti-receptor antisera. *Brain Res* 752: 26–34
159 Defagot MC, Malchiodi EL, Villar MJ, Antonelli MC (1997) Distribution of D_4 receptor in rat brain studied with sequence-specific antibodies. *Mol Brain Res* 45: 1–12
160 Meador-Woodruff JH, Grandy DK, Van Tol HHM, Damask SP, Little KY, Civelli O, Watson SJ (1994) Dopamine receptor gene expression in the human medial temporal lobe. *Neuropsychopharmacology* 10: 239–248
161 Matsumoto M, Hidaka K, Tada S, Tasaki Y, Yamaguchi T (1995) Full-length cDNA cloning and distribution of human dopamine D_4 receptor. *Mol Brain Res* 29: 157–162
162 Lanau F, Zenner MT, Civelli O, Hartman DS (1997) Epinephrine and norepinephrine act as potent agonists at the recombinant human dopamine D_4 receptor. *J Neurochem* 68: 804–812
163 Newman-Tancredi A, Audinot-Bouchez V, Gobert A, Millam MJ (1997) Noradrenaline and andrenaline are high affinity agonists at dopamine D_4 receptors. *Eur J Pharmacol* 319: 379–383
164 Sanyal S, Van Tol HHM (1997) Review the role of dopamine D_4 receptors in schizophrenia and antipsychotic action. *J Psychiat Res* 31: 219–232
165 Barr CL, Kennedy JL, Lichter JB, Van Tol HHM, Wetterberg L, Livak KJ, Kidd KK (1993) Alleles at the dopamine D_4 receptor locus do not contribute to the genetic susceptibility to schizophrenia in a large Swedish kindred. *Am J Med Gen* 48: 218–222
166 Macciardi F, Petronis A, Van Tol HHM, Marino C, Cavallini C, Smeraldi E, Kennedy JL (1994) Analysis of the D_4 dopamine receptor gene variant in an Italian schizophrenia kindred. *Arch Gen Psychiatry* 51: 288–292
167 Rao PA, Pickar D, Gejman PV, Ram A, Gershon ES, Gelernter J (1994) Allelic variation in the D_4 dopamine receptor (DRD4) gene does not predict response to clozapine. *Arch Gen psychiatry* 51: 912–917
168 Shaikh S, Collier D, Kerwin RW, Pilowsky LS, Gill M, Xu WM, Thornton A (1993) Dopamine D_4 receptor subtypes and response to clozapine. *Lancet* 341: 116
169 Seeman P, Guan H-C, Van Tol, HH (1995) Schizophrenia: elevation of dopamine D_4-like sites, using [^{3}H]nemonapride and [^{125}I]epidepride. *Eur J Pharmacol* 286: R3–5
170 Murray AM, Hyde TM, Knable MB, Herman MM, Bigelow LB, Carter JM, Weinberger DR, Kleinman JE (1995) Distribution of putative D_4 dopamine receptors in *post mortem* striatum from patients with schizophrenia. *J Neurosci* 15: 2186–2191
171 Sumiyoshi T, Kido H, Sakamoto H, Urasaki K, Suzuki K, Yamaguchi N, Mori H, Yokogowa K (1994) *in vivo* dopamine-D2 and serotonin 5-HT2 receptor binding study of risperidone and haloperidol. *Pharm Biochem Behav* 47: 553–557

172 Marzella PL, Hill C, Keks N, Singh B, Copolov D (1997) The binding of both [^{3}H]nemonapride and [^{3}H]raclopride is increased in schizophrenia. *Biol Psychiatry* 42: 648–654
173 Seeman P, Van Tol HHM (1995) Dopamine D_4-like receptor elevation in schizophrenia: cloned D_2 and D_4 receptors cannot be discriminated by raclopride competition against [^{3}H]nemonapride. *J Neurochem* 64: 1413–1415
174 Matsumoto M, Hidaka K, Tada S, Tasaki Y, Yamaguchi T (1996) Low levels of mRNA for dopamine D_4 receptor in human cerebral cortex and striatum. *J Neurochem* 66: 915–919
175 Meador-Woodruff JH, Haroutunian V, Powchik P, Davidson M, Davis KL, Watson SJ (1997) Dopamine receptor transcript expression in striatum and prefrontal and occipital cortex. *Arch Gen Psychiatry* 54: 1089–1095
176 Roberts DA, Balderson D, Pickering-Brown SM, Deakin JFW, Owen F (1996) The relative abundance of dopamine D_4 receptor mRNA in *post mortem* brains of schizophrenics and controls. *Schizophrenia Res* 20: 171–174
177 Patel S, Patel S, Marwood R, Emms F, Marston D, Leeson PD, Curtis NR, Kulagowski JJ, Freedman SB (1996) Identification and pharmacological characterization of [^{125}I]L-750,667, a novel radioligand for the dopamine D_4 receptor. *Mol Pharmacol* 50: 1658–1664
178 Lahti RA, Primus RJ, Gallager DW, Roberts R, Tamminga CA (1996) Distribution of dopamine D_4 receptor in human *post mortem* brain sections: autoradiographic studies with [^{3}H]-NGD-94-1. *Schizoph Res* 18: 173
179 Seeman P, Guan H-C, Nobrega J, Jiwa D, Markstein R, Balk J-H, Picetti R, Borrelli E, Van Tol HHM (1997) Dopamine D_2-like sites in schizophrenia but not in Alzheimer's, Huntington's, or control brains, for [^{3}H]benzquinoline. *Synapse* 25: 137–146
180 Seeman P (1992) Dopamine receptor sequences: therapeutic levels of neuroleptics occupy D_2 receptors, clozapine occupies D_4. *Neuropsychopharmacol* 7: 261–284
181 Kramer MS, Last B, Getson A, Reines SA (1997) The effects of a selective D_4 dopamine receptor antagonist (L-745,870) in acutely psychotic inpatients with schizophrenia. *Arch Gen Psychiatry* 54: 567–572
182 Reynolds GP (1996) The importance of dopamine D_4 receptors in the action and development of antipsychotic agents. *Drugs* 51: 7–11
183 Glase SA, Akunne HC, Georgic LM, Heffner, TG, MacKenzie RG, Manley PJ, Pugsley TA, Wise LD (1997) Substituted [(4-phenylpiperazinyl)-methyl]benzamides: selective dopamine D_4 agonists. *J Med Chem* 40: 1771–1772
184 Merchant KM, Gill GS, Harris DW, Huff RM, Eaton MJ, Lookingland K, Lutzke BS, McCall RB, Piercey MF, Schreur PJ (1996) Pharmacological characterization of U-101387, a dopamine D4 receptor selective antagonist. *J Pharmacol Exp Ther* 279: 1392–1403
185 Kula NS, Baldessarini RJ, Kebabian JW, Bakthavachalam V, Xu L (1997) RBI-257: a highly potent dopamine D_4 receptor-selective ligand. *Eur J Pharmacol* 331: 333–336
186 Van Vliet LA, De Boer P, Wikström H, Pugsley TA, Heffner TG, Wise LD Substituted N-(1-Benzyl-piperidin-4-yl)benzamides as dopamine D_4 preferring antagonists. Does dopamine D_4 antagonism contribute to atypical character of antipsychotics? *J Med Chem; in press*

Atypical Antipsychotics
ed. by B.A. Ellenbroek and A.R. Cools

Multireceptor atypical antipsychotic drugs

Herbert Y. Meltzer

Department of Psychiatry, Vanderbilt University School of Medicine, Suite 306, 1601 23rd Avenue S, Nashville, TN 37215, USA

Introduction

The atypical antipsychotic drugs are those antipsychotic agents which produce fewer extrapyramidal side-effects (EPS) at clinically effective antipsychotic doses than do the typical neuroleptic drugs [23]. This definition of an atypical antipsychotic drug is still controversial [3]. Various authorities have suggested that the term be dropped completely and some other general name be used, e.g. novel antipsychotics, while others propose that the definition be broadened to include features beyond antipsychotic efficacy and low EPS, e.g. specific pharmacological features such as multireceptor activity, efficacy in treatment-resistant schizophrenia, and ability to improve negative symptoms [3, 4]. Clozapine is the prototypical atypical antipsychotic drug [5]. It was designated as an atypical anti-psychotic because it differed from the neuroleptic agents that were available at the time of its introduction in 1960 in that the neuroleptics produced catalepsy in rodents and EPS in man at clinically relevant doses and clozapine did not [6]. This term was widely used by preclinical investigators to refer to clozapine in their efforts to understand the biological basis for the difference between it and the prototypical typical neuroleptic drug, haloperidol, with regard to their effects on the limbic and nigrostriatal dopaminergic systems, the probable sites of antipsychotic action and EPS, respectively [7]. Thus, there has been much historical precedent to the definition of atypicality that focuses on the extrapyramidal system differences between antipsychotic drugs. Furthermore, acute and chronic EPS are the most significant side-effects of the first generation of antipsychotic drugs because of their influence upon compliance, and its effect, in turn upon relapse and rehospitalization [8], as well as the sometimes fatal neuroleptic malignant syndrome, and the ability to cause tardive dyskinesia [9]. What has complicated the issue of the essence of an atypical antipsychotic is the discovery of the many advantages of clozapine other than low EPS, including no known ability to cause tardive dyskinesia, efficacy in treatment-resistant schizophrenia, improvement in negative symptoms, decreased risk of suicide, and improvement in cognition, to name the most important [10] (see Naber et al., this volume].

As mentioned above, the term novel antipsychotic has been suggested as a substitute for atypical antipsychotic but this time-dependent designation will not long survive the aging of the class of drugs referred to as atypical. It is clearly difficult to describe clozapine as novel 40 years after its discovery and 30 years after its clinical introduction. It is possible that if a clearly defining feature of the action of the atypical antipsychotic drugs emerges, e.g. a common ability to affect some second messenger system which is not produced by typical neuroleptics or to lack certain side-effects produced by the typical neuroleptics, that a more precise, biologically driven appellation could be substituted for atypical without confounding the original concept. For the time being, it seems most useful to retain the original meaning of an atypical antipsychotic and to consider other important features of the atypical antipsychotic drugs, e.g. effects on treatment-resistant patients, lack of prolactin secretion, stimulation, etc. as separate factors which may or may not be shared by some or all atypical antipsychotic agents.

The antipsychotic drugs designated as atypical are the prototypical agent, clozapine, and a group of drugs which have been approved in some countries for antipsychotic use: olanzapine, quetiapine, risperidone, sertindole and ziprasidone. There are other known agents which have similar clinical properties and are also related to this series of agents with regard to their pharmacology, i.e. they are more potent as serotonin $(5\text{-HT})_{2a}$ than as dopamine (DA) D_2 receptor antagonists [11]. These include fluperlapine, iloperidone, melperone and ORG 5222. M100907 and SR 46349B are selective 5-HT_{2a} antagonists which are currently being clinically studied to determine if they are atypical antipsychotic agents. Preliminary results are encouraging but further testing is needed. It is noteworthy that there are several preclinical studies which indicate that the combination of low-dose haloperidol and M100907 gives haloperidol an atypical profile but M100907 is ineffective in altering the typical neuroleptic effects of high-dose haloperidol, thus reinforcing the notion that the relative amount of D_2 and 5-HT_{2a} receptor blockade achieved by antipsychotic agents is a critical element of atypicality. Because there is limited published data, and because of space limitations, M100907 will not be further discussed here. Should further study establish that M100907 is a clinically effective antipsychotic, with atypical properties, this would provide considerate additional support for the hypothesis that 5-HT_{2a} receptor blockade is a critical component of the atypical antipsychotic profile of clozapine, olanzapine, quetiapine, risperidone, sertindole, and ziprasidone. Other drugs of different chemical classes have been found to produce low EPS. These include amisulpride, a selective $D_{2/3}$ antagonist [12], and remoxipride, a selective D_2 antagonist [13], both of which have no effective affinities for other DA receptors or other types of 5-HT receptors. These drugs are discussed in Den Boer and Korf, this volume. There are also novel pharmacologic agents which have been suggested to be atypical antipsychotics on the basis of their efficacy in standard animal models believed to predict antipsychotic efficacy, e.g. conditioned avoidance response, and which have no significant ability to produce EPS. The selective 5-HT_{1a} agonist 8-hydroxy-2-(di-n-propylamino)tetralin (8-OH-DPAT) is an example of this type of agent [14].

The purpose of this article will be to discuss some of the clinical and pharmacological features of the atypical antipsychotic drugs and to suggest some of the ways these drugs should be used clinically. Other uses of these agents will also be considered. The role of these agents in the treatment of schizophrenia *vis-à-vis* the typical neuroleptics will also be considered. Clozapine is considered in depth elsewhere in this volume. Detailed reviews of the clinical pharmacology of clozapine [15], risperidone [16], olanzapine [17], sertindole [18], quetiapine [19], and ziprasidone [20] should also be consulted.

An overview of the clinical role of the atypical antipsychotic drugs in the treatment of schizophrenia

Typical neuroleptic drugs such as haloperidol, loxapine, fluphenazine, perphenazine, molindone and thiothixene have been the first line treatments of schizophrenia since the introduction of chlorpromazine in 1954. These drugs share in common the ability to block D_2 receptors as the major basis for their efficacy. Blockade of D_2 receptors in the mesolimbic areas such as the nucleus accumbens and olfactory tubercle appears to be the basis for their major action, the control of positive symptoms such as delusions and hallucinations [21]. Blockade of D_2 receptors in the striatum appears to be the basis for their ability to produce EPS [21]. Chronic administration of these agents leads to tardive dyskinesia at the rate of 4–5% per year in younger patients and much higher rates in patients over the age of 60 due to declining dopaminergic function. Blockade of D_2 receptors in the anterior pituitary gland is the basis for their ability to stimulate prolactin secretion [21].

Typical neuroleptic drugs are able to reduce positive symptoms to no more than mild levels in about 70% of schizophrenic patients. About 10% of schizophrenic patients do not respond to typical neuroleptic drugs during the first episode [22]. Another 20% of patients with schizophrenia develop resistance to this action of these agents during the subsequent course of their illness [23]. Typical neuroleptic drugs do not significantly improve negative symptoms such as withdrawal, anhedonia, lack of motivation, lack of spontaneity and affective flattening. There is some evidence that these agents can, in fact, induce or worsen some negative symptoms [24]. This has led to the distinction between primary and secondary negative symptoms; the former are an intrinsic manifestation of the schizophrenia diathesis. The latter may be secondary to neuroleptics, positive symptoms, depression, and other factors as well. As will be discussed, a key difference between the atypical antipsychotic drugs and the typical agents is that at least some of the atypical agents appear to have a superior effect upon negative symptoms, be they primary or secondary. Typical neuroleptic drugs also do not improve cognitive function which is majorly impaired in schizophrenia [25]. Those typical neuroleptic drugs such as thioridazine and mesoridazine which have strong antimuscarinic properties may produce further impairment in some memory functions [25]. As mentioned above, major limitations of the typical neuroleptic drugs are their ability to produce EPS and tardive dyskinesia. Neuroleptic malignant syndrome is a rare and sometimes fatal side-effect of these agents. Typical neuroleptics produce sedation and modest weight gain as well as modest impairment in menstrual function in females and sexual function in males [26]. Advantages of these agents include the availability of long-acting forms, e.g. parenterally administered fluphenazine and haloperidol decanoate. These formulations permit weekly-monthly treatment and almost certain delivery of medication provided the dose is high enough. These long acting formulations are widely used for patients who are non-compliant with oral agents [27].

Risperidone

Pharmacology

Risperidone is a benzisoxazole compound which was specifically developed by Janssen Research Foundation because of its potent 5-HT_{2a} antagonism and somewhat less potent D_2 receptor antagonism [16]. As summarised by Megens et al. [16], the *in vitro* receptor binding profile of risperidone for a number of key receptors is as follows: Ki for the 5-HT_{2a} receptor, 0.16 nM; α_1, 0.81 nM; D_2 1.4 nM; H_1 2.1 nM; D_4, 7.0 nM; α_2, 7.5 nM; and D_3, 13 nM. It is also a potent 5-HT_7 receptor antagonist, Ki 1.39 nM and a weak 5-HT_{2c}, Ki 63 nM and 5-HT_6 antagonist, Ki 425 nM [28]. It must be understood that these values are dependent upon the conditions of the *in vitro* binding assays and should be considered as approximations and mainly of use for relative purposes (see also Leysen, this volume). Risperidone is a weak antimuscarinic agent [29]. Thus, there is approximately a 10-fold difference between the affinity of risperidone for the 5-HT_{2a} receptor and D_2 receptor *in vitro*. *In vivo*, it is a potent antagonist of the effects of 5-HT in a variety of systems, including head twitches induced by 5-HT_{2a} antagonists such as 2,5-dimethoxy-4-methylamphetamine (DOM) and quipazine [29]. The ED_{50} for risperidone to block 5-HT_{2a} receptors in the frontal cortex of rats is 0.037–0.12 mg/kg. The ED_{50} for blockade of DA-mediated effects *in vivo* is approximately 10-fold higher than that for blockade of serotonin-mediated effects. The ED_{50} for occupancy of D_2 receptors in various rat brain regions ranges between 0.22 and 1.3 mg/kg, which is approximately 10-fold higher than that for 5-HT_{2a} receptors [29]. The occupancy by risperidone of 5-HT_{2a} and D_2 receptors in cortex and basal ganglia of patients will be described subsequently. In summary, risperidone may be described as a potent 5-HT_{2a}, 5-HT_7, D_2, α_1, and H_1 antagonist. Notably, it lacks significant affinity for the 5-HT_{1a}, 5-HT_{2c} and muscarinic receptors, which is likely to have some bearing upon its impact on psychopathology, cognition and extrapyramidal side-effects.

Metabolism and pharmacokinetics

Risperidone is a prodrug in that is extensively metabolised in the liver by cytochrome P 450 2D6 to 9-hydroxyrisperidone in approximately 92–94% of Caucasians [30]. Thus, this metabolite is the active species in the majority of patients. About 6–8% of Caucasians and a small proportion of Asians have a polymorphism of the CYP 2D6 gene which leads to poor metabolism of risperidone. CYP 2D6 is the enzyme responsible for the metabolism of a variety of drugs, e.g. antidepressant, neuroleptics, antiarrhythmics and other drugs. This leads to the possibility of a significant number of drug interactions. For example, quinidine, which inhibits CYP 2D6, would convert all people who took it to poor metabolisers of risperidone. For poor metabolisers of risperidone, the active moiety is mainly the parent compound. The receptor binding profile of 9-OH-risperidone is very similar to that of risperidone itself. The half-life of the 9-hydroxy metabolite is about 21 h whereas the half-life of risperidone is about 3 h. Thus, risperidone can be used on a once a day schedule for normal metabolisers whereas multiple doses are needed for those who are poor metabolisers. Risperidone is well absorbed from the gut. A long acting formulation of risperidone is in clinical testing.

Clinical studies

The efficacy and side-effect profile of risperidone in the treatment of schizophrenia was established in a series of multicentre trials in which multiple doses of risperidone were compared with placebo and usually a single dose of risperidone. Perhaps the most influential of these studies was that of Marder and Meibach [31] which was carried out in the United States. This was a double-blind, multicentre, inpatient study in which 388 patients with schizophrenia were randomly assigned to 8 weeks' treatment with placebo, risperidone 2, 5, 10 or 16 mg/day or 20 mg of haloperidol daily. The patients were predominantly male with duration of illness averaging 15 years, and 8–10 prior hospitalisations. Patients had been in the hospital an average of 29 weeks prior to entry although some were more recent admissions with acute exacerbations. Thus, it is highly likely that this study included a mixture of neuroleptic-resistant and responsive patients, an issue that will be addressed subsequently. This study was the defining study in the early recommendations for the appropriate dose of risperidone so it is worthwhile to consider the results in some detail. Overall, statistically significant differences in clinical improvement were found between 6 and 16 mg of risperidone vs placebo and vs haloperidol. The 2 mg dose was not significantly superior to placebo although there were slightly more completers (46% vs 32%) and the percentage of patients who improved clinically (defined by a 20–43% reduction in total score on the Positive and Negative Syndrome Scale (PANNS) was 22% and 35% for the placebo and 2 mg dose group, respectively. The completer and responder rates for the patients receiving 6 mg/day were 55 and 57%, respectively. These were approximately the same for the patients receiving 16 mg/day of risperidone. Haloperidol was also superior to placebo with completer and responder rates of 42 and 30%, respectively. Improvement in positive symptoms was greater than placebo for patients who received 6, 10 or 16 mg risperidone or 20 mg haloperidol. Improvement in negative symptoms was greater than in the placebo group only for patients receiving 6 and 16 mg/day of risperidone. The 2 and 6 mg doses of risperidone were associated with EPS equivalent to placebo whereas the higher doses of risperidone and the single dose of haloperidol were associated with higher EPS ratings and more frequent use of anticholinergic medication. It was concluded that the "optimal daily dose of risperidone for most schizophrenic patient in this study was 6 mg." These results were consistent with a Canadian multicenter trial [32] and those of other multicenter trials [33]. One of the issues left unsettled in these studies was the possibility that the most effective doses for risperidone relative to side-effect potential might differ between neuroleptic-responsive and -resistant patients and as a function of duration of illness. There is evidence that the optimal dose of clozapine for neuroleptic-resistant patients is significantly higher for neuroleptic-resistant than for neuroleptic-responsive patients. Similarly, it is well known that first episode patients require lower doses of neuroleptic drugs for control of positive symptoms and are more likely to develop EPS at equivalent doses. The mean dose of risperidone in one open trial of a group of first episode schizophrenic patients was 4.7 (S.D. 1.5 mg)/day [34].

Negative symptoms

The issue of whether the improvement in negative symptoms by risperidone and other atypical antipsychotic drugs is due to an effect on so-called primary negative symptoms *vs* secondary negative symptoms has been much debated. Some have suggested that these agents only improve negative symptoms that are secondary to such factors as positive symptoms, depression, and EPS [24]. Moller et al. [35] used path analysis to determine if risperidone had a differential effect on negative symptoms compared to haloperidol after controlling for the effect of both drugs on positive symptoms, depression, and EPS. Data from the combined US and Canadian multicenter trials were utilized. It was found that there was a contribution of improvement in positive symptoms and EPS, but not depression, to the improvement in negative symptoms, but that there was still an effect on negative symptoms unaccounted for by the risperidone-treated group that could have been due to improvement in primary negative symptoms. The superiority of risperidone over haloperidol for the treatment of negative symptoms also emerged from a factor analysis of PANNS scores of the combined US and Canadian multicenter trial. This advantage of risperidone was not influenced by covarying changes in EPS ratings [36].

There has been one large multicenter trial comparing risperidone and olanzapine which has been published to date [37]. Another has been completed but not published. The study of Tran et al. [37] was an international, multicenter, double-blind, parallel groups, 28-week prospective study of 339 patients with schizophrenia, schizophreniform disorder or schizoaffective disorder. Both drugs were effective in the management of psychotic symptoms. Statistically significant advantages were noted for olanzapine in the improvement of negative symptoms on one of two rating scales as well as overall response rate using two of four criteria. The mean modal dose for the olanzapine treatment group was 17.2 ± 3.6 mg/day for olanzapine and 7.2 ± 2.7 mg/day for risperidone. The overall similarities between these two drugs with regard to efficacy appear greater than the differences, assuming that doses are properly adjusted. There are differences in side-effects and cost which may be more important in clinical choice for initiating treatment. This will be discussed subsequently.

Risperidone has been found to be clinically useful in the treatment of mood disorders with psychotic features, e.g. mania and psychotic depression [38]. There is, however, currently more evidence that clozapine is effective in treatment-resistant mood disorders, including rapid cycling mania [39]. Some patients with schizoaffective disorder or schizophrenia experience an activation with risperidone which may be indicative of its antidepressant action [40].

Effects upon cognition

There have been four studies of the effects of risperidone on cognition in schizophrenia. These have been reviewed by Meltzer and McGurk 1999 [40a]. Improvement in attention, executive function, verbal learning and memory, and working memory have been the most consistent findings [41–43].

Efficacy in neuroleptic-resistant patients

There have been numerous studies of risperidone in neuroleptic-resistant patients with mixed results [44–46]. Collectively, these papers suggest that some proportion of patients who fail to have an adequate response to typical neuroleptic drugs will respond to risperidone but the proportion appears to be less than that of clozapine. The studies of Jeste et al. [45] and Bondolfi et al. [46] are difficult to interpret because they did not clearly distinguish between neuroleptic-resistant and intolerant patients. The Bondolfi et al. study [46] compared clozapine and risperidone in a mixed population and found them equivalent. However, the dose of clozapine was not high enough to provide a fair comparison, the trial duration was brief, and the sample size was too small. There is anecdotal evidence that a number of patients who fail to respond adequately to risperidone will respond to clozapine [47]. It is not clear how many poor responders to risperidone will respond to olanzapine or *vice versa*. Controlled studies are needed to determine the effectiveness of treating with clozapine after a failed trial with either a typical neuroleptic or any of the atypical antipsychotics other than clozapine.

Extrapyramidal and other side-effects

The advantages of risperidone over haloperidol with regard to EPS have been evident in studies with low doses of risperidone vs relatively high doses of haloperidol. The incidence of EPS in patients treated with risperidone vs perphenazine [48], zuclopenthixol [49] and methotrimeprazine [50] were comparable. However, the doses of risperidone were relatively high in these studies. For example, in the Blin et al. study [50], the average dose of risperidone was 7.4 mg/day and there were fewer EPS at that dose of risperidone than in a haloperidol-treated group of patients, mean dose 7.6 mg/day. Simpson and Lindenmayer [51] have concluded that low doses of risperidone cause few or no EPS. Risperidone has been found to produce intolerable worsening of motor symptoms in some patients with Parkinson's disease given risperidone to treat L-DOPA-induced psychosis [52], although there are some more favorable reports. It clearly produces greater exacerbations of Parkinsonism in this group than clozapine or melperone, another atypical antipsychotic. Patients who are intolerant of the EPS-inducing side-effects of typical neuroleptics are more likely to be sensitive to the D_2 receptor blocking properties of risperidone as well [51]. These patients should be treated with very low doses of risperidone or possibly other atypical antipsychotic drugs with lower potential to produced EPS at clinically equivalent doses. It appears that clozapine, sertindole, quetiapine, and possibly ziprasidone have the least EPS among the atypical antipsychotic drugs with olanzapine intermediate. The combination of risperidone and a typical neuroleptic is likely to lead to increased EPS and may compromise some of the advantages of risperidone for EPS. Therefore, clinicians should usually prescribe 4 mg risperidone per day in the neuroleptic-responsive schizophrenic patient for up to 4–6 weeks before increasing the dose. This strategy should lead to fewer EPS and possibly greater efficacy.

There is some evidence that risperidone may cause as well the suppression of some of the symptoms of tardive dyskinesia [51]. Because it is more potent as a D_2 antagonist than is clozapine, it is likely that the risk is greater with risperidone and that it increases with dose. It is well known that the elderly are more vulnerable to develop tardive dyskinesia. There is now a widespread use of risperidone in elderly patients with organic psychoses. Clinical experience with patients of this type who are exposed only to risperidone will provide a good indication of risk for tardive dyskinesia. In the meantime, it is appropriate to caution patients that there is an unknown risk of tardive dyskinesia with risperidone.

Risperidone is also associated with moderate weight gain, comparable to that of typical neuroleptic drugs, but less than that of clozapine and olanzapine [16, 53]. Risperidone also produces some postural hypotension because of its α_1 blocking properties [16].

Risperidone produces greater increases in serum prolactin secretion than any of the other atypical antipsychotic drugs. The increases appear to be at least comparable to those of typical neuroleptics. Peuskens et al. [53] reported a dose-proportional increase in serum prolactin levels during an 8-week study of risperidone vs placebo and haloperidol. Clozapine, sertindole and quetiapine do not produce any increase in serum prolactin levels during clinical administration whereas olanzapine produces transient increases in serum prolactin levels [54]. The biological basis for this gross difference in effects on prolactin secretion is unclear. It suggests some qualitative difference between risperidone and the other atypical antipsychotic drugs rather than relative differences in potency as D_2 and 5-HT_{2a} receptor antagonists in vivo. These should not be grossly different between drugs such as olanzapine and risperidone, especially at lower doses of risperidone. It is possible that the particular mix of effects of risperidone on a variety of DA and 5-HT receptors produces a net inhibition of the dominant inhibitory effect of DA on prolactin secretion at the level of the lactotrophe. It is possible that some novel aspect of risperidone's action might be responsible that could help uncover some heretofore undescribed mechanism regulating prolactin secretion. This qualitative difference between risperidone and the other atypical antipsychotic drugs is particularly impressive evidence of the important differences between the atypical antipsychotic drugs which reflects their diverse and complicated pharmacology.

There is a long list of possible adverse effects of hyperprolactinemia. These include amenorrheoa, irregular menses, anovulation, gynecomastia, galactorrhoea, sexual dysfunction (including erectile or ejaculatory dysfunction, azospermia, and decreased libido), infertility, obesity, and hirsutism [54]. There is no evidence that hyperprolactinemia is associated with increased risk of breast cancer or any other type of cancer [55]. Despite the list of reported adverse effects of prolactin secretion, there is no strong evidence that risperidone is associated with marked problems of this nature. For example, in the study of Hoyberg et al. [48], which included 15 females treated with risperidone and an equal number treated with haloperidol, there was no difference in the rates of amenorrhoea between the two drugs (15 and 7%, respectively). There were also no differences in erectile dysfunction, ejaculatory dysfunction, orgastic dsyfunction or sexual desire between the two groups for males and females combined. None of these side-effects exceeded 10% incidence and none resulted in drug discontinuation.

Summary

Risperidone is a highly useful addition to the treatment of schizophrenia and other forms of psychosis. It may produce significant advantages over typical neuroleptic drugs with regard to negative symptoms, cognition, and EPS but it produces equivalent increases in serum prolactin levels. Its tolerability with regard to EPS is highly dose dependent so that it must be used at the lower doses where possible.

Olanzapine

Pharmacology

Olanzapine is a thienobenzodiazepine which has a binding profile similar to that of clozapine and has been shown to have a variety of preclinical effects comparable to clozapine [56]. The *in vitro* receptor binding profile of olanzapine for a number of key receptors is as follows: Ki for the 5-HT_{2a} receptor, 4 nM; D_2 11 nM; D_1, 31 nM; D_4, 27 nM; α_1, 19 nM; α_2, 230 nM; H_1 7 nM; M_1, 1.9 nM; and M_2, 18 nM [56]. It is also a potent 5-HT_6 (Ki 2.5 nM) and 5-HT_{2c}, (Ki 11 nM) receptor antagonist and a weak 5-HT_7 antagonist (Ki 205 nM) [28]. Utilising the binding data of Bymaster et al. [56], clozapine is relatively more potent as a 5-HT_{2a} antagonist than D_2 antagonist, followed by risperidone, olanzapine and quetiapine in that order. Olanzapine and risperidone are distinguished in their greater potency for the 5-HT_6 and 5-HT_7 receptors, respectively. Olanzapine and clozapine are the most potent antimuscarinic agents. Risperidone lacks H_1 receptor antagonism whereas all four compounds are potent α_1 antagonists.

Metabolism and pharmacokinetics

Olanzapine has a half-life of 24–30 h which indicates that single daily administration is adequate. The metabolic pathways of olanzapine involved CYP2D6, CYP1A2 and flavin-containing monooxygenases as well as N-glucuronidation [57]. It has a low potential for drug-drug interactions and requires extremely high concentrations not likely to be achieved under clinical conditions to inhibit cytochrome P-450 systems [58]. Plasma levels < 9.3 ng/ml have been reported to predict better clinical response to olanzapine in inpatients with an acute exacerbation [59].

Clinical studies

The efficacy of olanzapine in treating psychosis and negative symptoms in patients with an acute exacerbation of schizophrenia has been firmly established in a variety of large scale, multicenter trials [60–63]. In these trials, olanzapine at doses of 10–20 mg/day has been superior to placebo, and equivalent or superior to haloperidol, in some measures of total psychopathology, positive, or negative symptoms. For example, in the North American multicenter trial, high dose olanzapine (15 ± 5 mg/day) was superior to haloperidol (15 ± 5 mg/day) in the treatment of negative symptoms as assessed by the Scale for the Assessment of Negative Symptoms (SANS) [61]. In an international study of olanzapine vs haloperidol, involving nearly 2000 patients, olanzapine was statistically significantly superior to haloperidol on PANNS Total, Positive and Negative Symptom scale scores. For example, the mean change in the Total PANNS score was -17.7 ± 21.8 and -13.4 ± 20.6 for the olanzapine and haloperidol groups, respectively ($p = 0.05$). The overall response rate was also superior for olanzapine than for haloperidol. However, it should be noted that only one dose of haloperidol was studied and that was relatively high. Olanzapine has also been found to be efficacious as a maintenance treatment of schizophrenia [64, 65]. The estimated relapse rates, defined as the need for hospitalisation, during a 1-year period in three studies of patients receiving olanzapine for maintenance treatment ranged from 19.6–28.6%. These rates were significantly lower than those in patients receiving placebo, ineffective doses of olanzapine, or haloperidol.

The effect of olanzapine to improve negative symptoms was found to be on primary rather than secondary negative symptoms in a path analysis of the US Multicenter Trial described above [66]. High dose olanzapine had a significantly greater effect on SANS subscales: anergia, affective flattening, avolition-apathy but not anhedonia-asociality. The path analysis controlled for the effects of EPS, positive symptoms, and depression. The advantages of olanzapine for negative symptoms were also present in an analysis of a subgroup of 116 patients with predominantly negative symptoms and 117 patients who met criteria for the deficit state.

The average clinical dose of olanzapine is 12.5 – 15 mg/day but some patients respond to lower doses. Doses higher than 20 mg/day are rarely more effective than lower doses.

Augmentation of olanzapine with typical neuroleptic drugs should be done sparingly so as not to diminish the advantages conveyed by greater occupancy of 5-HT_{2a} receptors.

Olanzapine has some efficacy to treat the depression associated with schizophrenia or schizoaffective disorder. It is also effective in some cases of treatment-resistant depression, especially in conjunction with selective serotonin reuptake inhibitors. It is also useful in some forms of mania [67].

Effects upon cognition

There is minimal data available on the effect of olanzapine and cognition. In a study of 20 outpatients, Meltzer and McGurk 1999 [40 a] observed significant improvement in some measures of attention, executive function, verbal learning and memory, and verbal fluency. The effects were comparable to those with clozapine. Further studies are needed to establish the efficacy of olanzapine in this regard.

Efficacy in treatment-resistant schizophrenia

Olanzapine and chlorpromazine were compared in a double blind, parallel group trial in 84 patients who previously had failed to respond to haloperidol in a prospective 6-week trial [68]. Patients received either olanzapine 25 mg/day or chlorpromazine up to 1200 mg/day plus benztropine mesylate. Fifty-nine (70%) of the patients completed the study. There was no difference in efficacy between the two drugs. Only 7% of the olanzapine- and none of the chlorpromazine-treated patients were considered responders. EPS and akathisia were comparable in the two groups. Many of the patients who failed to respond to olanzapine subsequently responded to clozapine (Conley R, personal communication). However, there are other data which suggest a more favorable response to olanzapine in neuroleptic-resistant patients. For example, [69] Conley et al. reported significant improvement following switching to olanzapine in an open trial of 60 neuroleptic-resistant schizophrenic patients with and without substance abuse. Direct comparisons with clozapine are needed to evaluate the relative efficacy of olanzapine in these patients. Clinical experience suggests some partial responders to typical neuroleptics will respond better to olanzapine. Switching patients from clozapine to olanzapine often results in relapse unless careful cross titration is done. The proportion of patients on clozapine who may be switched to olanzapine without loss of efficacy has not been established.

Extrapyramidal and other side-effects

Olanzapine produces dose-dependent EPS, including some dystonic reactions in patients with schizophrenia, but these are less frequent and severe than those produced by typical neuroleptic drugs [61, 62]. Olanzapine is less well tolerated than clozapine in patients with Parkinson's disease [70]. Studies are ongoing to determine if low dose olanzapine may be more tolerable in this population. Olanzapine may be associated with a lower risk of tardive dyskinesia than haloperidol [71] but more data are required to know the extent to which the risk is reduced. It is unlikely that it is as risk free in this regard as clozapine.

With partial response to olanzapine (or risperidone), especially with regard to positive symptom control, clinicians will be tempted to raise the dose beyond the normal upper limit of 20 mg/day and to add a typical or atypical antipsychotic. There is no evidence that higher doses are useful. Addition of low dose haloperidol (≤ 5 mg/day) may be tried but the potential for greater EPS will be significantly increased. There is no evidence to support combined use of atypical antipsychotic drugs.

The major side-effect of olanzapine is weight gain [60, 62]. Increases in weight averaging 3.5 ± 3.9 kg have been reported after 6 weeks of treatment [60]. In another study, the increase was smaller: 1.88 ± 3.54 kg [62]. The increase was greater in those with low body weight and comparable in males and females. Some patients gain between 5–20 kg, however. Some patients develop adult-onset diabetes. Clozapine produces similar weight gain with occasional precipitation of adult onset diabetes. Olanzapine is also associated with some increase in liver enzymes, orthostatic hypotension, anticholinergic side-effects, and sedation [60, 62]. Olanzapine produces slight transient increases in serum prolactin levels which are smaller in magnitude than those produced by typical neuroleptic drugs [60].

Summary

Olanzapine has found wide acceptance as an atypical antipsychotic drug because of its once-a-day administration, efficacy for negative symptoms, improvement in cognitive function, and low EPS profile. Significant weight gain may be a problem for some patients.

Quetiapine (Seroquel)

Pharmacology

Quetiapine is a dibenzothiazepine antipsychotic, which like clozapine, olanzapine and risperidone, was specifically developed by its manufacturer, Zeneca, because of its relatively greater affinity for the 5-HT_{2a} than for the D_2 receptor [72]. Some of the published literature on quetiapine refers to it by its trade name, Seroquel. Quetiapine is a low potency agent. The *in vitro* receptor binding profile of quetiapine for a number of key receptors is as follows: Ki for the 5-HT_{2a} receptor, 13 nM; D_2 132 nM; D_1 321 nM; 5-HT_{1a}, 330 nM; muscarinic, 288 nM; α_1, 48 nM; and α_2, 37 nM [19, 72]. It is a weak 5-HT_{2c}, 5-HT_6 and 5-HT_7 antagonist. Its preclinical profile is that of an atypical antipsychotic drug. It does not upregulate striatal D_2 receptor density after chronic administration to rodents, indicative of a low tendency to cause EPS and possibly tardive dyskinesia [72]. Quetiapine blocks amphetamine-induced increase in catalepsy in rats at doses of 10–80 mg/kg and causes catalepsy in a similar dose range, suggesting only a modest advantage with regard to EPS [73]. However, in the haloperidol-sensitised cebus monkey model, quetiapine shows low potency to cause EPS, which is what has been noted clinically. Electrophysiological studies demonstrate a clozapine-like selectivity to diminish firing of the ventral tegmental dopamine neurons, sparing the nigro-striatal dopamine neurons, another indication of atypicality [74]. Quetiapine had a clozapine-like profile in two other tests of atypicality: the rat paw test and amphetamine-induced social isolation in monkeys [75].

Metabolism and pharmacokinetics

Quetiapine is well absorbed and is approximately 83% protein bound. It has a short half-life, 6 h. It is metabolised in the liver by CYP3A4 to inactive metabolites [76]. Quetiapine has significant interactions with phenytoin, carbamazepine, barbiturates, rifampin and glucocorticoids; co-administration with these agents may require dosage adjustment [77]. Despite the short half-life, a clinical trial compared three dosing regimens (450 mg/day given in two or three divided doses, and 50 mg/day given twice daily); both of the higher dose groups were superior to the low dose group and there were no differences between the two high-dose schedules [78]. Quetiapine is absorbed better after eating [77].

Clinical studies

There have been a number of phase II trials and open trials of the efficacy and tolerability of quetiapine which have suggested that it is as effective as typical antipsychotics with fewer extrapyramidal side-effects and that it has no effect on serum prolactin levels. These studies have been reviewed elsewhere [76, 77] and will not be discussed here. There have been several controlled studies that have been consistent with the generalisations noted above. [79] Small et al. conducted a multicenter trail of 286 chronic or subchronic patients with schizophrenia in an acute exacerbation who were randomised to 6 weeks of treatment with high-dose quetiapine (250–750 mg/day) or low dose quetiapine (< 250 mg/day) or placebo. The average clinical dose in the high-dose group during the double-blind phase of the study was 360 mg. For those who completed the study in this group, the average dose was 488 mg/day. There was a large number of dropouts in this study, with fewer occurring in those receiving high-dose quetiapine than the other two groups which were comparable. Most of the withdrawals were due to lack of efficacy. The high-dose group showed improvement in positive and negative symptoms on some but not all rating scales. In general, the improvement was modest using a last value carried forward analysis. According to *a priori* criteria, more patients responded to quetiapine (high-dose, 53%; low dose, 50%; placebo, 37%). Arvanitis and Miller studied the effect of five fixed doses of quetiapine (75, 150, 300, 600, and 750 mg/day), haloperidol, 12 mg/day and placebo in an inpatient parallel groups, double blind, 6-week study of schizophrenic patients in an acute exacerbation [80]. The four higher doses of quetiapine were significantly different from placebo on BPRS total, BPRS positive symptom cluster and Clinical Global Severity of Illness item scores. There was a trend for superior efficacy at 300 mg/day. There were no significant difference between quetiapine and haloperidol on any of the outcome measures. Both drugs showed greater but comparable improvement in positive and negative symptoms compared to placebo. There is anecdotal evidence that some neuroleptic-resistant patients respond to quetiapine, generally at higher doses, but no controlled studies have been conducted to our knowledge. There is also no evidence regarding efficacy of quetiapine in patients who fail to respond to risperidone or olanzapine. There are no data on the effect of quetiapine on cognition in schizophrenia.

Side-effects

Quetiapine appears to cause fewer EPS than either risperidone or olanzapine. Quetiapine is tolerable in patients with Parkinson's disease to a much greater extent than risperidone or olanzapine (Freedman J, personal communication). The incidence of EPS in the quetiapine-and placebo-treated groups in the study of Arvantis and Miller [80] were not significantly different. The use of anticholinergic medication was also comparable in the quetiapine and placebo-treated groups. The major side-effects with quetiapine are headache, agitation, dry mouth, dizziness, weight gain and postural hypotension [77, 80]. Decreased serum thyroid hormone levels, increased hepatic transaminases and elevated serum lipids have been reported. Animal studies suggest an increased risk of cataracts [81]. This does not appear to be a major problem in man, fortunately. No increases in serum prolactin levels have been reported in a review of all the clinical trial data available with quetiapine [82].

Summary

Quetiapine has been shown to be an effective antipsychotic with a low EPS profile. It has a flat dose response curve with some patients responding to 150 mg/day and others requiring 750 mg/day. Average clinical dose appears to be between 300–500 mg/day. There have not yet been data to suggest efficacy advantages over typical neuroleptic drugs but tolerability appears good because of its low side-effect profile.

Ziprasidone

Pharmacology

Ziprasidone is a benzisothiazolyl piperazine which has been shown to have atypical antipsychotic properties in man and laboratory animals. As with the compounds already discussed, ziprasidone has a higher affinity for the 5-HT_{2a} than D_2 receptor. The pKi values of ziprasidone for key receptors are 5-HT_{2a}, 9.4; 5-HT_{2c}, 8.88; 5-HT_{1a}, 8,47; D_2, 8.32; D_3, 8.13; α_1, 7.98; H_1, 7.33; and D_1, 6.28 [83]. It is important to note that ziprasidone is an agonist at the 5-HT_{1a} receptor. There is extensive evidence that 5-HT_{1a} agonism is able by itself to produce effects in brain that are consistent with an atypical antipsychotic action [84]. Just as 5-HT_{2a} antagonism when coupled to D_2 receptor antagonism may lead to an atypical antipsychotic, or even by itself have antipsychotic properties, e.g. M100907, 5-HT_{1a} agonism, in conjunction with various dopamine receptor blocking properties, e.g. D_2 or D_4, or by itself, e.g. 8-OH-DPAT, may also lead to an atypical antipsychotic profile. (See Millan et al. [84] for further discussion and references).

Metabolism and pharmacokinetics

The half-life of ziprasidone is 4–10 h. Twice daily administration is possible despite this relatively short half-life. Ziprasidone should be taken after eating in order to facilitate absorption. Ziprasidone is metabolised mainly by CYP 3A4 and has little interaction with any of the other CYP enzymes at clinically relevant dosages [20].

Clinical studies

Key papers concerning ziprasidone are in press or submitted and will only be summarised here. Ziprasidone, like quetiapine, has been shown to be superior to placebo for the reduction of total psychopathology, positive and negative symptoms. There is limited evidence to suggest superiority over typical neuroleptics with regard to improvement in positive and negative symptoms. However, there have been few direct comparisons. Ziprasidone was compared to placebo in a 1-year maintenance study in stable, hospitalised chronic schizophrenic patients [85]. Ziprasidone significantly reduced the risk of relapse (from 71% to about 40%, depending on dose). Ziprasidone was associated with significant improvement in negative symptoms and global functioning. The dose range of ziprasidone for acute treatment appears to be between 40–160 mg/day. Maintenance doses appear to be at the lower end of this range. There is anecdotal evidence for efficacy of ziprasidone in some neuroleptic-resistant schizophrenic patients. Preliminary data on the cognitive effects of ziprasidone are encouraging (P. Harvey, personal communication). Ziprasidone does not increase serum prolactin levels and is virtually devoid of EPS and weight gain. Its major side-effects are nasal congestion and somnolence. There has been some concern of cardiovascular side-effects, e.g. increased QTc interval; however, perusal of the available data does not reveal a significant problem in this regard. However, further study is underway. A parenteral formulation of ziprasidone has been developed which should be useful in situations where oral medication is unacceptable or more rapid action is needed. However, no long-acting formulation is available.

Summary

Ziprasidone appears to be a useful additional atypical antipsychotic agent because of its very favorable side-effect profile, including no weight gain, major problems with olanzapine and clozapine, and no prolactin elevation, a less serious side-effect of risperidone. Possible cardiovascular side-effects of ziprasidone need to be further studied but the available evidence is not disturbing as is the case with sertindole. Its overall efficacy must be clarified in additional studies. Comparisons with the other atypical antipsychotics and clozapine are necessary. It also has a parenteral formulation which should be useful in emergency situations.

Sertindole

Sertindole, like the drugs already considered, is an atypical antipsychotic drug which fits the model of a relatively more potent 5-HT_{2a} than D_2 antagonist [86]. Several large-scale clinical trials confirmed its efficacy in schizophrenia with virtually no EPS [87–88]. However, it produced a prolongation of the QTc interval, leading to serious cardiovascular complications, in sufficient numbers of patients to require close EKG monitoring at the initiation of treatment. It is approved for use in some European countries but not in the United States. It appeared to have the lowest EPS potential of any agent other than clozapine.

Iloperidone

Iloperidone is a benzisoxazole which shares the overall pharmacology of the agents already considered, i.e. potent 5-HT_{2a} compared to D_2 receptor antagonism [89]. It also has a relatively high affinity for the 5-HT_6, 5-HT_7, 5-HT_{2c}, D_4 and D_3 receptors, which is clozapine-like. It has actions in animal models which are characteristic of an atypical antipsychotic [90]. Clinical trials are currently in place to determine its efficacy and side-effect profile in schizophrenia.

Conclusions

The atypical antipsychotic drugs reviewed here, together with clozapine, represent a major advance in the treatment of schizophrenia. Considerations of their efficacy and side-effect profiles are needed to determine the extent to which they should replace the typical neuroleptic drugs. This discussion has not considered cost effectiveness issues to any extent, although an analysis of the new and old treatments based on their cost effectiveness is necessary in a time of scarce resources for treatment. The atypical antipsychotics have clear advantages for EPS of the acute and subacute types. Clozapine and possibly the other atypical drugs have a reduced risk of tardive dyskinesia which should be a major factor in the decision to use these medications. The evidence for atypical antipsychotic drugs to improve cognition is steadily increasing and this should be one of the driving forces behind the substitution of these agents for the typical neuroleptic drugs. Because of the compliance problem that is less with the atypical than the typical antipsychotics, it is important to develop a long acting atypical antipsychotic. While the current group of atypical antipsychotic drugs is predominantly characterised by relatively more potent 5-HT_{2a} than D_2 receptor antagonism, it is likely that a number of different strategies will emerge for compounds which produce fewer EPS than the typical neuroleptics. Because these compounds are so effective in that regard, the real challenge is to develop agents which address other key features of schizophrenia, especially cognitive impairment and negative symptoms without the side-effect burden of this group of compounds. Clozapine stands out among the atypicals as a unique compound because of its clear effectiveness in treatment-resistant patients [91]. The other atypical antipsychotics discussed here all have their benefits and drawbacks but are clearly the best choice for first line treatment. Extensive research remains to be done to determine how best to use these agents with regard to specific patients.

Side-effects such as weight gain and prolactin stimulation are helpful considerations but they are not usually as powerful determinants of compliance as EPS has been in the past. Clinicians will likely find all the atypical antipsychotics useful and necessary to provide optimal management.

Acknowledgement
Supported, in part, by grants from the Warren Foundation, the Essel Foundation and the Lattner Foundation.

References

1 Hippius H (1989) The history of clozapine. *Psychopharmacol* 99: S3–S5
2 Meltzer HY (1995) The concept of atypical antipsychotics. In: JA den Boer, HGM Westenberg, HM van Praag (eds) *Advances in the Neurobiology of Schizophrenia, Volume 1.* Wiley & Sons, Ltd., England, pp 265–273
3 Gerlach J, Casey DE (1996) New antipsychotics: preclinical and clinical research. *Psychopharmacology* 124: 1
4 Nutt DJ (1990) Specific anatomy, non-specific drugs: the present state of schizophrenia. *J Psychopharmacol* 4: 171–175
5 Baldessarini R, Frankenberg F (1991) Clozapine: A novel antipsychotic agent. *New Eng J Med* 324: 746–754
6 Moore, NC, Gershon S (1989) Which atypical antipsychotics are identified by screening tests? *Clin Neuropharmacol* 12: 167–184
7 Chiodo LA, Bunney BS (1983) Typical and atypical neuroleptic: differential effects of chronic administration of the activity of A_9 and A_{10} midbrain dopaminergic neurons. *J Neurosci* 3: 1607–1619
8 Marder SR (1998) Facilitating compliance with antipsychotic medication. *J Clin Psychiatry* 59 Suppl 3: 21–25
9 Hansen TE, Casey DE, Hoffman WF (1997) Neuroleptic intolerance. *Schiz Bull* 23: 567–582
10 Meltzer HY (1997) Treatment-resistant schizophrenia: the role of clozapine. *Curr Med Res Opinion* 14: 1–20
11 Meltzer HY, Matsubara S, and Lee, M (1989) Classification of typical and atypical antipsychotic drugs on the basis of dopamine 5-HT_{2a} and serotonin 2 pKi values. *J Pharmacol Exp Thera* 251: 238–246
12 Schoemaker H, Claustre Y, Fage D, Rouquier L, Cherqui K, Curet O, Oblin A, Gonon F, Carter C, Benavides J, Scatton B (1997) Neurochemical characteristics of amisulpride, an atypical dopamine D_2/D_3 receptor antagonist with both presynaptic and limbic selectivity. *J Pharm Exp Thera* 280: 83–97
13 Ogren SO, Florvall L, Hall H, Magnusson O, Ångeby-Møller K (1990) Neuropharmacological and behavioural properties of remoxipride in the rat. *Acta Psych Scand* 358: S21–S26
14 Ahlenius S (1989) Antipsychotic-like properties of the 5-HT_{1a} agonist 8-OH-DPAT in the rat. *Pharmacol Toxicol* 64: 3–5
15 Fitton A, Heel RC (1990) Clozapine: a review of its pharmacological properties, and therapeutic use in schizophrenia. *Drugs* 40: 722–747
16 Megens AAHP, Awouters FHI, Schotte A, Meert TR, Dugovic C, Niemegeers CJE, Leysen JE (1991) Survey on the pharmacodynamics of the new antipsychotic risperidone. *Psychopharmacology* 114: 9–23
17 Moore NA, Tye NC, Axton MS, Risius FC (1992) The behavioral pharmacology of olanzapine, a novel "atypical" antipsychotic agent. *J Pharmacol Exp Thera* 262: 545–551
18 Dunn CJ, Fitton A (1996) Sertindole. *CNS Drugs* 5: 224–230
19 Gunasekara NS, Spencer CM (1998) Quetiapine-a review of its use in schizophrenia (review). *CNS Drugs* 9: 325–340
20 Davis R, Markham A (1997) Ziprasidone. *CNS Drugs* 8: 153–162

21 Meltzer HY, Stahl SM (1976) The dopamine hypothesis of schizophrenia: a review. *Schiz Bull* 2: 19–76
22 Mayerhoff DI, Loebel AD, Alvir JM, Szymanski SR, Geisler SH, Borenstein M, Lieberman JA (1994) The deficit state in first-episode schizophrenia. *Am J Psychiatry* 151: 1417–1422
23 Meltzer HY, Lee M, Cola P (1998) The evolution of treatment resistance: biologic implications. *J Clin Psychopharmacology* 18 (2 Suppl 1): 5S–11S
24 Carpenter WT Jr, Heinrichs DW, Wagman AM (1988) Deficit and nondeficit forms of schizophrenia: the concept. *Am J Psychiatry* 145: 578–583
25 Heaton, RK, Crowley TJ (1981) Effect of psychiatric disorders and their somatic treatments on neuropsychological test results. In: S Filskov, TJ Boll (eds) *Handbook of clinical neuropsychology*, John Wiley and Sons, New York, pp 481–525
26 Gitlin MJ (1994) Psychotropic medications and their effects on sexual function: Diagnosis, biology, and treatment approaches. *J Clin Psychiatry* 55: 406–413
27 Kane JM, Aguglia E, Altamura AC, Ayuso Guiterrez JL, Brunello N, Fleischhacker WW, Gaebel W, Gerlach J, Gukelfi JD, Kissling W, Lapierre YD, Lindstrom E, Mendlewicz J, Racagni G, Carulla LS, Schooler NR (1998) Guidelines for depot antipsychotic treatment in schizophrenia. *Eur Neuropsychopharmacol* 8: 55–66
28 Roth BL, Craigo SC, Choudhary MS, Uler A, Monsma FJ, Shen Y, Meltzer HY, Sibley DR (1994) Binding of typical and atypical antipsychotic agents to 5-hydroxytryptamine 6 (5-HT_6) and 5-HT hydroxytryptamine 7 (5-HT_7) receptors. *J Pharmacol Exp Thera* 268: 1406–1410
29 Schotte A, Janssen PFM, Gommeren W, Luyten W, Van Grompel P, Lesage AS, De Loore K, Leysen JE (1996) Risperidone compared with new and reference antipsychotic drugs: *in vitro* and *in vivo* receptor binding. *Psychopharmacology* 124: 57–73
30 Huang ML, Van Peer A, Woestenborghs R, De Costger R, Heykants J, Jansen AAI, Zylick Z, Visscher HW, Johkman JHG (1993) Pharmacokinetics of the novel antipsychotic agent risperidone and the prolactin response in healthy subjects. *Clin Pharmacol Ther* 54: 247–268
31 Marder SR, Meibach RC (1994) Risperidone in the treatment of schizophrenia. *Amer Psychiatry* 151: 825–835
32 Chouinard G, Jones B, Remington G, Bloom D, Addington D, MacEwan GH, Labelle A, Beauclair L, Arnott W (1993) A Canadian multicenter placebo-controlled study of fixed doses of risperiodone and haloperidol in the treatment of chronic schizophrenic patients. *J Clin Psychopharmacol* 13: 25–40
33 Claus A, Bollen J, DeCuyper H, Eneman M, Malfroid M, Peuskens J, Heylen S (1992) Risperidone *vs* haloperidol in the treatment of chronic schizophrenic inpatients: A multicentre double-blind comparative study. *Acta Psychiatrica Scandinavica* 85: 295–305
34 Kopala LC, Fredrikson D, Good KP, Honer WG (1996) Symptoms in neuroleptic-naive, first episode schizophrenia: response to risperidone. *Biol Psychatry* 39: 296–298
35 Moller HJ, Muller H, Borison RL, Schooler NR, Chouinard G (1995) A path-analytical approach to differentiate between direct and indirect drug effects on negative symptoms in schizophrenic patients. A re-evaluation of the North American risperidone study. *Euro Arch Psych Clin Neuro* 245: 45–49
36 Marder S, Davis JM, Chouinard, G (1997) The effects of risperidone on the five dimensions of schizophrenia derived by factor analysis: combined results of the North American trials. *J Clin Psychiatry* 58: 538–546
37 Tran PV, Hamilton SH, Kuntz AJ, Potvin JH, Andersen SW, Beasley C, Tollefson GD (1997) Double-blind comparison of olanzapine *vs* risperidone in the treatment of schizophrenia and other psychotic disorders. *J Clin Psychopharmacol* 17: 407–418
38 Segal J, Berk M, Brook S (1998) Risperidone compared with both lithium and haloperidol in mania: A double-blind randomized controlled trial. *Clin Neuropharmacol* 21: 176–180
39 Frye MA, Ketter TA, Altshuler LL, Denicoff K, Dunn RT, Kimbrell TA, Cora-Locatelli G, Post RM (1998) Clozapine in bipolar disorder: treatment implications for other atypical antipsychotics. *J Aff Dis* 48: 91–104
40 Dwight MM, Keck PE Jr, Stanton SP, Strakowski SM, McElroy SL (1994) Antidepressant activity and mania associated with risperidone treatment of schizoaffective disorder. *Lancet* 344: 554–555

40a Meltzer HY, McGurk SR (1999) The effects of clozapine, risperidone, and olanzapine on cognitive function in schizophrenia. *Schiz Bull* 25: 233–256
41 Stipp E, Lussier I (1996) The effect of risperidone on cognition in patients with schizophrenia. *Can Psych* 41 (suppl 2): S35–S40
42 Green MF, Marshall BD Jr, Wirshin WC, Ames D, Marder SR, McGurk SR, Kern RS, Mintz, J Does risperidone improve verbal working memory in schizophrenia. *Am J Psychiatry* 154 (6): 799–804
43 McGurk SR, Green MF, Wirshing WC, Ames D, Marshall BD, Marder SR, Mintz J (1997) The effects of risperidone vs haloperidol on cognitive functioning in treatment-resistant schizophrenia: the trail making test. *CNS Spectrums* 2: 60–64
44 Smith RC, Chua JW, Lipetsker B, Bhattacharyya A (1996) Efficacy of risperidone in reducing positive and negative symptoms in medication-refractory schizophrenia: an open prospective study. *J Clin Psychiatry* 57: 460–466
45 Jeste DV, Klausner M, Brecher M, Clyde C, Jones J (1996) A clinical evaluation of risperidone in the treatment of schizophrenia: A 10-week, open-label, multicenter trial. *Psychopharmacology* 131: 239–247
46 Bondolfi G, Dufour H, Patris M, May JP, Billeter U, Eap CB, Baumann P (1998) Risperidone vs clozapine in treatment resistant chronic schizophrenia: A randomized double-blind study. *Am J Psychiatry* 155: 499–504
47 Ganguli R, Brar JS (1998) The effects of risperidone and olanzapine on the indications for clozapine. *Psychopharmacol Bull* 34 (1) 83–87
48 Hoyberg OJ, Fensbo C, Remvig J, Lingjaerde O, Sloth-Nielsen M, Salvesen I (1993) Risperidone *vs* perphenazine in the treatment of chronic schizophrenic patients with acute exacerbations. *Acta Psych Scand* 88: 395–402
49 Huttenenen MO, Piepponen T, Rantanen H, Larmo I, Nyholm R, Raitasuo V (1995) Risperidone vs zuclopentihoxl in the treatment of acute schizophrenic episodes; a double-blind parallel-group trial. *Acta Psychiatr Scand* 91: 271–277
50 Blin O, Azorin JM, Bouhours P (1996) Antipsychotic and anxiolytic properties of risperidone, haloperidol, and methotrimeprazine in schizophrenic patients. *J Clin Psychopharmacol* 16: 38–44
51 Simpson GM, Lindenmayer JP (1996) Extrapyramidal symptoms in patients treated with risperidone. *J Clin Psychopharmacol* 17/3: 194–201
52 Rich SS, Friedman JH, Ott BR (1995) Risperidone vs clozapine in the treatment of psychosis in six patients with Parkinson's disease and other akinetic-rigid syndromes. *J Clin Psychiatry* 56: 556–559
53 Peuskens J (1995) Risperidone in the treatment of patients with chronic schizophrenia: A multinational, multicentre, double-blind, parallel-group study vs haloperidol. *Br J Psychiatry* 166: 712–726
54 Hamner MB, Arana GW (1998) Hyperprolactinaemia in antipsychotic-treated patients: Guidelines for avoidance and management. *CNS Drugs* 209–222
55 Schyve P, Smithline F, Meltzer HY (1978) Neuroleptic-induced prolactin elevation and breast cancer: an emerging clinical issue. *Arch Gen Psychiatry* 25: 1291–1330
56 Bymaster FP, Calligaro DO, Falcone JF, Marsh RD, Moore NA, Tye NC, Seeman P, Wong DT (1996) Radioreceptor binding profile of the atypical antipsychotic olanzapine. *Neuropsychopharmacol* 14: 87–96
57 Ring BJ, Catlow J, Lindsay TJ, Gillespie T, Roskos LK, Cerimele BJ, Swanson SP, Hamman MA, Wrighton SA (1996) Identification of the human cytochromes P450 responsible for the *in vitro* formation of the major oxidativ metabolites of the antipsychotic agent olanzapine. *J Pharmacol Exp Thera* 276: 658–666
58 Ereshefsky L (1996) Pharmacokinetics and drug interactions: Update for new antipsychotics. *J Clin Psychiatry* 57 Suppl 11: 12–25
59 Perry PJ, Sanger T, Beasley C (1997) Olanzapine plasma concentrations and clinical response in acutely ill schizophrenic patients. *J Clin Psychopharmacol* Vol 17/6: 472–477
60 Beasley CM Jr, Sanger T, Satterlee W, Tollefson G, Tran P, Hamilton S (1996a) Olanzapine *vs* placebo: results of a double-blind, fixed-dose olanzapine trial. *Psychopharmacology* 124: 159–167
61 Beasley CM Jr, Tollefson G, Tran P, Satterlee W, Sanger T, Hamilton S (1996b) Olanzapine vs placebo and haloperidol acute phase results of the north american double-blind olanzapine trial. *Neuropsychopharmacol* 14: 111–123

62 Tollefson GD, Beasley CM Jr, Tran PV, Street JS, Krueger JA, Tamura RN, Graffeo KA, Thieme ME (1997) Olanzapine vs haloperidfol in the treatment of schizophrenia and schizoaffective and schizophreniform disorders: results of an international collaborative trial. *Am J Psychiatry* 154: 457–465
63 Hamilton SH, Revicki DA, Genduso LA, Beasley CM (1998) Olanzapine vs placebo and haloperidol – quality of life and efficacy results of the North American double-blind trial. *Neuropsychopharmacol* 18: 41–49
64 Dellva MA, Tran P, Tollefson GD, Wently AL, Beasley CM Jr (1997) Standard olanzapine vs placebo and ineffective-dose olanzapine in the treatment of schizophrenia. *Psychiatric Services* 48: 1571–1577
65 Tran PV, Dellva MA, Tollefson GD, Wentley AL, Beasley CM Jr (1998) Oral olanzapine *vs* oral haloperidol in the maintenance treatment of schizophrenia and related psychoses. *Brit J Psychiatry* 172: 499–505
66 Tollefson GD, Sanger TM (1996) Negative symptoms: a path analytic approach to a double-blind, placebo-and haloperidol-controlled clinical trial with olanzapine. *Am J Psychiatry* 154: 466–474
67 McElroy SL, Frye M, Denicoff K, Altshuler L, Nolen W, Kupka R, Suppes T, Keck PE, Jr, Leverich GS, Kmetz GF, Post RM (1998) Olanzapine in treatment-resistant bipolar disorder. *Aff Dis* 49: 119–122
68 Conley RR, Kelly DL, Gale EA (1998b) Olanzapine response in treatment-refractory schizophrenic patients with a history of substance abuse. *Schiz Res* 33: 95–101
69 Conley RR, Kelly DL, Gale EA (1998b) Olanzapine response in treatment-refractory schizophrenic patients with a history of substance abuse. *Schiz Res* 33: 95–101
70 Friedman JH, Goldstein S, Jacques C (1998) Substituting clozapine for olanzapine in psychiatrically stable Parkinson's disease patients: results of an open label trial. *Clin Neuropharmacol* 21: 285–288
71 Tollefson GD, Beasley CM Jr, Tamura RN, Tran PV, Potvin JH (1997b) Blind, controlled, long-term study of the comparative incidence of treatment-emergent tardive dyskinesia with olanzapine or haloperidol. *Am J Psychiatry* 154: 1248–1254
72 Saller CF, Salama AI (1993) Seroquel: biochemical profile of a potential atypical antipsychotic. *Psychopharmacol* 112: 285–292
73 Migler BM, Warawa EJ, Malick JB (1993) Seroquel:behavioral effects in conventional and novel tests for atypical antipsychotic drug. *Psychopharmacology* 112: 299–307
74 Goldstein JM, Litwin LC, Sutton EB, Malick JB (1993) Seroquel: electrophysiological profile of a potential atypical antipsychotic. *Psychopharmacology* 112: 293–298
75 Ellenbroek BA, Lubbers LJ, Cools AR (1996) Activity of "seroquel" (ICI 204,636) in animal models for atypical properties of antipsychotics: A comparison with clozapine. *Neuropsychopharmacol* 15: 406–416
76 Casey DE (1996) "Seroquel" (quetiapine): preclinical and clinical findings of a new atypical antipsychotic. *Exp Opin Invest Drugs* 5: 939–957
77 Misra LK, Erpenbach JE, Hamlyn H, Fuller WC (1998) Quetiapine: a new atypical antipsychotic. *South Dakota J Med* 51: 189–193
78 King DJ, Link CG, Kowalcyk B (1998) A comparison of bd and tid dose regimens of quetiapine (seroquel) in the treatment of schizophrenia. *Psychopharmacol* 137: 139–146
79 Small JG, Hirsch SR, Arvanitis LA, Miller BG, Link CG (1997) Quetiapine in patients with schizophrenia: a high and low-dose double-blind comparison with placebo. *Arch Gen Psychiatry* 54: 549–557
80 Arvanitis LA, and Miller BG (1997) Multiple fixed dose of "Seroquel" (queitapine) in patients with acute exacerbation of schizophrenia: A comparison with haloperidol and placebo. The Seroquel Trial 13 Study Group. *Biological Psychiatry* 42: 233–246
81 Caley CF, Rosenbaum S (1998) Focus on quetiapine-the fourth atypical antipsychotic. *Hospital Formulary* 33: 105–117
82 Hamner MB, Arvanitis LA, Miller BG, Link CG, Hong WW (1996) Plasma prolactin in schizophrenia subjects treated with seroquel. *Psychopharmacol Bull* 32: 107–110
83 Seeger TF, Seymour PA, Schmidt AW, Zorn SH, Schulz DW, Lebel LA, McLean S, Guanowsky V, Howard HR, Lowe JA 3rd, et al. (1995) Ziprasidone: a new antipsychotic with combined dopamine and serotonin receptor antagonist activity. *J Pharmacol Exp Thera* 275: 101–113

84 Millan MJ, Gobert A, Newman-Tancredi A, Audinot V, Lejeune F, Rivet J-M, Cussac D, Nicolas JP, Muller O, Lavielle G (1998): S 16924 ((R)-2-{1-[2-(2,3-dihydro-benzo[1,4] dioxin-5-yloxy)-ethyl]-pyrrolidin-3yl}-1-(4-fluoro-phenyl)-ethanone), a novel potential antipsychotic with marked serotonin 5-HT_{1A} agonist properties: 1. Receptorial and neurochemical profile in comparison with clozapine and haloperidol. *J Pharmacol Exp Ther* 286: 1341–1355
85 Arato M, O'Connor R, Meltzer HY (Submitted) The ziprasidone extended use in schizophrenia (Zeus) study: a prospective, double-blind, placebo-controlled, 1-year clinical trial.
86 Perregaard J, Arnt J, Bogeso KP, Hyttel J, Sanchez C (1992) Noncataleptogenic, centrally acting dopamine D-2 and serotonin 5-HT_2 antagonists within a series of 3-substituted 1-(4-fluorophenyl)-1H-indoles. *J Med Chem* 35: 1092–1101
87 VanKammen DP, McEvoy JP, Targum SD, Kardatzke SD, Sebree TB (1996) A randomized, controlled, dose-ranging trial of sertindole in patients with schizophrenia. *Psychopharmacology* 124: 168–175
88 Zimbroff DL, Kane JM, Tamminga CA, Daniel DG, Mack RJ, Wozniak PJ, Sebree TB, Wallin BA, Kashkin KB (1997) Controlled, dose-response study of sertindole and haloperidol in the treatment of schizophrenia. *Am J Psychiatry* 154: 782–791
89 Kongsamut S, Roehr JE, Hartman HB, Weissensee P, Kerman LL, Tang L, Sandrasagra A (1996) Iloperidone binding to human and rat dopamine and 5-HT receptors. *Eur J Pharmacol* 317: 417–423
90 Szewezak MR, Corbett R, Rusk DK, Wilmot CA, Conway PG, Strupczewski JT, Cornfeldt M (1995) The pharmacological profile of iloperidone, a novel athypical antipsychotic agent. *J Pharmacol Exp Thera* 274: 1404–1413
91 Kane J, Honigfeld G, Singer, J, Meltzer HY, and the Clozaril Collaborative Study Group (1988) Clozapine for the treatment-resistant schizophrenic: a double-blind comparison with chlorpromazine. *Arch Gen Psychiatry* 45: 789–796

Atypical Antipsychotics
ed. by B.A. Ellenbroek and A.R. Cools

New discoveries in the development of antipsychotics with novel mechanisms of action: beyond the atypical antipsychotics with serotonin dopamine antagonism

Stephen M. Stahl and Darius K. Shayegan

Department of Psychiatry, University of California San Diego and Clinical Neuroscience Research Center, 8899 University Center Lane, Suite 130, San Diego, CA 92122, USA

Introduction

Antipsychotic innovation can be divided into three eras. The first era began with the serendipitous discovery of the classical antipsychotic neuroleptics, later found to mediate their therapeutic actions by blocking D_2 dopamine receptors, particularly in the mesolimbic dopamine pathway [1]. From the late 1950s through the 1980s, a large number of effective compounds sharing this mechanism of action were thus discovered and marketed. The use of such classical antipsychotic compounds has now given way to the era of "atypical antipsychotics" which began in the late 1980s when the atypical properties of clozapine were observed, and attributed at least in part to the simultaneous blockade of serotonin 2A receptors as well as D_2 dopamine receptors [1–3]. We are currently nearing the end of this era now that several SDAs (serotonin dopamine antagonists) have been discovered and marketed, with a few more in the late stages of clinical development. These compounds have been discussed and emphasised in many of the preceding chapters of this book.

Here we will introduce the possibilities of what might be next in store for the treatment of psychosis. A number of potential pharmacological mechanisms are under investigation at the current time. These range from conceptual drug targets for which compounds have not yet been identified, to preclinical discoveries of agents with novel mechanisms of action, to the early clinical evaluation of some of these new agents in patients with schizophrenia. Some of the information about these compounds is published in the scientific and clinical literature, and other information is available through unpublished communications as well as through newsletters and publications which monitor the activities of the pharmaceutical industry (e.g. [4]). The earlier the compound is in the discovery process, the less reliable the information. Nevertheless, this overview will attempt to sample the most up-to-date information available about the progress regarding the most innovative of the contemporary drug development strategies in this third era of antipsychotic discovery, namely "beyond the serotonin dopamine antagonists and the atypical antipsychotics".

Novel serotonergic and dopaminergic mechanisms

Overview: serotonin 2A/dopamine 2 antagonists (SDAs) more or less

No atypical antipsychotic is merely a serotonin 2A/dopamine 2 antagonist (SDA) although every member of this group does have these properties, including clozapine, risperidone, olanzapine, quetiapine (all marketed in the US and many other countries), sertindole (marketed outside the US), and ziprasidone (in late clinical development at this writing) (e.g. [2, 3]). The older agents zotepine (marketed in Europe and not in the US) and loxapine (marketed world-wide and generic in many countries) might also be able to be added to this list of agents with SDA properties [2]. As has been discussed extensively in other chapters of this book, simultaneous binding to 5HT2A receptors appears to endow dopamine 2 antagonism with both improved tolerability (fewer EPRs (extrapyramidal reactions), less tardive dyskinesia, less prolactin elevation) and improved efficacy (enhanced action on negative symptoms, and possibly efficacy in reducing depressive and cognitive symptoms in schizophrenia). The SDA/atypical antipsychotics, however, bind to more than a dozen known neurotransmitter sites, spawning at least two different strategies for improving their safety and efficacy.

The first strategy to improve the safety and tolerability of the current atypical antipsychotics is to combine several of their known pharmacological properties in a more desirable "cocktail," with perhaps other pharmacological properties added as well. Thus, novel mixtures of serotonin 2A/dopamine 2 antagonism with high affinity for other receptors such as alpha 1 receptors, or norepinephrine reuptake, or $5HT_{1A}$, $5HT_{1D}$, or serotonin reuptake are examples of this approach.

The second strategy is to target selectively just one of these additional properties, hoping that this would lead to an improved clinical profile. Thus, for the serotonin system, this has led to selective targeting of 5HT receptors such as $5HT_{2A}$ receptors, $5HT_{2C}$ receptors and $5HT_6$ receptors. For the dopamine system, that means selective targeting of D_1, D_3, D_4 or presynaptic D_2 autoreceptors. Later we will discuss novel approaches which target neurotransmitter systems other than serotonin and dopamine.

More than SDA pharmacology

SDA plus potent alpha 1 antagonism

Iloperidone (in clinical development) is an agent with SDA properties, but has even more potent actions as an alpha 1 antagonist [5]. Whether this will prove to be an asset or a liability remains to be determined. Thus, one could look at this compound as similar to risperidone, but with unwanted alpha 1 antagonism, predicting a high incidence of orthostatic hypotension. On the other hand, the alpha 1 antagonist properties may have unique effects upon CNS noradrenergic systems associated with unique efficacy.

SDA plus $5HT_{1A}$ agonist properties
Although selective $5HT_{1A}$ agonists or antagonists are not theoretically attractive candidates for novel antipsychotic actions, when these properties are part of a pharmacological cocktail, this may lead to desirable ancillary properties in the treatment of psychosis, particularly in the reduction of anxiety and depression associated with psychosis. Thus, clozapine is known to have $5HT_{1A}$ partial agonist properties, and ziprasidone (also an SDA) also has $5HT_{1A}$ agonist effects [2].

SDA plus $5HT_{2C}$ agonist, $5HT_{1D}$ agonist and serotonin reuptake inhibitor properties
The SDA ziprasidone has several unique pharmacologic properties associated with SDA. It is also a $5HT_{2C}$ agonist, a $5HT_{1D}$ agonist and a serotonin reuptake inhibitor [2, 6]. Early clinical results suggest less weight gain with ziprasidone than other atypical antipsychotics [6]. Perhaps $5HT_{2C}$ antagonist properties of other atypical antipsychotics as well as histamine 1 antagonist properties of atypical antipsychotics account for the weight gain, sometimes quite significant, of many of these compounds. As ziprasidone not only lacks potent antihistamine actions, but is in fact a $5HT_{2C}$ agonist rather than $5HT_{2C}$ antagonist, this could explain data suggesting it has little or no weight gain associated with chronic treatment. The $5HT_{1D}$ agonist properties and serotonin reuptake inhibition could perhaps be theoretically attractive as an antidepressant or anxiolytic for such associated symptoms in psychotic illnesses.

SDA plus norepinephrine reuptake blockade
Two SDA compounds are known to have norepinephrine reuptake blocking properties, namely ziprasidone and zotepine [2, 6, 7]. Theoretically, this could endow these compounds with favorable ancillary antidepressant properties, although this has not yet been proven. As mentioned above, ziprasidone also has serotonin reuptake blocking properties [2, 6].

Other serotonin/dopamine cocktails

D_2 antagonist but $5HT_{1A}$ agonist
Mazapertine (in clinical development) is a D_2 agonist, but rather than $5HT_{2A}$ antagonist properties, has $5HT_{1A}$ agonist properties [4]. The ability of this pharmacologic mixture to yield the improved side effect profile and

improved efficacy profile of the SDAs are in still the process of being determined.

D_2, D_3 and D_4 antagonist but $5HT_{1A}$ agonist

Nemonapride (in clinical development in Japan) is a D_2 antagonist with potent $5HT_{1A}$ agonist properties [8]. It also has potent actions as an antagonist at both D_3 and D_4 receptors as well. Early clinical results support efficacy as an antipsychotic in schizophrenia, but no special efficacy features have yet been confirmed.

Less than SDA pharmacology

Selective $5HT_{2A}$ antagonists

No agent lacking D_2 antagonist properties has yet been proven effective as an antipsychotic. One agent entering Phase III clinical development which is a selective antagonist of the $5HT_{2A}$ receptor, but not the dopamine 2 receptor is MDL-100,907 [4, 9, 10]. Past studies with the $5HT_{2A/C}$ antagonist ritanserin (dropped from clinical development) suggested efficacy in lowering extrapyramidal side-effects in the presence of a dopamine 2 antagonist, and some efficacy for negative symptoms, but limited efficacy for positive symptoms. More recent preliminary results from the $5HT_{2A}$ selective antagonist MDL-100,907 suggest efficacy for both positive and negative symptoms in schizophrenia. Clinical development with this compound is continuing.

Selective $5HT_{2C}$ agonist/antagonist

Both selective agonists and antagonists for the $5HT_{2C}$ receptor are in development for a number of indications, including obesity, anxiety and psychosis [4]. Already mentioned is the association of $5HT_{2C}$ receptor antagonism with weight gain [11]. However, most studies of the $5HT_{2C}$ receptor have been with rodents and not humans, and the acute effects of drugs are sometimes the opposite of their long-term effects. Thus, short-term stimulation of the $5HT_{2C}$ receptor may lead to down regulation and desensitisation of this receptor with diminished receptor activity with chronic administration. Whether a selective $5HT_{2C}$ compound, either agonist or antagonist will prove effective in treating some of the symptoms of schizophrenia remains quite speculative, although some basic science studies suggest a rationale to this approach [12]. Some $5HT_{2C}$ agonists are PNU 22394E, PNU-15267A and PNU-57378 (preclinical development stage), and antagonists are Org-12962 (Phase I) and SB-200646A (Phase I) and SB-242084 (Phase II for anxiety).

Selective $5HT_6$ antagonists

Some of the atypical antipsychotics (notably clozapine, olanzapine, quetiapine and sertindole) block the $5HT_6$ receptor [2]. Now that this receptor has been cloned, selective antagonists for this receptor are being pursued to determine their psychotropic properties.

Selective $5HT_3$ or $5HT_7$ antagonists
On the basis of promising preclinical results, several indications for $5HT_3$ antagonists were pursued all with disappointing results in clinical trials. This includes anxiety, dementia and schizophrenia. Further development is not known to be continuing for psychosis for the $5HT_3$ selective compounds at the present time.

Several atypical antipsychotics block the $5HT_7$ receptor including clozapine, quetiapine, risperidone and sertindole [2]. Thus, it is theoretically possible to target this receptor selectively, just as several other serotonin receptors subtypes such as the $5HT_{2A}$ and $5H_{T6}$ receptors are being targeted. However, no known compounds are in preclinical or clinical development at the present time.

D_2-like receptor antagonists

Selective D_4 antagonists
There are at least five subtypes of dopamine receptor, namely D_1 through D_5. Sometimes they are clustered into two larger subgroups, the D_1-like (i.e. D_1 and D_5 receptors) and the D_2-like (i.e. D_2, D_3 and D_4). All known antipsychotic drugs to date block both the D_2 and the D_3 receptor, but only some block the D_4 receptor as well. Due to the fact that clozapine blocks the D_4 receptor, and some preclinical studies and *post mortem* studies of brains from schizophrenics have suggested a prominent role for the D_4 receptor, antagonists for this site have been developed. Nonselective antagonists include YM-43611 (D_3 and D_4 antagonist in preclinical development) and nemonapride (D_4, but also D_2, D_3 and $5HT_{1A}$). Nemonapride has been reported to be effective in schizophrenia in Japanese studies [13], but any special properties attributable to its D_4 actions remain unknown.

On the other hand, the truly D_4 selective compounds L-745,870 [14] and fananserin have yielded disappointing results in early Phase II clinical trials of schizophrenia [4]. Lack of efficacy for positive symptoms has been reported, including possible worsening of these symptoms. However, it is possible that targeting other symptom dimensions in schizophrenia such as cognitive symptoms may result in favorable pharmacologic actions. Thus, the D_4 selective antagonists PNU-101387G (Phase II), NGD 94-4 (Phase I), LU-111995 (Phase I/II) are currently in clinical trials in schizophrenia [4]. Given the disappointing early clinical results for positive symptoms of schizophrenia, some of these trials are proceeding with an emphasis on monitoring cognitive symptoms such as working memory.

Selective D_3 antagonists

As mentioned above, another member of the D_2-like receptor group is the D_3 receptor, which nearly every D_2 antagonist also blocks [2, 3]. Theoretically, the D_3 receptor may act in opposition to the D_2 receptor and the D1 receptor in that it inhibits psychomotor behaviour in rodents. That is, whereas D_2 antipsychotics (which also are D_3 antagonists) induce powerful hypomotility and even catalepsy in rodents, but D_3 selective antagonists do not, and may actually increase psychomotor behaviour. Thus, it is theoretically possible that D_3 antagonism without D_2 antagonism would active behaviours in schizophrenic patients and thus reduce negative symptoms, such as social withdrawal, anhedonia, and apathy without causing cognitive side-effects of the D_2 antagonists.

Only recently have the D_3 properties been selectively targeted with low D_2 properties, such as E-2030, GR-218.321. GR-103,691, PNU 170413, LU-201640, S-14297, and PD-152255, all in early preclinical development). It will indeed be interesting to see if the preclinical behavioural profiles of such agents play out as therapeutic advantages in clinical testing of schizophrenia.

Presynaptic D_2 autoreceptor agonist

It is theoretically possible to reduce dopaminergic activity at post-synaptic D_2 receptors by shutting off the presynaptic dopamine terminal *via* stimulation of its presynaptic D_2 autoreceptors. Various strategies for targeting this receptor are to exploit any possible separation in binding affinities of the presynaptic vs the postsynaptic D_2 receptors. Aripiprazole is one example of this approach and this compound has proceeded to clinical development with some interesting and encouraging clinical results. The compound CI-1007 is also a novel but nonselective dopamine autoreceptor agonist which also has partial agonist properties at D_2 and D_3 receptors. It is in early clinical testing [15].

D_2 modulator/"normalizer" and D_2 partial agonists

Dopamine presents a theoretical quandary to the drug development scientist: namely, how to decrease theoretically overactive dopamine at D_2 mesolimbic receptors which are mediating positive psychotic symptoms, while simultaneously increasing theoretically underactive dopamine at D_2 receptors in the cortex (especially dorsolateral prefrontal and limbic cortex) which are mediating negative symptoms of schizophrenia. One potential pharmacological solution to this problem is a partial agonist at D_2 receptors. Thus, finding a compound on the agonist/antagonist/inverse agonist spectrum with sufficient full agonist properties to enhance activity in dopamine deficient brain areas with sufficient partial agonist properties to antagonise activity in dopamine excess brain areas would be the goal. Two such compounds which attempt to embody such theoretically desirable properties are the partial agonists terguride (clinical testing in Parkinson's

Disease) and CI-1007 (preclinical and early clinical testing) [15]. Whether either of these compounds will simultaneously treat both positive and negative symptoms by their partial D_2 agonist properties remains to be determined.

A related but different action is exemplified by the compound PNU 9639 also known as OSU 6162 [16]. Although the mechanism of action of this compound is still somewhat obscure, it acts somewhat like a partial agonist at D_2 receptors, yet has such low binding affinity for these receptors that this cannot readily account for its pharmacological activity. Studies have referred to it as a "dopamine normalizer" since it seems to inhibit high dopaminergic tone and activate low dopaminergic tone. Thus, PNU-9639 blocks overactive dopamine neurons mediating l-DOPA dyskinesias in MPTP primates [16], blocks d-amphetamine-induced hyperactivity in rodents, yet produces behavioural stimulation in habituated rates, increases immediate early genes in cortical areas affected in schizophrenia, and increases dopamine release. Although this compound is still at the preclinical stage, this relatively exciting portfolio of properties could be quite interesting to test in schizophrenia.

D_1-like antagonists

Selective D_1 antagonists

As mentioned above, the D_1-like family of dopamine receptors includes both D_1 and D_5 receptors. Although there are no known selective D_5 antagonists, there is some interest in targeting the D_1 receptor selectively. Since clozapine has D_1 antagonist properties, this receptor has been targeted selectively in order to determine whether any of clozapine's atypical clinical properties can be accounted for by D_1 antagonism. Early D_1 selective antagonists have served as preclinical tools, but clinical testing has shown poor oral bioavailability in man, and they have not been extensively tested clinically. NNC-010687 is proceeding in preclinical development.

Novel neurotransmitter mechanisms other than serotonin and dopamine

Sigma antagonists

The physiological functions of the sigma receptor remain poorly characterised, thus, these receptors constitute the "sigma enigma." Originally discovered as one of the opiate receptors, it is now associated with the actions of the psychotomimetic agent phencyclidine (PCP) and the activity of NMDA glutamate receptors. Theoretically, a sigma antagonist could block the actions of PCP and thus the mechanism of psychosis in schizophrenia as well. Sigma receptors may also modulate the activity of dopaminergic and cholinergic neurons as well as glutamate neurons, and have regulatory input to learning, memory and aggressive behavior on the basis of studies in rodents. Early clinical testing of the sigma antagonist BMY-14,802 did not result in impressive efficacy and had some associated liver function test abnormalities, and was dropped from further development. Other sigma antagonists include panamesine, also known as EMD-57445 [17], PD-144418 [18], BD-1047, and BD-1063 [19]. Panamesine has recently been reported to have modest efficacy in a Phase II study of schizophrenia [19], yet further clinical development is said to be discontinued. PD-144418 is selective for sigma 1 receptors, and reverses NMDA actions in rats. Clinical studies are not yet underway.

Sanofi SR 31742A is yet another selective sigma antagonist with promising preclinical results and which is now in clinical testing of schizophrenia [4]. Another sigma ligand is OPC-14523, a combination sigma agonist, $5HT_{1A}$ agonist and 5HT reuptake inhibitor. This compound is in Phase II testing for depression [4]. As it is difficult to extrapolate from experiments in rodents to humans especially for sigma receptors, it is not clear where on the agonist/partial agonist/antagonist spectrum an ideal sigma compound for schizophrenia would be. Thus, study of sigma agonists defined in preclinical studies of rodents may nevertheless be interesting hypothesis-generating tools for new therapeutic strategies in schizophrenia.

Cannabinoid antagonists

The psychoactive ingredient in marijuana has long been characterised as delta-9-tetrahydrocannabinol (THC), but only recently have receptors for cannabinoids been identified in the central nervous system (cannabinoid CB1 receptors) and in the immune system (CB2 receptors) [20, 21]. CB1 receptors are coupled to G proteins and modulate adenylate cyclase and ion channels. Not surprisingly, a candidate for the endogenous modulator of CB1 receptors was described following the characterisation of the CB1 receptors. This "endogenous marijuana" is known as anandamide, a member of a family of fatty acid ethanolamide that may represent a novel class of naturally occurring lipid neurotransmitters. Its actions are mimicked not only by THC, by also by a recently discovered synthetic agonist CP-55,940, and antagonised by SR 141716A [20–22].

Since most psychotropic drugs with reinforcing properties, including marijuana, mediate their actions through the mesolimbic dopamine pathway, an antagonist of the cannabinoid receptors could theoretically reduce the activity of this pathway. This may not only reduce substance-induced reinforcing behaviour, especially for marijuana; by reducing the activity of the mesolimbic dopamine pathway which is theoretically hyperactive in psychosis, it may also reduce the positive symptoms of psychosis in schizophrenia [23]. This very novel approach is currently in testing of schizophrenia with SR 141716A [4].

Selective noradrenaline reuptake inhibition

Recently the first truly selective noradrenaline reuptake inhibitor reboxetine, has been marketed in Europe for the treatment of depression. Lacking the undesirable anticholinergic, antihistaminic, and alpha-1 antagonist properties of noradrenaline selective tricyclic antidepressants such as desipramine, nortriptyline and maprotilene, reboxetine can cause very robust inhibition of the noradrenaline transporter without the tricyclic side-effects [24]. This is analogous to the situation when the SSRIs replaced the tricyclic antidepressants as more potent serotonin transporter inhibitors without the undesirable tricyclic side-effects.

As noradrenaline plays a major role in cognitive functions which are abnormal in schizophrenia, such as attention, working memory, and information processing, it is possible that boosting noradrenaline would enhance these cognitive functions in schizophrenia. Testing of these concepts is now proceeding in schizophrenia and other disorders characterised by cognitive dysfunctioning.

Developing future antipsychotic agents by modulating peptide receptors

Several neuropeptides are believe to "modulate" dopamine neurotransmission. Those which can attenuate dopamine activity without blocking D_2 receptors are theoretically attractive candidates as antipsychotics without extrapyramidal symptoms, including tardive dyskinesia.

Neuropeptide Y

This neuropeptide enhances NMDA-stimulated dopamine release in the rat nucleus accumbens, which suggests that a neuropeptide Y antagonist would be interesting to test in schizophrenia. No such compounds which stimulate or block neuropeptide Y receptors have yet been identified for preclinical drug development.

Neurotensin

Neurotensin is co-localised with dopamine in the mesolimbic dopamine pathway, but is much lower in concentration in nigrostriatal and mesocortical dopaminergic pathways [25–27]. Neurotensin can alter dopaminergic activity preferentially in the mesolimbic dopamine pathway. It has the opposite effect of amphetamine on dopamine release, leading some to hypothesise that a neurotensin agonist would be the compound to study in schizophrenia. On the other hand, neurotensin increases the release of dopamine in the mesolimbic system, and a neurotensin antagonist may also be theoretically preferred for schizophrenia. Although some synthetic peptide agonists have been identified as preclinical research tools, a non-peptide neurotensin antagonist, SR-142948 is currently in Phase II clinical testing in schizophrenia. Theoretically, a neurotensin antagonist could reduce positive symptoms of psychosis without producing extrapyramidal symptoms by exploiting differential actions on the mesolimbic rather than the nigrostriatal dopamine systems.

Cholecystokinin

Cholecystokinin (CCK) is also co-localised with dopaminergic neurons, and has two receptor subtypes, with CCK-A being predominantly outside the CNS and CCK-B within the CNS [28–29]. CCK mimics the action of antipsychotics in inhibiting dopamine firing in the mesolimbic system in rodents, suggesting a role for CCK-B agonists in schizophrenia. On the other hand, CCK has been described as both inhibiting and facilitating dopamine-mediated behaviours in the mesolimbic pathway, making it just as confusing whether an agonist or antagonist of CCK is desired as whether an agonist or antagonist of neurotensin is desired for the novel treatment of schizophrenia [28, 29].

The nonselective CCK antagonist proglumide has been studied in rats and shown to selectively antagonise CCK-induced excitation of midbrain dopamine neurons, but was not impressive as an antipsychotic in a clinical study of schizophrenic patients already on haloperidol [30]. The nonpeptide CCK-B antagonist L-365,260 has been studied in patients with panic disorder, failing to antagonise CCK-4 induced panic attacks [31]. Another CCK-B antagonist in preclinical and early clinical studies is LY 262691. The CCK-A antagonist SR 27897 is in Phase II testing for appetite disorders and irritable bowel syndrome, but not for schizophrenia. Although targeting the CCK system may be a provocative idea, results to date have been disappointing and lack a solid preclinical rationale for agonist or antagonist, for CCK-A or CCK-B receptors.

FMRF-amide

The neuropeptide FMRFamide (Phe-Met-Arg-Phe-NH_3) was discovered in molluscs, then found in vertebrates, and demonstrated to exert neuromodulatory effects on serotonergic and monoaminergic systems in mammals. One study suggests behavioural effects in rodents consistent with anti-psychotic actions [32]. No preclinical compounds have been identified for drug development for this peptide system, but this is a theoretical target for schizophrenia.

Substance P and the neurokinins

An interesting chapter in psychopharmacology has been unleashed by the publication of antidepressant actions of a substance P antagonist MK-869 comparable to the SSRI paroxetine and significantly better than placebo [33]. This finding has focussed attention on the potential behavioral actions mediated by the tachykinin peptides, of which substance P is perhaps the best known member. Tachykinins are also called neurokinins, and there are several such peptides, known as substance P, neurokinin A, neurokinin B, neuropeptide K and neuropeptide gamma [34]. There are also several receptor subtypes for the neurokinins, including a substance P-preferring subtype (i.e. neurokinin (NK-1 receptors), neurokinin A-preferring (i.e. NK-2 receptors) and neurokinin B-preferring (i.e. NK-3). Selective antagonists for all three receptor subtypes have been identified and are in clinical trials for a wide range of indications [4]. On the basis of the distribution of substance P, it was originally hypothesised that substance P would have a prominent role in pain, peripherally-mediated inflammation, migraine and emesis [34]. NK-1 antagonists were tested clinically in these indications and yielded disappointing results [34].

As characterisation of the endogenous ligands and receptor subtypes proceeded, however, it was determined that some of the preclinical studies were misleading. That is, there is an apparent mismatch between endogenous ligand distribution and the preferred receptor distribution for that ligand, leading to confusion in the determination of the physiological or potential pathological roles of the neurokinins [34]. Furthermore, most early studies of tachykinins were not surprisingly done in rats, but it is now known that there are marked phylogenetic differences in the distribution of NK receptors within the central nervous system of different species [34]. In fact, the rat may be a poor model for human NK receptors, whereas gerbil, guinea pig and primates may be better models.

As findings from more relevant species have evolved, and the results of an empirical trial in depression was reportedly positive, this has spawned a race for finding the best clinical applications for various neurokinin antagonists. Thus, several companies have taken older compounds which failed earlier clinical trials in pain, migraine, inflammation and emesis, and have begun clinical testing in CNS indications ranging from depression to anxiety to schizophrenia. A flurry of new compounds from many compounds selective for each NK receptor subtype are coming forward, and many are being tested in schizophrenia. Although indications of neurokinin control of dopaminergic neurons is beginning to evolve, clinical testing in fact is proceeding rather empirically, hoping for serendipity as much as testing a hypothesis which has evolved from preclinical neurobiology.

NK-1 antagonists

Nevertheless, several NK-1 antagonists are in clinical trials [4], and at least one is in testing for use in schizophrenia (SR-140333). Other NK-1 antagonists largely being studied in depression but also candidates for testing in schizophrenia include CP-99,994 (nonselective), RPR-100893 (poorly brain penetrant), lanepitant (LY-303870, also poorly brain penetrant), RP-67,580, MK-869, L-760,735, L-733,060, CP-96,345, L-743,310 (poorly brain penetrant), CGP 49823 (poorly brain penetrant), and CP-122,721. Numerous patents are being issued in this field and one can expect to see several additional compounds soon.

NK-2 antagonists

Several NK-2 antagonists are also progressing to clinical testing [4] including GR-159,897 and SR-48968. Only SR-144,190 is currently being tested in schizophrenia. As for NK-1 antagonists, numerous patents are being filed and several additional compounds selective for NK2 receptors can be expected in the near future.

NK-3 antagonists

Originally, this receptor was thought to be only in rat and not in man, but subsequent research has shown this to be wrong. The best known NK-3 antagonist is SR-142-801, in clinical testing both for depression and schizophrenia [4]. Other NK-3 antagonists in preclinical testing include a large number of newly patented compounds in very early preclinical testing as well as DuP 753, EXP 3174, SR 48968, L-158,809, and PD 161182.

Novel long-term strategies for the treatment of schizophrenia

Overview

The following section provides a brief overview of some of the most "cutting-edge" strategies for developing new treatments for schizophrenia. As such, their underlying hypotheses may be less well developed, and there are often only drug targets, and not yet any drug development candidates.

Nevertheless, peering into these activities can give one a glimpse of the possibilities in the longer range future.

Alpha 7-nicotinic cholinergic agonists

The role of cholinergic neurotransmission in memory and cognition is well established with the introduction of the acetylcholinesterase inhibitors tacrine and donepezil for Alzheimer's Disease [1, 35]. Since pro-cholinergic actions of cholinesterase inhibition enhances acetylcholine activity at both nicotinic and muscarinic receptors, this has encouraged testing of the relative roles of these two receptor subtypes in mediating the promnestic (memory enhancing) actions of acetylcholine [35]. Muscarinic selective agonists have shown some efficacy in Alzheimer's Disease, as have nicotinic agonists [35]. Moreover, the alpha7-nicotinic cholinergic receptor has been implicated in the familial transmission of sensory gating deficits in families with schizophrenia [36]. Deficits in activity at this receptor could theoretically predispose patients to problems with learning efficiency and accuracy, and underlie delusional thinking and social dysfunction. In addition, heavy smoking in many schizophrenics (about two-thirds of a North American population of schizophrenics compared to about one-fourth of smokers among nonschizophrenics) is consistent with the high concentration of nicotine necessary to activate the receptor and with the receptor's rapid desensitisation.

Thus, there are numerous theoretically appealing hypotheses to targeting this receptor to improve particularly the cognitive functioning of schizophrenia (and Alzheimer's Disease as well). Furthermore, this may reduce smoking among schizophrenics, and the health hazards associated with this. Several companies are targeting this approach [4], but specific compounds are not yet identified.

Blocking neurodegeneration and apoptosis

One hypothesis for the pathophysiology of schizophrenia, and especially for the process underlying its onset and somewhat progressive course, is excitotoxic neuronal destruction by glutamate [1, 2]. Overexcitation by glutamate at NMDA subtype receptors may mediate neuronal destruction leading to schizophrenia. Theoretically, too much glutamate is released, or too much of its co-transmitter glycine is released, leading to excessive calcium inflow to the neuron, activation of free radicals, and ultimate destruction of the cell. A similar idea has been put forth for many neurodegenerative disorders ranging from Parkinson's Disease to Alzheimer's disease to amyotrophic lateral sclerosis to stroke.

Theoretically, glutamate antagonists such as ipenoxazone or LY-235,050 may be helpful in interrupting the excitotoxic cascade by preventing the activation of NMDA receptors by glutamate. The NMDA receptor is also modulated by glycine, so glycine antagonists at the NMDA non-strychnine sensitive glycine receptor are being pursued. Another glutamate receptor subtype which may be involved in undesirable actions of overly active glutamate is the AMPA receptor subtype, for which antagonists such as CX-516 are being developed.

Free radical scavengers such as vitamin E and the lazaroids could possibly be developed to act as chemical sinks to soak up the toxic consequences of excessive glutamate activation [1, 2].

One particularly novel idea is to block the process of apoptosis which may be activated by glutamate over-activation (or by other mechanisms). That is, if neurons are persuaded to commit suicide by activating the process of apoptosis, their progressive destruction could lead to some of the clinical consequences of schizophrenia as well as other neurodegenerative disorders. One enzyme system which may be necessary for the process of apoptosis to occur are the caspase enzymes. Inhibitors of this enzyme system may prevent the initiation of apoptosis and thus prevent the consequences of unwanted neuronal death in schizophrenia and other neurodegenerative disorders.

Adenosine A2A antagonists/partial agonists

Adenosine is not only involved in the cAMP second messenger system, but it also has neurotransmitter functions itself. In particular the adenosine A2A receptor subtype is a target for antagonists to treat Parkinson's Disease. Such early preclinical compounds include KW 7002, Sch-58621 and others. Perhaps partial agonists or even agonists at this site would be useful for some of the symptoms of schizophrenia.

Signal transduction pathway and transcription factors

An area of intense interest for the long-term targeting of drug actions are events distal to the receptor binding sites for neurotransmitters [37, 38]. Thus, targeting various different G proteins wherever they have selective properties, is one approach "beyond the receptor." A still more interesting long-range proposal is to produce or induce the production of specific transcription factors which cause the expression (or stop the expression) of specifically-targeted genes. This would lead to theoretically desirable production of certain gene products, or the inhibition of production of undesirable gene products. This is a very long-range possibility, for we are a long way from understanding which genes are expressed by the current antipsychotic drugs, and what genes would be desirable to turn on or turn off in schizophrenia.

Molecular phenotyping and orphan receptors

Another long-term possibility is to understand whether there are certain genotypes of schizophrenic patients which respond selectively to one antipsychotic drug over another. We already know that different patients can have vastly different responses to individual antipsychotic drugs. Perhaps a certain genotype would match with the phenotype of drug responsiveness, and help guide psychotropic drug selection [39, 40].

Another long-range possibility is to target "orphan receptors." That is, there are numerous G-protein linked receptors which have been identified in the human genome but for which no known neurotransmitter acts. Since the majority of effective drugs in psychiatry act at such G-protein linked receptors, it is possible that agonists or antagonists to these receptors without a known neurotransmitter (i.e. the orphans waiting to be adopted by one of the neurotransmitters) might lead to a novel psychotropic drug, specifically for schizophrenia.

Neurodevelopmental approaches and growth factor modulation

Neuronal development may go awry in schizophrenia, and lead to its expression in late adolescence and early adulthood with further progressive changes in the adult architecture of the brain [1, 2, 41, 42]. This idea of neurodevelopmental aetiology to schizophrenia suggests that redirecting neurons appropriately might prevent or treat symptoms of the disorder. There are growth factors which can trigger neuronal cell division, axonal sprouting, neuronal migration, and axonal growth and innervation [43–45]. If these could ever be harnessed, this may produce a strategy for neurodevelopmental disorders. Currently, such growth factors are being investigated in neurodegenerative disorders such as amyotrophic lateral sclerosis, but we are a long way from any application to schizophrenia [46].

Conclusion

We have entered the third era of discovery of new agents for schizophrenia, beyond both the first era of conventional neuroleptics and the second era of atypical antipsychotics with serotonin dopamine antagonist properties. The possibilities are numerous and exciting. Perhaps the richest and most promising era for schizophrenia is now upon us, giving hope for the possibility that symptoms of this disorder cannot only be reduced, but eliminated and with return of schizophrenic patients to normal, productive lifestyles.

References

1 Stahl SM (1996) *Essential psychopharmacology.* Cambridge University Press, London
2 Stahl SM *Psychopharmacology of antipsychotics.* Martin Dunitz Ltd., London; *in press*
3 Arnt J, Skarsfeldt T (1998) Do novel antipsychotics have similar pharmacological characteristics? A review of the evidence. *Neuropsychopharmacol* 18: 63–101
4 Pharmaceutical Companies Analysis. (1998) MDIS Publications Ltd. Chichester
5 Szewczak MR, Corbett R, Rush DK, Wilmot CA, Conway PG, Strupczewski JT, Cornfeldt M (1996) The pharmacological profile of iloperidone, a novel atypical antipsychotic agent. *J Pharmacol Exp Ther* 274: 1404–1413
6 Tandon R, Harrigan E, Zorn S (1997) Ziprasidone: a novel antipsychotic with unique pharmacology and therapeutic potential. *J Serotonin Res* 4: 159–177
7 Rowley HL, Kilpatrick, IC, Needham PL, Heal DJ (1998) Elevation of extracellular cortical noradrenaline may contribute to the antidepressant activity of zotepine: an *in vivo* microdialysis study in freely moving rats. *Neuropharmacol* 37: 937–944
8 Assie MB, Cosi C, Koek W (1997) 5-HT_{1A} receptor agonist properties of the antipsychotic, nemonapride: comparison with bromerguride and clozapine. *Europ J Pharmacol* 334: 141–147
9 Sorenson SM, Kehne JH, Fadayel GM, Humphreys TM, Ketteler HJ, Sullivan CK, Taylor VL, Schmidt CJ (1993) Characterization of the 5-HT_2 receptor antagonist MDL 100907 as a putative atypical antipsychotic: behavioral, electrophysiological and neurochemical studies. *J Pharmacol Exp Ther* 266: 684–691
10 Grunder G, Yokoi F, Offord SJ, Ravert HT, Dannals RF, Salzmann JK, Szymanski S, Wilson PD, Howard DR, Wong DF (1997) Time course of 5-HT_{2A} receptor occupancy in the human brain after a single oral dose of the putative antipsychotic drug MDL 100,907 measured by positron emission tomography. *Neuropsychopharmacol* 17:175–185
11 Stahl SM (1998) Neuropharmacology of obesity: My receptors made me eat it. *J Clin Psychiat* 59: 447–448
12 Martin P (1998) *5-HT_2 receptor antagonism and antipsychotic drugs; a behavioral and neurochemical study in a rodent hypoglutamatergia model.* Goteborg University, Sweden
13 Satoh K, Someya T, Shibasaki M (1997) Nemonapride for the treatment of schizophrenia. *Am J Psychiat* 154: 292
14 Kramer MS, Last B, Getson A, Reines SA (1997) The effects of a selective D_4 dopamine receptor antagonist (L-745-870) in acutely psychotic inpatients with schizophrenia. *Arch Gen Psychiat* 54: 567–572
15 Sramek JJ, Elton MA, Posvar EL, Feng MR, Jhee SS, Hourani J, Sedman AJ, Cutler NR (1998) Initial safety, tolerability, pharmacodynamics and pharmacokinetics of C1-1007 in Patients With Schizophrenia. *Psychopharmacol Bull* 34: 93–99
16 Ekesbo A, Andren POE, Gunne LM, Tedroff J (1997) (–)-OSU 6162 inhibits levodopa-induced dyskinesias in a monkey model of Parkinson's disease. *Clin Sci Neuropathol neurorep* 8: 2567–2570
17 Frieboes RM, Murck H, Wiedemann K, Holsboer F, Steiger A (1997) Open clinical trial of the sigma ligand panamesine inpatients with schizophrenia. *Psychopharmacology* 132: 82–88
18 Akunne HC, Whetzel SZ, Wiley JN, Corbin AE, Ninteman FW, Tecle H, Pei Y, Pugsley TA, Heffner TG (1997) The pharmacology of the novel and selective sigma ligand, PD 144418. *Neuropharmacology* 36: 51–62
19 Tran TT, de Costa BR, Matsumoto RR (1998) Microinjection of sigma ligands into cranial nerve nuclei produces vacuous chewing in rats. *Psychopharmacology* 137: 191–200
20 Stahl SM (1998) Getting stoned without inhaling: anandamide is the brain's natural marijuana. *J Clin Psychiat* 59 (11): 566–567
21 Axelrod J, Felder CC (1998) Cannabinoid receptors and their endogenous agonist nandamide. *Neurochem Res* 23: 575–581
22 Carriero D, Aberman J, Linn SY, Hill A, Makriyannis A, Salamone JD (1998) A detailed characterization of the effects of four cannabinoid agonists on operant lever pressing. *Psychopharmacology* 137: 147–156

23 Emrich HM, Leweke FM, Schneider U (1997) Towards a cannabinoid hypothesis of schizophrenia: cognitive impairments due to dysregulation of the endogenous cannabinoid system. *Pharmacol Biochem Behav* 56 (4): 803–807
24 Burrows GD, Maguire KP, Norman TR (1998) Antidepressant efficacy and tolerability of the selective norepinephrine reuptake inhibitor reboxetine: a review. *J Clin Psychiat* 59: (Suppl)
25 Gudasheva TA, Voronina TA, Ostrovskaya RU, Zaitseva NI, Bondarenko NA, Briling VK, Asmakova LS, Rozantsev GG, Seredenin SB (1998) Design of N-acylprolyltyrosine "tripeptoid" analogues of neurotensin as potential atypical agents. *J Med Chem* 41: 284–290
26 Sarhan S, Hitchcock JM, Grauffel CA, Wettstein JG (1997) Comparative antipsychotic profiles of neurotensin and a related systemically active peptide agonist. *Peptides* 18: 1223–1227
27 Betancur C, Cabrera R, de Kloet ER, Pelaprat D, Rostene W (1998) Role of endogenous neurotensin in the behavioral and neuroendocrine effects of cocaine. *Neuropsychopharmacol* 19: 321–332
28 Gracey DJ, Bell R, King DJ, Trimble KM, McDermott BJ (1998) Enhancement of latent inhibition in the rat by the CCK antagonist proglumide. *Pharmacol Biochem Behav* 59: 1053–1059
29 Mauri MC, Rudelli R, Vanni S, Panza G, Sicaro A, Audisio D, Sacerdote P, Panerai AE (1998) Cholecystokinin, B-endorphin and vasoactive intestinal peptide in peripheral blood mononuclear cells of drug-naive schizophrenic patients treated with haloperidol compared to healthy controls. *Psychiat Res* 78: 45–50
30 Whiteford HA, Stedman TJ, Welham JW, Csernansky, JG, Pond SM (1992) Placebo-controlled, double-blind study of the effects of proglumide in the treatment of schizophrenia. *J Clinical Psychopharmacol* 12: 337–340
31 Bradwejn J, Koszycki D, Couetoux du Teretre A, Van Megen HJGM, Westenberg HGM, Den Boer JA, Karkanias C, Haigh J (1994) The Panicogenic effects of cholecystokinin tetrapeptide are antagonized by L-365,260, a central cholecystokinin receptor antagonist in patients with panic disorder. *Arch Gen Psychiat* 51: 486–493
32 Muthal AV, Mandhane SN, Chopde CT (1997) Central administration of FMRFamide produces antipsychotic-like effects in rodents. *Neuropeptides* 31 (4): 319–322
33 Kramer MS, Cutler N, Feighner J, Shrivastava R, Carman J, Sramek JJ, Reines SA, Liu G, Snavely D, Wyatt-Knowles E, et al. (1998) Distinct mechanism for antidepressant activity by blockade of central substance p receptors. *Science* 281: 1640–1645
34 Longmore J, Hill RG, Hargreaves RJ (1997) Neurokinin-receptor antagonists: pharmacological tools and therapeutic drugs. *Can J Physiol Pharmacol* 75: 612–621
35 Stahl SM (1998) Cholinesterase inhibitors for Alzheimer's disease. *Hosp Pract* 33 (11): 131–136
36 Adler LE, Olincy A, Waldo M, Harris JG, Griffith J Stevens K, Flach K, Nagamoto H, Bickford P, Leonard S, Freedman R (1998) Schizophrenia, sensory gating, and nicotinic receptors. *Schizophr Bull* 24: 189–202
37 Jope RS, Song L, Grimes CA, Pacheco MA, Dilley GE, Li X, Meltzer HY, Overholser JC, Stockmeier CA (1998) Selective increases in phosphoinositide signaling activity and G protein levels in post mortem brain from subjects with schizophrenia or alcohol dependence. *J Neurochem* 70: 763–771
38 Hudson CJ, Lin A, Cogan S, Cashman F, Warsh JJ (1997) The niacin challenge test: clinical manifestation of altered transmembrane signal transduction in schizophrenia? *Soc Biol Psychiat* 41: 507–513
39 Sorbi S, Nacmias B, Tedde A, Latorraca S, Forleo P, Guarnieri BM, Petruzzi C, Daneluzzo E, Ortenzi L, Piacentini S, Amaducci L (1998) No implication of apolipoprotein E polymorphism in Italian schizophrenic patients. *Neurosci Lett* 244: 118–120
40 Arnold SE, Joo E, Martinoli MG, Roy N, Trojanowski JQ, Gur RE, Cannon T, Price RA (1997) Apolipoprotein E genotype in schizophrenia: frequency, age of onset, and neuropathologic features. *Clin Neurosci Neuropathol Neurorep* 8: 1523–1526
41 Turner EE, Fedtsova N, Jeste DV (1997) Cellular and molecular neuropathology of schizophrenia: new directions from developmental neurobiology. *Schizophr Res* 27: 169–180
42 Conceits DM, Ragland JD, Gur RC, Gur RE (1997) Neuropsychological evidence supporting a neurodevelopmental model of schizophrenia: a longitudinal study. *Schizophr Res* 24: 289–298

43 Stahl SM (1998) Brain tonics for brain sprouts: how neurotrophic factors fertilize neurons. *J Clin Psychiat* 59: 149–150

44 Stahl SM (1998) Recognition molecules are trailblazers for axon pathways. *J Clin Psychiat* 59: 215–216

45 Stahl SM (1998) When neurotrophic factors get on your nerves: therapy for neurodegenerative disorders. *J Clin Psychiat* 59: 277–278

46 Thome J, Foley P, Riederer P (1998) Neurotrophic factors and the maldevelopmental hypothesis of schizophrenic psychoses. *J Neural Transm* 105: 85–100

Subject index